Trauma Care
Manual

Trauma Care Manual

Edited by

Ian Greaves
Consultant in Emergency Medicine, British Army,
Peterborough District Hospital and Honorary Lecturer in
Conflict Medicine, University College, London, UK

Keith M. Porter
Consultant Trauma Surgeon, Selly Oak Hospital,
Birmingham, UK

and

James M. Ryan
Leonard Cheshire Professor of Conflict Recovery and
Honorary Consultant in Accident and Emergency Medicine,
University College London Hospitals, London, UK

On behalf of

Trauma Care®

A member of the Hodder Headline Group
LONDON
Co-published in the USA by
Oxford University Press Inc., New York

First published in Great Britain in 2001 by
Arnold, a member of the Hodder Headline Group
338 Euston Road, London NW1 3BH

http://www.arnoldpublishers.com

Co-published in the United States of America by
Oxford University Press Inc.,
198 Madison Avenue, New York, NY10016
Oxford is a registered trademark of Oxford University Press

Whilst the advice and information in this book are believed to be true and accurate at the date of going to press, neither the authors nor the publisher can accept any legal responsibility or liability for any errors or omissions that may be made. In particular (but without limiting the generality of the preceding disclaimer) every effort has been made to check drug dosages; however it is still possible that errors have been missed. Furthermore, dosage schedules are constantly being revised and new side-effects recognized. For these reasons the reader is strongly urged to consult the drug companies' printed instructions before administering any of the drugs recommended in this book.

British Library Cataloguing in Publication Data
A catalogue record for this book is available from the British Library

Library of Congress Cataloging-in-Publication Data
A catalog record for this book is available from the Library of Congress

ISBN 0 340 75979 8

1 2 3 4 5 6 7 8 9 10

Commissioning Editor: Joanna Koster
Production Editor: James Rabson
Production Controller: Iain McWilliams
Cover design: Terry Griffiths

Typeset in Great Britain by Phoenix Photosetting, Chatham, Kent
Printed and bound in Great Britain by MPG Books Ltd, Bodmin, Cornwall

Contents

The **Trauma Care Manual** has been prepared for Trauma Care, a registered charity dedicated to improving the care of the victims of trauma.

Editors

Dr Ian Greaves
Mr Keith Porter
Prof Jim Ryan

With contributions from

Prof David Alexander*
Mr Gavin Bowyer*
Mr Adam Brooks*
Dr Gregor Campbell-Hewson
Dr Otto Chan
Mr Charles Cox
Mr Peter Driscoll*
Dr Michael Elliott
Dr Ian Greaves*
Dr Carl Gwinnutt*
Dr Karen Heath*
Prof Tim Hodgetts*
Mr Andrew Jacks

Mr Alan Kay*
Prof Rod Little*
Dr Ian Machonochie*
Dr Roderick Mackenzie*
Mr Steven Mannion*
Mr David Patton*
Mr Keith Porter*
Dr Bernard Riley
Dr Rob Russell
Prof Jim Ryan*
Dr Nick Sherwood
Dr Jo Sibert
Mr Lee Wallis

*Member of the Trauma Care Council or Trauma Care Advisory Board

Trauma Care would also like to thank:

Mr Keith Allison, Dr D Black, Mr Munchi Chocksi, Dr E Dykes, Mr Tim Graham, Mr Jonathon Hyde,
Dr RJ Kendall, Mr M Revell, Dr P Statham, Mr Richard Steyn, Mr Andrew Thurgood, Mr RJ Williams,
Dr A Naraghi and Dr P Mcalinden for their assistance with this project.

Preface

Trauma Care®, a registered charity, was founded in 1996 by a group of clinicians with an interest in the area, to promote and define best practice in the management of the victims of trauma. This aim has been furthered by a series of successful conferences which have, uniquely, brought together all the professions and specialities involved in trauma care. This programme of conferences continues and is expanding.

The *Trauma Care Manual* has been prepared by Trauma Care in order to begin the process of establishing United Kingdom guidelines for best practice in the management of major trauma. A structured approach is offered which takes into account current British and European clinical practice and is, wherever possible, supported by the available evidence.

We recognize that this is an ambitious project, but believe that the current volume is the first step on a road which will, hopefully, see the regular revision and re-issue of this manual. Future editions will take into account new developments and be based on a reading of the ever-increasing evidence base. As a consequence working groups have been set up, charged with the responsibility of maintaining and developing a current evidence base in their own areas of expertise and working towards the next edition of this manual.

We believe that the establishment of clear practical guidelines reflecting British practice is long overdue and hope that this first edition will grow into – and become recognized as – the definitive statement of best practice.

Dr Ian Greaves
Mr Keith Porter
Prof Jim Ryan

Trauma Care 2000

The trauma epidemic

OBJECTIVES

- To describe the most important causes of traumatic injury
- To illustrate the conditions promoting these injuries

INTRODUCTION

Trauma was estimated to have caused 10% of all deaths occurring in 1990 world-wide.[1] Truly, it may be described as an epidemic.

The details of this epidemic differ according to location. The causes of traumatic death in the developed world are different to those in the developing world. Nonetheless, trauma remains the third largest cause of death in all regions of the world, regardless of these differences.[2] If young people only are considered, trauma becomes the leading cause of death and is thus the greatest source of potential years of life lost.[3]

It is well recognized that for every death due to injury, there are many more people who are left disabled. For each of the 165 000 trauma deaths in the United States of America in 1982, there were at least two cases of permanent disability.[3] The Global Burden of Disease Study developed the concept of Disability Adjusted Life Years (DALYs). It was calculated that in 1990, intentional and unintentional injuries caused 10% of mortality world-wide, but 15% of DALYs.[4]

Changing demographics have an influence on patterns of injury. The population of the world is still increasing – earlier this year it reached 6 billion. However, the rate of population growth has been steadily slowing for the past 20 years. Between 1990 and 1994, the annual growth rate fell to 1.57%, but again, there is a marked difference between rates in developed and developing countries. In the developing world between 1990 and 1995, the population growth rate was 2.8% per annum, compared to 0.4% in the industrialized nations.[5] Throughout the world, birth rates are falling and life expectancy is improving.

In addition, the world is becoming more urbanized. In 1975, 38% of the total population lived in urban areas, but by 1988 this had increased to 42%. By the year 2000, it is predicted that 47% of the world's population will be living in cities.[5]

The net effect of these changes is to produce a population with a smaller proportion of young people, a greater proportion of the elderly, and a growing proportion of people living in cities. This, in turn, affects patterns of injury around the world, although the relationship between increasing urbanization and injury rates is far from straightforward. It has been claimed that the recent decrease in homicides in the USA can be attributed, in part, to the diminishing number of young men.[6] Meanwhile, the enlarging elderly population is more likely to have domestic accidents and to be more severely injured in any accident.

Another influential factor affecting patterns of injury all over the world is the increasing use of alcohol and other drugs. In one study, about 50% of people dying from injury tested positive for blood alcohol.[7] Some 56% of all the trauma admissions to the orthopaedic department of a New Orleans hospital during 1993 and 1994 tested positive for drugs or alcohol, rising to 71% of those admitted with gunshot wounds.[8] In the UK, the Department of Transport estimated that in the 11 months before October 1996, 25% of road fatalities had taken drugs, 20% of which were illicit substances.[9] A pedestrian who has been drinking is two-and-a-half times more likely to be involved in a road traffic accident (RTA) than one who has not.[10] Despite this undoubted association, the involvement of alcohol and other drugs in homicides, assaults and suicides is extremely complex, and is associated with other factors such as mental or physical illness, deviant personality types, poverty and cultural acceptance of violence.

Alcohol consumption has certainly increased during the past three decades, particularly in the developing countries. In the developed world, however, there is some evidence that increased public awareness has led to safer behaviour patterns. Stinson and De Bakey[11] found that alcohol-related deaths in the USA actually fell during the 1980s, largely due to an improvement in the drink-driving figures.

Increase in alcohol consumption 1960–1981

- **Canada 95%**
- **Japan 169%**
- **The Netherlands 243%**
- **Korea 762%**

(Source: Ref. 12)

THE DEVELOPED WORLD

In the developed world, absolute numbers of deaths due to injury have been falling for the past 20 years. Despite this decrease, trauma is playing a proportionately more important role because infectious and parasitic diseases have become so much less prominent. During the past decade, trauma has become the third largest cause of death across all ages, after diseases of the circulatory system and malignancies.[2]

In these countries, the three greatest causes of violent death are road traffic accidents (RTAs), falls and suicides. Generally, death rates from RTAs and falls are declining, while that from suicide is increasing. With the exception of the USA and Northern Ireland, the rate of homicide is stable and relatively minor.[2]

Road traffic accidents

During the past 20 years, motor vehicle density has increased everywhere. For example, between 1976 and 1994, the number of cars in the UK increased from nearly 18 million to 25 million. In the USA, the rise over the same period was from 142 to 202 million, while in Japan, the number of cars per thousand population increased by 426% between 1970 and 1994.[13]

In developed countries, the past 20 years have seen increased legislation and public effort with regard to seat belts, motor-cycle helmets, airbags, speed limits and drink-driving campaigns. These initiatives appear to be paying off. In the UK in 1977, young men between the ages of 15 and 24 years suffered a mortality rate of 605 deaths per million as a result of trauma, with 65% of these deaths being due to road accidents. By 1992 in the same age group, not only had the number of deaths resulting from trauma fallen to 487 per million, but only 46% of these were caused by RTAs.[14] On the whole, this is reflected in other developed countries around the world. The repeal of safety legislation, as has happened from time to time in the USA and elsewhere, reverses this trend.

In the USA, this reduction in mortality from road deaths has been levelling off for the past four years and mortality, in fact, started to rise again in the late 1990s. In 1995, traffic accidents superseded guns as the leading cause of death among children and young adults. The abolition of the nation-wide 55 mph speed limit last year may blacken the picture further.[5]

Intentional injuries: suicides and homicides

Currently, numbers of suicides are increasing, and there are few countries where this is an exception. In many established market economies where the rate of road deaths is decreasing and the homicide rate is at least stable, suicides are forming a larger proportion of violent deaths. This would appear to parallel the large increase in mental illness, and particularly unipolar depression, reported by the World Health Organization (WHO) during the past decade. Between 60% and 80% of suicides are associated with depression.[15]

Some facts about suicide remain constant over time and place. More men commit suicide than women, the ratio being at least 3:1 (often much higher). More older people commit suicide than younger people, with people aged over 75 years having a suicide rate about three times that of younger groups. Nonetheless, suicide has been one of the top five causes of death for the 15- to 24-year age group for many years, and the number is still increasing.[15]

Generally, suicide is under-reported, perhaps because it often goes unrecognized. Many road fatalities among young male pedestrians may be suicides rather than accidents. Sometimes, however, there is a reluctance to classify deaths as suicides. For example, in Roman Catholic countries, where suicide is regarded as a mortal sin by the Church, many such deaths are classified as accidental or of undetermined cause. Greece, Italy and Spain have among the lowest suicide rates in Europe.[15]

The USA and Europe has shown a general increase in suicide over the last three decades, particularly among 15- to 24-year-old men. There are one or two exceptions to this. For example, Hungary has had one of the highest suicide rates in the world for many years, but among Hungarian adolescents and young adults the rate has actually decreased slightly over the past 35 years. The UK has experienced the same increase in young suicides as the rest of Europe, but is the only country to record a fall in the suicide rate among the over-75s during the last 35 years.[15]

With few exceptions, the level of homicide in developed countries over the last two decades has shown little change.[16]

The USA is unusual in that it is an established market economy with a relatively high homicide rate. Between 1975 and 1992, the overall annual male homicide rate remained steady at about 16 per 100 000 population, yet at the same time the rate for 15- to 24-year-old men rose from 21 to 37 per 100 000 population.[17,18] However, in the last decade the rates appear to be stabilizing. The National Center for Health Statistics reports firearm death rates reaching a peak of 15.6 per 100 000 in 1993, and then falling to 13.9 per 100 000 in 1995, a decrease of 11%. This fall in fatal shootings is variously attributed to stricter laws and their enforcement, changes in public attitudes, and the fact that there are now fewer young men in the highest risk age group.[6]

Falls and other domestic deaths

Between 20% and 30% of all accidental deaths occur in the home.[19,20] For every death, there may be as many as four cases of permanent impairment.[20] The two age groups particularly at risk of domestic injury are children over the age of 1 year and adults over 65 years.[21] However, the elderly have a far higher mortality rate than the young; for example, in the UK, 12–13% of all domestic accidents occur in the over-65 age group, but these people suffer at least 70% of domestic deaths.[22] Children may have most of their accidents at home, but motor vehicles cause most of their deaths.[23]

The leading causes of deaths at home are falls, fires, suffocation, drowning and poisoning. Because of the high mortality rate in the elderly, falls account for the highest number of deaths – about 62%.[21] The proportions differ according to age group. In 1977 in the UK, suffocation caused most deaths in children up to 4 years old, while falls was overwhelmingly the leading cause of death in the over-75s, followed by fires.[19] At least 40% of falls in the elderly are associated with other medical factors.[24]

The 15- to 64-year-old age group suffer far fewer domestic accidents and deaths. Overdoses cause about one-half of the deaths, and of the remainder the majority can be ascribed to falls and fires. Alcohol/drug use is involved in 71% of domestic deaths in this age group.[24]

Deaths caused by falls in women aged >75 years (per 100 000 population)		
	1975	1994
USA	97.8	57.1
UK	165.4	71.3
Source: Refs 17 and 18.		

Occupational injuries

In developed countries, significant changes have occurred in the labour force over the past 20 years. In general, there has been a broad movement away from the primary (agriculture and energy) and manufacturing sectors towards the service sector. In Britain in 1973, 45% of employment was in the manufacturing, energy, agricultural and construction industries, while service industries made up the other 55%. By 1993, the service sector formed 71% of employment, with the primary industries reduced to 29%. Even within the primary industries, administrative and managerial workers now form a larger proportion of the workforce.[25]

In the UK, the annual fatal injury incidence rate has been declining for many years. It is currently well under 2 per 100 000 employees, which is less than half the rate of the early 1970s and less than one-quarter of the rate of the early 1960s. A large proportion of this change is probably because of the demographic changes mentioned.[25] However, it is also felt that there have been significant improvements in safety standards in many industries.[26] Over the past 10 years, the most frequent causes of death across industry as a whole have remained falling from a height, and being struck by a moving vehicle.

The same improvements are seen throughout the developed world. The WHO's International Classification of Diseases, Ninth Revision (ICD-9) has a category of deaths due to 'accidents caused by machinery and by cutting and piercing instruments'. The numbers are small but the changes are consistent.

Male deaths per 100 000 population from accidents caused by machinery		
	1979	1992
USA	1.5	0.9
Australia	1.2	0.8
The Netherlands	0.7	0.4
England/Wales	0.7	0.4
Source: Refs 18, 27–30.		

THE DEVELOPING WORLD

In developing countries, the situation is more difficult to summarize, not least because of the paucity of reliable data. Infectious and parasitic diseases have not yet been beaten, and accident rates are not declining. Again, trauma appears to be the third largest killer of men across all ages, and the fourth largest killer of women.[2]

In these countries, RTAs and suicides are currently less important, although rising in number. Accidental deaths form the largest group, although in Latin America and South Africa homicide remains a significant problem.[2]

Occupational injuries

Developing countries have also seen significant changes in the work force, although these differ from those that have occurred in the developed world. In Asia in particular, countries have shifted from a predominantly rural agricultural economy to one that depends on mechanization and industrialization. At the same time, the number of reported accidents has increased sharply. Some of this increase can be attributed to improvements in the reporting systems, but there is no doubt that there has also been a genuine rise in the occurrence of accidents. In 1988, the Republic of Korea reported a total of 116 deaths classified as 'accidents caused by machinery and by cutting and piercing instruments'. In 1994, the total number of deaths in the same category had increased to 514.[18,30] These rates are far higher than in the UK and other established industrial nations.

Natural disasters

'In disaster, the poor lose their lives while the rich lose their money'.[31]

The incidence of natural disasters is increasing, a fact which generally can be attributed to greater numbers of hydrometeorological disasters (such as tropical cyclones and flash floods) and bushfires. The incidence of geophysical hazards (earthquakes, volcanic eruptions) appears to be constant.[31]

However, deaths caused by natural disaster appear to be rising disproportionately. For example, between 1975 and 1994 there were three million such deaths world-wide.[32] There are, broadly speaking, two reasons for this: first, natural disasters and their attendant casualties are being more and more accurately monitored and reported; and second (and more importantly), as the world population rises, greater numbers of people are becoming exposed to natural hazards. Increasing urbanization means that many more people are living in shanty towns and squatter camps which afford little protection against the vagaries of Nature. For those in rural areas, population pressures force many to live in high-risk areas or on unsustainable land vulnerable to environmental hazards.[31]

Thus, the majority of deaths from natural hazards occur in developing countries. Between 1947 and 1981, the average annual death rate from natural disaster in Bangladesh was nearly 4000 per million population, and in Guatemala it was over 3000. The equivalent figure for the UK was 89, for the USA 51, and for Australia 11. Developing countries with two-thirds of the world's population suffer 90% of disaster-related deaths. Conversely, about 75% of all the economic loss is in developed countries.

The United Nations designated the 1990s the International Decade for Natural Disaster Reduction, the objective being:

'. . . to reduce through concerted international action, especially in developing countries, the loss of life, property damage, and social and economic disruption caused by . . . calamities of natural origin'.

It will be interesting to see how effective this has been.

Road traffic accidents

Until recently, RTAs have not contributed significantly to traumatic deaths in the developing countries, but this is changing. The number of cars in many developing countries is rising rapidly, without much attention being paid to safety matters. It is also thought that alcohol is increasingly implicated. In Zimbabwe, for instance, road deaths increased from 477 in 1965 to 1113 in 1989, making it the largest cause of death across all ages.[33] In China, the number of cars has increased from well under 1 million in 1970 to nearly 6 million in 1989. Interestingly, the Chinese still have relatively few cars, but their accident rate is already approaching that of the USA.[34]

Intentional injuries: suicides and homicides

Few data are available that document the suicide rate in Africa. Asia and the South Americas show the same general increases as have been seen in the developed world, with particular increases having been seen again in young adults and the elderly.[15]

In Latin American and Caribbean countries, the rate of homicide is generally higher than in the developed countries, but does not appear to be getting worse.[17,18,35,36]

COUNTRIES OF CENTRAL AND EASTERN EUROPE/NEWLY INDEPENDENT SOVIET STATES (CCEE/NIS)

These countries fall neither into the developed nor developing categories, but form a distinct and rapidly changing region of their own. In some of the countries of Central and Eastern Europe and the newly independent states of the USSR (CCEE/NIS), the number of violent deaths has been rising since the mid-1980s, mainly due to an increase in homicides and, to a lesser extent, road accidents.

Road traffic accidents

Up to the time of liberalization of these countries, death rates from RTAs followed the same downward trend as in the developed countries. However, since liberalization many of these countries have recorded increases both in vehicle density and road death rates. In the former East Germany, road deaths increased from 12 per million population in 1980 to 19.3 in 1994.[13] After the reunification of Germany, the rise in vehicle ownership and the inexperience of the drivers lead to a four-fold increase in death rates for car occupants between 1989 and 1990. It was the young who were most at risk, the death rate (per 100 000) increasing 11-fold for those aged 18–20 years and eight-fold for those aged 21–24 years.[37] Estonia had a road death rate of 26 per 100 000 population in 1987, but by 1994 this had increased to 44.[18]

Homicide

Within the past decade, a similar change has occurred in homicide rates. For many of these countries, homicides declined in the early 1980s, but increased dramatically in the latter half of that decade or the early 1990s.[17,18,35,36]

WARFARE

Traumatic deaths caused by warfare are not restricted to any one region. Since 1945, 22 million people have been killed and three times as many injured during war or violent conflict. In the 1960s on average, there were 11 active conflicts in any one year. In the 1970s, there were 14 and in 1996, there were at least 50.[38] Modern warfare differs significantly from wars in the first half of the century. Between 1989 and 1992, only three out of 82 violent conflicts were between nation states, the rest being internal.[38] The aim of modern war is to destabilize the political, social, cultural and psychological foundation of one's opponent, with exemplary torture, execution and rape being used routinely as methods of social intimidation.[39] Weapons designed to maim rather than kill are used against civilians as well as combatants, deliberately or otherwise.[40] Modern weapons and tactics extend the battlefield to the entire society.[41]

Combatants in warfare

The risk of wounding and death to combatants has decreased, mainly because far fewer troops are now actually exposed to combat – the so-called 'empty battlefield' of modern warfare. However, those that do see combat are at a greatly increased risk of injury from the high-velocity projectiles and antipersonnel weapons. Improved evacuation times and medical care have contributed to decreased mortality. In the First World War, 6% of the wounded died, compared with 3.6% in Vietnam.[41]

Civilians in warfare

Some 50% of casualties in the Second World War were civilians, compared with >80% in the United States war in Vietnam, and >90% currently. The distinction between combatants and civilians is diminishing,[37] and crowded, vulnerable areas such as shelters or hospitals are now often deliberately targeted.[39] UNICEF states that during the past ten years 2 million children have died and 4–5 million children have been injured or disabled. The deliberate destruction of health centres with the internment or execution of health personnel exacerbates the problem.[38] Because most violent conflicts now are internal, the number of people killed is often relatively small; nonetheless, such people may form a significant proportion of the population of a country. In 1994, 14% of the Rwandan population was slaughtered in the space of three months.[38] Moreover, very often civilians are disabled rather than killed, with one in every 236 Cambodians being an amputee.[39] This continued morbidity has grave implications for the financial well-being of the victim, and for the economy of their country as a whole.

Weapons and patterns of injury

Recent wars have been marked by an increase in the number of explosive wounds caused by fragmenting antipersonnel weapons such as rockets, artillery shells, mortar bombs and mines. Fragment wounds are usually to the soft tissues and carry a lesser mortality than bullet wounds, which frequently include fractured bones and damaged vital structures.[39] However, explosive weapons can be used against large groups of people. Antipersonnel mines combine these two patterns of injury, and cause the most devastation in terms of morbidity and long-term effects. Head injuries have the highest mortality, but lower-extremity injury causes the most morbidity. There has also been an increase in the number of burns and inhalation injuries, with as many as one in four modern war injuries being burns.[39]

Antipersonnel mines are the most well-known of weapons causing 'superfluous injury or unnecessary suffering'; that is, injury greater than that necessary to put the combatant *hors de combat*. Another example is the laser designed to blind rather than to kill. These weapons are deemed abhorrent by the International Committee of the Red Cross (ICRC), and the blinding lasers were banned by a Geneva convention in 1995. As yet there is no legal definition of 'superfluous injury or unnecessary suffering' (SInUS); this being a concept that the SIrUS project of the ICRC is aiming to clarify.[40]

> **SUMMARY**
>
> - Death rates due to injury are falling in developed countries, but increasing in many developing countries.
> - Deaths due to road traffic accidents, intentional injuries and war injuries are likely to increase in number.
> - Prevention of injury remains neglected and must be improved.

REFERENCES

1. Murray CJL, Lopez AD. The Global Burden of Disease. In: Murray CJL, Lopez AD (eds). (1st ed.) *Global Burden of Disease and Injury*; Vol. 1. The Harvard School of Public Health, 1996.
2. Bourbeau R. Analyse comparative de la mortalite violente dans les pays developpes et dans quelques pays en developpement durant la periode 1985–1989. *World Health Statistics Quarterly* 1993; **46**: 4–32.
3. Trunkey DD. Trauma. *Scientific American* 1983; **249**: 20–7.

4. Murray CJL, Lopez AD. Mortality by cause for eight regions of the world: global burden of disease study. *Lancet* 1997; **349**: 1269–76.
5. Global socio-economic development trends (1985–1988). *World Health Statistics Quarterly* 1989; **42**: 190–6.
6. Dejevsky M. Gun deaths fall in US – as road toll picks up speed. *The Independent*, 26th July, 1997: 10.
7. Goodman RA, Istre GR, Jordan FB, Horndon JL, Kelaghan J. Alcohol and fatal injuries in Oklahoma. *Journal of Studies on Alcohol* 1991; **52**: 156–61.
8. Levy RS, Hebert CK, Munn BG, Barrack RL. Drug and alcohol use in orthopaedic trauma patients: a prospective study. *Journal of Orthopaedic Trauma* 1996; **10**: 21–7.
9. English S. 'Lollipop' may lick problem of drivers on drugs. *The Times*, 9th October, 1997.
10. Irwin ST, Patterson CC, Rutherford WH. Association between alcohol consumption and adult pedestrians who sustain injuries in road traffic accidents. *British Medical Journal* 1983; **286**: 522.
11. Stinson FS, DeBakey SF. Alcohol-related mortality in the US, 1979–1988. *British Journal of Addiction* 1992; **87**: 777–83.
12. Walsh B, Grant M. International trends in alcohol production and consumption: implications for public health. *World Health Statistics Quarterly* 1985: **38**: 130–41.
13. HMSO. 1997. *International Comparisons of Transport Statistics, 1970–1994*. (1st ed.) London.
14. HMSO. 1993. *Office of Population Censuses and Surveys. Mortality Statistics – Cause*. London.
15. Diekstra RFW, Gulbinat W. The epidemiology of suicidal behaviour: a review of three continents. *World Health Statistics Quarterly* 1993; **46**: 52–68.
16. Wolfgang ME. Homicide in other industrialised countries. *Bulletin of the New York Academy of Medicine* 1986; **62**: 400–12.
17. World Health Organization, 1976. *World Health Statistics Annual, 1973–1976*, Geneva.
18. World Health Organization, 1996. *World Health Statistics Annual, 1995*, Geneva.
19. Waters E, Cliff K. Accidents will happen. *Nursing Mirror* 1981; **153**: 46–7.
20. Lang-Runtz H. Preventing accidents in the home. *Canadian Medical Association Journal* 1983; **129**: 482–5.
21. Department of Trade and Industry, 1987. *Home Accident Surveillance System. Home and Leisure Accident Research: Eleventh Annual Report*, London.
22. Poyner B. *Home and Leisure Accident Research – The Elderly*. London: Department of Trade and Industry, 1986.
23. Mazurek AJ. Epidemiology of paediatric injury. *Journal of Accident and Emergency Medicine* 1994: 9–16.
24. Poyner B, Hughes N. *Home and leisure accident research: personal factors*. London: Department of Trade and Industry, 1990.
25. Drever F. *Occupational Health Decennial Supplement*. (1st ed.) London: HMSO, 1995.
26. Lees FP. *Loss Prevention in the Process Industries*. (2nd ed.) Oxford: Butterworth-Heinemann, 1996, vol. 1.
27. World Health Organization, 1983. *World Health Statistics Annual, 1983*, Geneva.
28. World Health Organization, 1995. *World Health Statistics Annual, 1994*, Geneva.
29. World Health Authority, 1981. *World Health Statistics Annual, 1981*, Geneva.
30. World Health Authority, 1994. *World Health Statistics Annual, 1993*, Geneva.
31. Smith K. *Environmental Hazards*. (2nd ed.) London, New York: Routledge, 1996.
32. International Decade for Disaster Reduction. *Journal of the American Medical Association* 1994; **271**: 1822.
33. Zwi A, Msika B, Smetannikov E. Causes and remedies. *World Health* 1993 (1): 18–20.
34. Roberts I. China takes to the roads. *British Medical Journal* 1995; **310**: 1311–13.
35. World Health Organization, 1977. *World Health Statistics Annual, 1977*. (1st ed.), Geneva.
36. World Health Organization, 1978. *World Health Statistics Annual, 1978*, Geneva.
37. Winston FK, Rineer C, Menon R, Baker SP. The carnage wrought by major economic change: ecological study of traffic-related mortality and the reunification of Germany. *British Medical Journal* 1999; **318**: 1647–50.
38. Summerfield D. The social, cultural and political dimensions of contemporary war. *Medicine, Conflict and Survival* 1997; **13**: 3–25.
39. Aboutanos MB, Baker SP. Wartime civilian injuries: epidemiology and intervention strategies. *J Trauma* 1997; **43**: 719–26.

40. Coupland RM. Abhorrent weapons and 'superfluous injury or unnecessary suffering': from field surgery to law. *British Medical Journal* 1997; **315**: 1450–2.

41. Garfield RM, Newgut AI. Epidemiologic analysis of Warfare – a historical review. *Journal of the American Medical Association* 1991; **266**: 688–92.

2

Mechanism of injury

OBJECTIVES

- To demonstrate how the mechanism of injury affects injury patterns
- To demonstrate the importance of determining the mechanism of injury

INTRODUCTION

Each episode of trauma will have its own unique characteristics and consequences for the patient. However, patterns of injury emerge depending on the mechanisms which have been involved in causing the incident. For this reason all the information that can be gained about the causative mechanism of an injury is useful, and trauma team leaders must obtain as much information as possible. The importance of a proper handover can not be overemphasized. Where possible, photographs or videos of the incident scene will allow the hospital team a greater appreciation of what has happened. This appreciation allows the recognition of important clues as to what injuries are likely. These injuries can then be actively sought and excluded.

> **Always speak to the pre-hospital team**

Some mechanisms are highly predictive of serious injury,[1-4] and the victims of such incidents should – where possible – be taken to the hospital which is best able to manage them. Ideally, the hospital will have been informed of their impending arrival, which will allow the appropriate specialties to have been warned and to be waiting to receive them. These mechanisms are shown in Table 2.1.

Table 2.1 *Mechanisms predictive of serious injury*

- Fall of >6 m
- Pedestrian or cyclist hit by car
- Death of other occupant in same vehicle
- Ejection from vehicle/bike
- Major vehicular deformity or significant intrusion into passenger space
- Extrication time >20 min
- Vehicular roll-over
- Penetrating injury to head or torso
- All shotgun wounds

Mechanisms of injury can be divided into:

- blunt;
- penetrating;
- thermal; and
- blast.

A single incident may include elements of all of these. The common factor is that the damage done depends on the energy transfer to the body tissues. Thermal injury demonstrates this well; the more heat (or cold) experienced by the tissues, the larger and deeper the burn.

Other factors that affect the damage sustained are the surface area and length of time over which the force is applied. The type of tissue affected will also play a role. Whatever the mechanism, children are likely to be more seriously injured than adults because their smaller size increases the chance of vital organs being involved.

BLUNT TRAUMA

In blunt trauma the energy transfer to the patient occurs over a large area. Blunt trauma can be further divided either by the forces produced, or the type of incident (Table 2.2). The forces are often found in combination. Blunt trauma is by far the most common mechanism of injury in most parts of the UK.

Table 2.2 *Subclassification of blunt trauma*

Forces	Incident type
Direct impact/compression	RTA: vehicle occupants
Shear	vehicle versus vehicle
Rotation	vehicle versus stationary object
	(motor)cyclists
	pedestrians
	Fall
	Assault with blunt object

Direct impact/compression

This is the commonest type of force which results in blunt trauma, and causes injury by direct pressure. Superficial tissues are most affected, but deeper tissues are involved as the energy transfer increases. Direct force produces contusion and haemorrhage, increasing to organ rupture and fractures. A minor blow to the head may cause a scalp haematoma with or without laceration. A harder blow will produce skull fractures, cerebral contusions and extra- or subdural haematomas. Another example of a direct force injury is duodenal rupture caused by compression between the lap segment of a seat belt and the lumbar spine. Pattern bruising over the abdomen or chest from a seat belt suggests significant force, and should raise the index of suspicion for internal injury. 'Reading the wreckage' extends to the patient, and not just the scene.

Shearing

Shearing forces make organs and tissue planes move relative to each other, tearing communicating structures and blood vessels. The force can be caused by deceleration or acceleration and as a result is most often associated with high-speed road traffic accidents (RTAs) and high falls. After impact, organs continue to move forward on their points of attachment causing them to tear. Aortic rupture in a high-speed RTA is a good example, the descending aorta being fixed but the arch being free and unsupported. Severe deceleration can make the arch shear off from the descending aorta, causing an injury that is most often fatal within seconds.

Rotation

Similar effects to shearing forces are produced when a body part is twisted relative to adjoining parts. Rotational forces produce spiral and oblique fractures, ligament damage and dislocations, and are also responsible for degloving injuries. In these, the soft tissue of a limb is rotated while the bone remains stationary; for example, when a limb is run over or trapped in machinery. As a result, the blood and nervous supplies to the soft tissue may be lost. These injuries are often very difficult to identify at first, but can have devastating results.

Road traffic accidents

VEHICLE OCCUPANTS

At the scene of an RTA, the process of 'reading the wreckage' can provide a large amount of information regarding the amount of energy involved, and how it was directed. This information should be sought from members of the pre-hospital team who attend the accident and emergency department.

- Was the collision head-to-head, a side impact ('T-bone'), from behind, or oblique?
- Did the vehicle roll over?
- How much intrusion into the passenger space has there been?
- Where was each patient, and were they restrained?
- Were there any other occupants of the same vehicle, and what has happened to them?
- How long was the extrication time?

Frontal impacts cause shortening of the front of the car as the bonnet buckles and the engine is forced rearward into the passenger compartment which, together with the occupants, is still moving forwards. The lower limbs of the front seat occupants may be trapped and injured by the engine or pedals, and contact with the dash board may cause knee, femoral or hip fractures/dislocations. The torso can be injured by striking the steering wheel or by the seat belt restraining it, and at high speed, deceleration injuries may result as internal organs are subjected to shearing forces. Head, facial and cervical spine injuries can result from contact with the steering wheel or windscreen, and forearm fractures may occur as the driver attempts to brace against the steering wheel.

Side-on impacts will cause one pattern of injuries on the side of the vehicular contact due to the direct force, typically comprising a fractured pelvis and ribs with associated internal injuries, but the patient may then be flung into the occupant on the other side of the car; this causes further injuries to both patients. This is seen clearly in the neck and head, the neck initially abducting to the side of impact causing compression on that side and stretching on the other. A head injury will also occur as the head hits the side window. As the patient is flung across the car, the same pattern occurs, but the head injury is caused by contact with the other occupant's head.

Oblique and rotational impacts will cause combinations of frontal and side-on injuries. A vehicle may roll over as the result of any impact, but this event suggests increased energy and damage to the car and occupants.

When a stationary object has been hit, the nature of that object can have an important effect on the outcome. If there has been movement or deformation of the object, for example a parked car, then some of the impact energy will have been dissipated in this. If, however, there has been no movement or deformation, for example an impact with a tree, then the whole of the impact energy will be channelled into the vehicle and its occupants.

Damage within the passenger compartment will provide an indication of how much force may have been transmitted to the patient. If the steering wheel is bent or the windscreen has a bull's-eye pattern, they have been deformed by contact with the patient's chest or head, and therefore a significant force will have been applied to the patient.

Cars may have considerable safety features built in, such as airbags, crumple zones, side-impact bars and head restraints. The age and type of car may therefore be important in determining the injuries suffered by the occupants. Compulsory seat belt legislation has considerably changed the pattern of injuries which are seen.[5] It is worth remembering that both seat belts and airbags are responsible for causing certain injuries in collisions, as well as preventing others. Pattern bruising across the chest and abdomen is evidence of significant trauma.

Look for pattern bruising across the chest and abdomen

Any patient who has been ejected from a vehicle must be assumed to have suffered severe injury, since sufficient force has obviously been applied to them to thrust them out through a window or door. They will then have hit the ground at considerable speed. Injury patterns are difficult to predict in ejectees, but there is a higher incidence of severe injury and death. Similarly, any occupant from a passenger compartment in which there has been an ejection or death should be treated with a very high index of suspicion for serious injury, as the same forces that caused the ejection or death have also been applied to them.

MOTORCYCLISTS AND CYCLISTS

Motorcyclists and pedal cyclists experience similar patterns of injury, although the injuries to the former tend to be more serious due to the greater speeds involved. The injuries suffered will be determined by the speed and direction of impact. Both groups are relatively unprotected compared with motorists, and may have their legs crushed between the car bumper and the bike. Separation, or ejection, from the bike suggests significant trauma, and both groups are vulnerable to secondary injuries from impact with the road after the collision. The distance the victim is found from their bike and the condition of the bike will both provide significant clues to the degree of the forces involved.

Motorcyclists have, by law, to wear a helmet. If this is removed at the scene, it should be transported to hospital with the patient, because examination of it can provide invaluable information regarding the forces involved. Cyclists are not required to wear helmets, even though their use has been shown to reduce injury morbidity and mortality,[6] and is strongly encouraged as part of accident-prevention campaigns. If a helmet has been worn, once again, it should stay with the patient.

Motorcyclists are more likely to be wearing protective clothing to reduce friction burns and abrasions. These may act like an anti-shock garment in pelvic fractures, and the pelvis should be assessed before such clothing is cut off in the resuscitation room. Motorcycle leathers may also have a beneficial effect in controlling bleeding from lower-limb long bone fractures, and they should therefore be removed as part of the C component of the primary survey as a controlled procedure.

> **Do not rush to remove lower-limb motorcycle leathers**

If cycle leathers were worn, this should be clearly recorded in the medical notes.

PEDESTRIANS

In road traffic accidents involving pedestrians, the size of the patient, as well as the speed and size of the vehicle, will affect the injuries sustained.

Adults
An adult stuck by a car is usually hit side-on, either because they did not see the vehicle or as a result of trying to move out its way. The car bumper makes the primary impact with the victim's legs, and the victim is then thrown up onto the bonnet, windscreen or even over the car depending on the speed. The legs and pelvis take the first impact of the bumper and the front of the bonnet. This produces the typical bumper fracture of the lateral tibial plateau and fibula with disruption of the medial co-lateral ligament. Femoral and pelvic fractures are also common. Secondary injuries are caused by subsequent impacts. If hit by a vehicle with a high front such as a bus or lorry, an adult will be thrown either to the side or under the vehicle.

Children
The smaller size of the child means that the car bumper will impact somewhere on the torso, throwing the child to the side or forwards and then under the car. Thus, the primary impact is likely to cause thoracic, abdominal or pelvic injuries. Head, facial and cervical spine injuries may result as the child's head then strikes the bonnet. Children will often turn to face the car before impact, thereby changing the pattern to a frontal one.

SECONDARY INJURIES

Secondary injuries occur as a result of impacts after the first contact with the bumper. The faster the speed of the car, the higher up the bonnet and windscreen the victim is thrown. At around 45 k.p.h. (28 m.p.h.) they are likely to be thrown right over the car, landing on the rear of the vehicle or on the road. Secondary impact with the bonnet causes pelvic fractures and thoracoabdominal injuries. The head is then likely to hit the windscreen causing head, facial and cervical spine injuries. The victim who is thrown over the car is likely to suffer multiple injuries, depending on how they land. If they are very unfortunate they may also be struck by a following vehicle.

Running-over injuries

Running-over injuries are suffered by those who are thrown under a vehicle or forwards and then run over by it. The wheels may run over the limbs, head or body, resulting in severe direct and rotational injuries. Other parts of the underside of the vehicle may cause direct trauma on contact and the victim may be dragged along the road for some distance.

Falls

Factors affecting the pattern of injury suffered in a fall include:

*   the height of the fall (and therefore the speed of impact);
*   the surface fallen onto; and
*   the position of the body on impact.

Victims landing on their feet are likely to suffer calcaneal fractures, femoral neck or acetabular fractures and vertebral compression fractures as direct force is transmitted up the body. Shear forces may produce aortic and intestinal rupture. Similarly, falls onto the head or arms will produce direct injuries at the point of first impact, with both direct and shear forces transmitted to the rest of the body.

Assaults with blunt objects

The material and surface area of the implement used, as well as the strength with which it is wielded, will determine the energy transfer, and therefore the severity of the injuries sustained. It is difficult to predict an overall pattern of injury; however, defensive manoeuvres may produce increased trauma to limbs, hands and back. The same medicolegal requirements as for penetrating trauma should be borne in mind when recording the history and examination.

PENETRATING TRAUMA

Penetrating trauma is most often the result of assault in civilian practice, and the need for subsequent forensic and medicolegal reports should be remembered when recording the history and clinical findings in these cases. In the UK penetrating trauma is rare outside a few city centres. Penetrating trauma can be subdivided depending on the energy transfer involved (Table 2.3).

Table 2.3 *Types of penetrating trauma*

Low-energy:	knife (and similar wounds)
Medium-energy:	conventional handguns
High-energy:	assault rifles

Low-energy wounds

Stab wounds are low-energy transfer injuries that cause direct tissue damage along a straight track. Knives are the commonest weapon, but many other (often seemingly innocuous) implements have been used. If the weapon is still *in situ*, it must be left until removed in theatre, where any resultant haemorrhage from tamponade release can be swiftly controlled. Any information from the pre-hospital carers or the victim regarding the type and size of the weapon, the time and angle of attack, the range at which it was thrown or fired (where appropriate), and the condition of the patient and blood loss at the scene is useful.

Medium- and high-energy wounds (see Chapter 16)

The injuries caused by these projectiles depend on their physical make-up, the speed, range and characteristics of their flight, and the nature of the tissues impacted.[7] All of these variables determine how much energy is transferred to the tissues, and how rapidly. As the missile penetrates the body, the transfer of energy expands the tissues and forces them out of the way, creating a temporary cavity which then collapses in on itself. The size of the cavity depends on the amount of energy transferred, and is more closely related to the velocity than to the size of the missile. Cavities produced by military or hunting rifles are much larger than the bullets fired, and create a temporary vacuum that sucks pieces of clothing and debris into the wound from outside. To compound this, the tissues displaced to form the cavity may be devitalized and may require extensive débridement.

Bullets fired from conventional 9-mm handguns are not usually associated with extensive cavitation, although some modern specialist handguns can fire bullets with sufficient energy to produce these effects.

The physical characteristics of missiles that are important are profile and composition. The profile determines the surface area that initially impacts with the target. The larger the surface area, the greater the immediate energy transfer; however, more energy is expended in flight, reducing range and penetrating power. A bullet made to be heavy will also increase energy transfer but will again expend more energy in flight. Some bullets are made to fragment or expand on impact. This ensures maximum energy transfer to the tissues as the surface area is increased, and the fragments spread into the tissues causing further damage. Shotgun wounds at short to medium range can be particularly devastating because of the large surface area created by the pellets.

Yaw, pitch and tumble all describe characteristics of the flight of a missile. The accuracy and range of a gun is improved by the 'rifled' barrel. This makes the bullet spin around its longitudinal axis, increasing stability. Yaw describes horizontal angulation and pitch describes vertical angulation in flight. Both will increase as the range lengthens, thereby increasing the surface area on impact and the chance of tumbling. Tumble is caused by loss of stability in flight as the heavier base overtakes the point producing end-over-end spin. This can occur as the result of a ricochet or on impact with the target, again increasing surface area and energy transfer to the tissues.

The density and elasticity of the tissues involved also plays a role. Solid organs, especially if they are surrounded by a rigid or semi-rigid capsule (e.g. the liver and brain), absorb a lot of energy and have very little elastic recoil. They, therefore, are likely to be very badly damaged by medium- to high-energy gunshots. Because they have no elastic recoil, bones may shatter as a result of the impact, creating splinters that act as secondary missiles and cause further damage. The lungs are much less dense, have a great deal of elasticity, absorb less energy, and are therefore less affected by cavitation. Clearly, if any essential organ is hit by a bullet, however little energy it carries, the results are likely to be devastating.

Missiles may not follow straight tracks through the body. It is not immediately important as to whether a wound is an entrance or exit point, and what its exact track was. Wrong assumptions can be made by premature labelling, and other injuries and projectiles missed as a result. The precise passage can be worked out later once the patient has been assessed and stabilized.

During initial resuscitation do not waste time trying to match supposed entrance and exit wounds

---

BLAST

Blast combines the actions of blunt, penetrating and thermal trauma with some of its own. In the United Kingdom, blast injuries are usually the result of terrorist activity or industrial accidents. Munitions are often designed to fragment, and terrorist bombs may have 'shipyard confetti' packed around them. This creates a hail of medium- and high-energy fragments designed to injure as many people as possible.

The actions of blast can be divided into:

- primary – direct effects of the blast wave;
- secondary – due to fragments;
- tertiary – gross displacement of the body with amputation and potential disintegration;[8]
- crush injuries;
- burns; and
- psychological effects.

The subject of blast injuries is discussed in detail in Chapter 16. A summary is given below.

Primary effects

The massive release of energy in an explosion creates an instantaneous increase in the pressure of the surrounding air. This shock front spreads out faster than the speed of sound in all directions. Its force decreases with distance from the centre of the explosion, but waves may reflect off solid surfaces and tissue planes. This sets up further pressure that augments or works at angles to waves still coming in, causing increased damage.

Tympanic membrane rupture is a common injury as a result of the shock front, and a reliable indicator that significant blast exposure has occurred. However, as shock-wave patterns are unpredictable, the absence of this injury does not exclude significant exposure. The lungs and intestines are also particularly vulnerable to the shock front because they have a large air/soft tissue interface. Haemorrhage, membraneous and viscous rupture and perforation may all be caused. Simple and tension pneumothoraces are frequent and air embolus can occur. 'Blast lung' may present as acute respiratory failure up to 48 h after the explosion.

Secondary effects

These are caused by flying debris and may cause blunt or penetrating injury depending on the nature of the fragments. The fragments may be part of the explosive device or energized components of the environment such as broken glass.

Tertiary effects

Mass movement of air following the detonation is known as the 'blast wind'. This is responsible for tertiary blast effects, which include displacement of the body (and consequent impact injuries), amputation and total bodily disruption.

Crush injuries

Crush injuries may result from the collapse of surrounding buildings.

Burns

As well as producing pressure, the energy released in the explosion produces heat, causing flash burns to exposed skin and setting light to flammable materials in the environment.

Psychological effects

Due to the devastating nature of the injuries, explosions – particularly those due to terrorist activity – may produce severe psychological problems in victims and carers.

SUMMARY

An understanding of the mechanisms involved in the production of traumatic injuries allows the early activation of trauma resources, and prompts the carers to search for both obvious and occult injuries. By actively seeking injuries suggested by the mechanism, injuries will not be missed and their treatment not delayed. Aggressive intervention based on the mechanism of injury will save lives and decrease the degree of disablement suffered by survivors.

REFERENCES

1. Bond RJ, Kortbeek JB, Preshaw RM. Field trauma triage: combining mechanism of injury with the pre-hospital index for an improved trauma triage tool. *Journal of Trauma* 1997; **43**: 283–7.
2. Ochsner MG, Schmidt JA, Rozycki GS, Champion HR. The evaluation of a two-tier trauma response system at a major trauma center: is it cost effective and safe? *Journal of Trauma* 1995; **39**: 971–7.
3. Rowe J-A. Incorporating mechanism of injury into an emergency department's trauma triage tool. *Journal of Emergency Nursing* 1996; **22**: 583–5.
4. Tinkoff GH, O'Connor RE, Fulda GJ. Impact of a two-tiered trauma response in the Emergency Department: promoting efficient resource utilisation. *Journal of Trauma* 1996; **41**: 735–40.
5. Thomas J. Road traffic accidents before and after seat belt legislation – study in a District General Hospital (comment in *Journal of the Royal Society of Medicine* 1990 August; **83**(8): 536). *Journal of the Royal Society of Medicine* 1990 February; **83**(2):79–81.
6. American College of Surgeons' Committee on Trauma. *Advanced Trauma Life Support for Doctors – course manual*. Chicago, Illinois: American College of Surgeons, 1997.
7. Kirby NG (ed.): *Field Surgery Pocket Book*. London: HMSO, 1981.
8. Maynard R, Cooper G, Scott R. Mechanisms of injury in bomb blasts and explosions. In: Westerby S (ed.). *Trauma; Pathogenesis and Treatment*. Oxford: Heinemann Medical Books, 1989.

3

Patient assessment

OBJECTIVES

- To explain the tasks of the trauma reception team
- To demonstrate the systematic approach to initial trauma care
- To demonstrate a method of seamless transition to definitive care

INTRODUCTION

Trauma care covers a spectrum starting from the scene of the accident right through to the end of rehabilitation. Each link is vitally important so that the patient (and their relatives) receives the best possible result. This chapter will concentrate on the initial reception of the trauma patient in the resuscitation room.

The errors that occur in the early management of the trauma patient are not made by uncaring people. Doctors and nurses are often distracted by obvious problems (e.g. the painful deformed leg) and miss the subtly developing critical condition (e.g. the bleeding pelvis). Another common mistake is to overlook a non-fatal problem (such as a carpus dislocation) in the desire to save the patient's life. Nevertheless, if these non-fatal injuries are not appropriately managed, at the correct time, the patient could develop a life-long impairment.[1]

What is required is a systematic approach that aims to identify and treat both immediately and potentially life-threatening conditions before the limb-threatening ones, but does not omit the latter. As far as the doctor and nurse in the resuscitation room are concerned, this usually starts with a call from Ambulance Control.

PRE-HOSPITAL COMMUNICATION

A warning from ambulance control or, ideally direct from the scene, enables essential information to be transmitted so that the receiving personnel can prepare for the patient's arrival (Table 3.1). Without such a system delays occur and key personnel may not be present when the patient arrives.

Table 3.1 *Essential pre-hospital information*

- The mechanism of injury
- Number, age and sex of the casualties
- The airway, breathing and circulatory status of the patient
- The conscious level
- Recognized injuries
- What care has been provided, and its effect
- Estimated time of arrival

The mechanism of the injury provides invaluable information about the forces the patient was subjected to, and the direction of impact. Further help comes from a description of the damage to the car or the weapon used (see Chapter 16). For example, in a road traffic accident (RTA) a frontal impact can result in damage to the head, face, airway, neck, mediastinum, liver, spleen, knee, shaft of femur and hips. Similarly, ejection from a vehicle is another predictor of serious injury, this victim having a 300% greater chance of sustaining a serious injury compared with those who remained in the car. Fatalities at scenes following RTAs should raise concerns, as it it significantly increases the likelihood of serious or life-threatening injuries in those who reach hospital alive.

Once this information has been received, the trauma reception team should be summoned to the resuscitation room.

THE TRAUMA RECEPTION TEAM

The make-up of this team varies between hospitals, depending upon resources and the time of the day. Nevertheless, it is recognized that resuscitation is carried out more effectively if the team has certain key features (Table 3.2).

Table 3.2 *Essential features of a trauma reception team*[2-6]

• Medical personnel trained in trauma management*
• Each person is assigned specific tasks
• There is senior team leadership

*For example, ATLS certification.

Each member of the team needs to be immunized against hepatitis and wearing protective clothing. In the UK, the latter consists of latex gloves, aprons and goggles. However, ideally universal precautions should be taken because all blood and body fluids must be assumed to carry HIV and hepatitis viruses.[7] While putting on their protective clothing, team members should be given the pre-hospital information and told their specific tasks during the resuscitation (Table 3.3). Ideally these duties should be carried out simultaneously under the direction of a team leader. In this way any life-threatening conditions can be

Table 3.3 *Tasks of the trauma reception team*

Role 1   Leader
- Coordinates the specific tasks of the individual team members
- Questions the ambulance personnel
- Assimilates the clinical findings
- Determines the investigations in order of priority
- Liaises with specialists who have been called
- Carries out particular procedures if they cannot be delegated to other team members

Role 2   Airway management
- Clears and secures the airway while taking appropriate cervical spine precautions
- Establishes a rapport with the patient giving psychological support throughout his/her ordeal in the resuscitation room

Role 3   Circulation management
- Establishes peripheral intravenous infusions and takes bloods for investigations
- Brings extra equipment as necessary
- Carries out other procedures depending on skill level (e.g. catheterization)
- Connects the patient to the monitors and records the vital signs
- Records intravenous and drug infusion

Role 4   Communications
- Cares for the patient's relatives when they arrive
- Liaises with the trauma team to provide the relatives with appropriate information and support
- Calls specialists on instruction from team leader

treated in the shortest possible time.[2,3] It is recognized, however, that in the UK the team may (at least initially) consist of only a single doctor and nurse. In such situations the key tasks must be carried out in the correct sequence (see below) until further help arrives.

RECEIVING THE PATIENT

In most units in the UK the ambulance bay is close to the resuscitation room. In these circumstances the patient can be rapidly transferred by the paramedic personnel. However, when the distance is great, or an airway problem has been identified, a doctor should quickly assess the patient in the ambulance to see if immediate intervention is required.

If the patient arrives in the resuscitation room on a long spine board, transfer to a hospital trolley will be straightforward, although the board will still need to be removed at the earliest suitable moment (usually during the log-roll). When this is not the case, five people will be required in order to achieve a safe transfer; this can usually be achieved by a combination of paramedic and departmental staff. This must be a well-practised procedure in order to protect the spinal cord if it is intact, and to prevent further injury if it is already compromised. During this transfer the patient's head and neck needs to be stabilized by one member of the team while three others lift from the side. This allows the fifth member to replace the ambulance trolley cot with a resuscitation trolley.

The team can now carry out a primary survey and resuscitation of the patient.

PRIMARY SURVEY AND RESUSCITATION

The objectives of this phase are to identify and correct any immediately life-threatening conditions. To do this, the activities listed in Table 3.4 need to carried out. The activities should be performed simultaneously if there are enough personnel, but if this is not the case the tasks should be carried out in alphabetical order. While this is going on the paramedics need to be asked about their pre-hospital findings (see Table 3.1).

Table 3.4 *The primary survey and resuscitation*

A – Airway and cervical spine control
B – Breathing
C – Circulation with haemorrhage control
D – Disability
E – Exposure

> **It is essential that problems are anticipated, rather than reacted to once they develop**

Airway and cervical spine control

A cervical spinal injury should be assumed if the patient has been the victim of significant blunt trauma, or if the mechanism of injury indicates that this region may have been damaged. Consequently, none of the activities described to clear and secure the airway must involve movement of the neck.

One member of the team needs manually to immobilize the cervical spine while talking to the patient. This not only establishes supportive contact, but also assesses the airway. If the patient replies in a normal voice, giving a logical answer, then the airway can be assumed to be patent and the brain adequately perfused. When there is an impaired or absent reply, the airway could be obstructed. In these cases the procedures described in Chapter 4 need to be carried out in order to clear and secure the airway.

The complications of alcohol ingestion and possible injuries of the chest and abdomen increase the chance of the patient vomiting. Consequently, constant supervision is required because it is impractical to nurse the trauma victim in any position other than supine. If vomiting does start, no attempt should be made to turn the patient's head to one side unless a cervical spine injury has been ruled out radiologically and clinically. If a spinal board is in place the whole patient can be turned; however, in the absence of this equipment, the trolley should be tipped head down by 20° and the vomit sucked away as it appears in the mouth.

Oxygen (100%) needs to be provided once the airway has been cleared and secured. When the breathing is adequate, the oxygen should be provided at a rate of 15 l/min via a mask with a reservoir bag attached. With a well-fitting mask an inspired oxygen concentration of approximately 85% can be achieved using this method. A pulse oximeter should then be connected to the patient. In cases where the SaO_2 cannot be maintained, ventilatory support must be provided mechanically. In these cases an end-tidal CO_2 monitor must be fitted to confirm tracheal intubation and provide some indication of pulmonary perfusion (see Chapter 4).

The neck should then be inspected for five features which could indicate the presence of an immediately life-threatening thoracic condition (Table 3.5).

Table 3.5 *Signs in the neck indicating possible life-threatening thoracic conditions*

Sign	Condition
Swellings and wounds	Vascular and airway injury
Distended neck veins	Cardiac tamponade, tension pneumothorax
Tracheal deviation	Tension pneumothorax
Subcutaneous emphysema	Pneumomediastinum
Laryngeal crepitus	Laryngeal cartilage fracture

When the presence of these signs has been checked, the neck can then be immobilized with an appropriately sized semi-rigid collar and a commercial head block and straps or sandbags and tape. The only exception to this rule is the restless patient who will not keep still. Since it is possible to damage the neck if the head is immobilized while the body moves, a suboptimal state is accepted; this consists of using a semi-rigid collar on its own.

Breathing

When assessing the trauma victim's chest in the primary survey, the doctor needs to keep in mind six immediately life-threatening thoracic conditions (Table 3.6).

Table 3.6 *Immediately life-threatening thoracic conditions*

- Airway obstruction
- Tension pneumothorax
- Open chest wound
- Massive haemothorax
- Flail chest
- Cardiac tamponade

Since these conditions require immediate treatment, the examination must be selective but efficient. The examination of the chest begins by inspection to see if there are any marks or wounds. The respiratory rate, effort and symmetry of breathing are then assessed. Percussion and auscultation in the axillae should then be carried out to assess ventilation of the periphery. Listening over the anterior chest mainly detects air movement in the large airways which can drown out sounds of pulmonary ventilation. Consequently, differences between the two sides of the chest can be missed, especially if the patient is being artificially ventilated.

> **The respiratory rate and effort are very sensitive indicators of underlying lung pathology. They should therefore be monitored and recorded at frequent intervals**

If there is no air entry to either side then there is either a complete obstruction of the upper airway, or an incomplete seal between the face and mask. The airway and ventilation technique should therefore be checked and treated appropriately (see Chapter 4). A local thoracic problem is more likely if there is asymmetry in air entry and the percussion note. The immediately life-threatening conditions capable of producing this are a tension pneumothorax, an open chest wound, and a massive haemothorax. Their diagnosis and management are discussed in detail in Chapter 5.

Examination of the back of the chest requires the patient to be turned onto their side. Normally this is carried out at the end of the primary survey (see below), but it can be useful to turn the patient at this stage in order to exclude a posterior chest injury if there are clinical suspicions.

Circulation

The key objectives regarding circulatory care are to stop any haemorrhage, assess for hypovolaemia, obtain vascular access and provide appropriate fluid resuscitation.

HAEMORRHAGE CONTROL

Bleeding can result from long-bone fractures, associated vascular injuries and soft tissue trauma. Irrespective of its source, such bleeding needs to be controlled. Direct pressure is the preferred way of managing external haemorrhage. In contrast, attempting to clamp vessels in the resuscitation room wastes time and may lead to further tissue damage. This applies particularly in cases of life-threatening internal or external haemorrhage. Associated hypothermia, acidosis and coagulopathy in these cases will enhance blood loss by preventing haemostatic control other than by direct pressure. It is therefore essential that these patients are identified early so that their appropriate management can be discussed by the surgeons, intensivists and emergency medical personnel.

Tourniquets increase intraluminal pressure, distal ischaemia and tissue necrosis, and should therefore only be used in cases where the limb is deemed unsalvageable or no other method has been effective in controlling bleeding, for example, major arterial bleeding. If this decision is taken, it is important to note the time that the tourniquet was applied so that neighbouring soft tissue is not jeopardized.

Long bones should be splinted and external fixation considered in certain pelvic fractures. When used appropriately the latter can be a life-saving manoeuvre as it can stop exsanguination, but it is only of use in particular types of pelvic fracture. Consequently, orthopaedic assessment of the patient and their radiographs is essential. In the meantime, pelvic binding or application of the pneumatic anti-shock garment (PASG) can be used to help reduce pelvic bleeding.

ASSESSMENT FOR HYPOVOLAEMIA

Once any overt haemorrhage has been stemmed, signs of hypovolaemia need to be sought. As with the thoracic examination this is best done in a systematic fashion. The skin should be observed for colour, clamminess and capillary refill time. The heart rate, blood pressure and pulse pressure are then measured, and the conscious level assessed. An automatic blood pressure recorder and ECG monitor should also be connected to the patient at this time so that these vitals signs can be recorded frequently.

It is important to be aware that patients have an altered cardiovascular response to haemorrhage after significant skeletal trauma.[8-10] The blood pressure and heart rate tends to be maintained even with significant blood loss, but this is at a cost of increased tissue oxygen debt and higher incidences of multiple organ failure. Isolated vital signs are therefore unreliable in estimating the blood loss or the physiological impairment of the patient, especially at the extremes of age.[10,11] Consequently, when assessing blood loss in the early stages of the resuscitation the functions of several essential organs need to be taken into account. In this way reliance is not simply placed on a single vital sign such as blood pressure. Later on, depending upon the clinical situation, these clinical assessments can be augmented by recordings from invasive monitoring devices.

By this time, the presence of significant amounts of blood in the thorax should have been suspected, established or excluded, a gentle palpation of the abdomen and a single attempt at compressing the pelvis will assist in the location of haemorrhage. The common sites of occult bleeding are:

- the chest;
- the abdomen and retroperitoneum;
- the pelvis;
- long-bone fractures; and
- external into splints and dressings.

VASCULAR CANNULATION

Trauma victims require large-bore intravenous access in areas which are not distal to vascular or bony damage. Once cannulation has been obtained, 20 ml of blood must be taken to allow for grouping and cross-match, analysis of the plasma electrolytes and a full blood count. A BM stix® should also be taken. If peripheral intravascular access is not possible, then a femoral line should be inserted or a venous cut-down carried out. Intra-osseous access is an effective alternative in children (see Chapter 13).

> **If the patient's name is not known, some system of identification is required, so that drugs and blood can be administered safely**

FLUID RESUSCITATION

The rate of fluid infusion needs to take into account the mechanism of injury. Evidence for this approach comes from clinical and animal studies.[12–15] Workers have shown an increase in survival by limiting fluid resuscitation, until surgery, in cases of unrepaired vascular injury following penetrating trauma. In contrast, infusing fluids to achieve a normal blood pressure will increase blood loss. The reasons for this are not precisely known, but it is probably due to a combination of impaired thrombus formation and inhibition of the body's physiological compensatory response to blood loss. It follows that patients who are shocked as a consequence of uncontrollable haemorrhage (for example, from penetrating trauma to the torso) need surgery rather than aggressive fluid resuscitation.

As described previously, the altered cardiovascular response to haemorrhage following blunt trauma means that a significant hemorrhage may have occurred by the time the blood pressure falls. Therefore, once any overt bleeding has been stemmed, enough warm crystalloid should be infused to maintain a radial pulse. Depending on the patient's response, warmed blood may also be needed. Further clinical assessment and more sophisticated monitoring will then be needed to ensure there is adequate tissue perfusion (see Chapter 6).

Disability

In the primary survey and resuscitation phase the AVPU response or, if time permits, the Glasgow Coma Score and pupillary response need to be recorded. These tests represent a baseline for the more detailed mini-neurological examination which is carried out in the secondary survey. It is essential that these assessments are monitored frequently to detect any deterioration. There are many possible causes for this, but the most common in the trauma patient are:

- hypoxia;
- hypovolaemia;
- hypoglycaemia (especially in the alcoholic and paediatric trauma victim); and
- raised intracranial pressure.

Exposure

The patient's remaining clothes should now be removed so that a full examination can be carried out. The presence of injuries, and the possibility of spinal instability, mean that garments must be cut along seams so that there is minimal patient movement. It is important to note that the rapid removal of tight trousers can precipitate sudden hypotension due to the loss of the tamponade effect in the hypovolaemic patient. These garments should only be removed when effective intravenous access has been established.

> **Once stripped, trauma victims must be kept warm and covered with blankets when not being examined**

It is important to be aware that trauma victims often have sharp objects such as broken glass and other debris in their clothing, hair and on their skin. Because ordinary surgical gloves provide no protection against this, the personnel undressing the patient must initially wear more robust gloves.

At this stage, a log-roll should be carried out after the removal of neck immobilization devices and the substitution of manual immobilization. This assesses the spine from the base of the skull to the coccyx, and a rectal examination is carried out at the same time (Table 3.7). In addition, the back of the patient is carefully examined for signs of injury.

Table 3.7 *Information from a rectal examination*

- Is sphincter tone present?
- Has the rectal wall been breached?
- Can spicules of bone be felt?
- Is the prostate in a normal position?
- Is there blood on the examiner's finger?

When the primary survey has been completed, the team leader should pause to carry out a quick mental check (Table 3.8). Using the information available so far it is then important to consider if the patient is getting better or worse and this also helps to determine if urgent surgical intervention is required. For example, the patient may need to be taken directly to the operating theatre to gain control of a source of bleeding if there is no response to aggressive intravenous resuscitation.

Table 3.8 *Mental check at the end of the primary survey and resuscitation phase*

- Is the airway still secure?
- Is the patient receiving high-flow oxygen?
- Are all the tubes and lines secure?
- Have the blood samples been sent to the laboratories?
- Are all the monitors functioning?
- Are the vital signs being recorded every 5 min?
- Is an arterial blood gas sample needed?
- Has the radiographer been called?

> **Only when all the ventilatory and hypovolaemic problems have been corrected can the team continue the more detailed secondary survey**

In the UK, relatives and friends often arrive at the same time as the patient. It is best that these people are met by a nurse who is not involved in the resuscitation. Then, depending upon their wishes, they can be accompanied to the resuscitation room or to a private room which has all necessary facilities. The decision to admit relatives to the resuscitation room will depend on local policy. If relatives are not admitted to the resuscitation room, information can be passed to them from the resuscitation on a regular basis, while at the same time information can be sought about the patient's past medical history and current medication.

SECONDARY SURVEY

Once the immediately life-threatening conditions have been either excluded or treated, the whole of the patient should be assessed. This requires a head-to-toe, front-to-back assessment along with a detailed medical history and appropriate investigations. In this way all the injuries can be detected and appropriately prioritized. The common error of being distracted before the whole body has been inspected must be avoided, as potentially serious injuries can be missed – especially in the unconscious patient.

If the patient deteriorates at any stage, their airway, breathing and circulatory state must be immediately re-assessed in the manner described in the primary survey

---

Examination

THE SCALP

The entire scalp needs to be examined for lacerations, swellings or depressions. This requires the neck support to be removed (when required) and the head to be immobilized manually. The front and sides of the scalp can then be checked. The occipital region should already have been examined during the log-roll. Blind probing of wounds should be avoided, as further damage to underlying structures can result.

It is important to remember that in small children, scalp lacerations can bleed sufficiently to cause hypovolaemia; consequently haemostasis is crucial in these cases, and this is best achieved either by applying direct pressure or by using a self-retaining retractor.

NEUROLOGICAL STATE

An assessment of the Glasgow Coma Score, the pupillary responses and the presence of any lateralizing signs should now be recorded. These constitute a 'mini-neurological' examination which acts as a robust assessment of the patient's neurological state (see Chapter 8). These parameters should be measured frequently so that any deterioration can be detected early.

BASE OF SKULL

The skull base lies along a diagonal running from the mastoid to the eye. Consequently, the signs of a fracture are also found along this line (Table 3.9).

Table 3.9 *Signs of a base of skull fracture*

- Bruising over the mastoid (Battles's sign)
- Haemotympanum
- Blood and CSF ottorrhoea
- Blood and CSF rhinorrhaea
- 'Panda eyes'
- Scleral haemorrhage with no posterior margin
- Sub-hyloid haemorrhage

Because Battle's sign and 'panda eyes' usually take 12–36 h to appear, they are of limited use in the resuscitation room. A cerebrospinal fluid (CSF) leak may be missed as it is invariably mixed with blood. Fortunately, the presence of CSF in this bloody discharge can be detected by noting the delay in clotting of the blood, and the double ring pattern when it is dropped onto an absorbent sheet. This should preclude auroscopy of the external auditory canal because of the risk of meningitis. As there is a small chance of a nasogastric tube passing into the cranium through a base of skull fracture, these tubes should be passed orally when this type of injury is suspected.

EYES

Inspection of the eyes must be carried out before significant orbital swelling makes examination too difficult. It is important to check for haemorrhages, both inside and outside the globe, for foreign bodies under the lids (including contact lenses), and for the presence of penetrating injuries. If the patient is conscious, the visual acuity can be tested by asking them to read a name badge or fluid label. If they are unconscious, the pupillary response and corneal reflexes must be determined.

THE FACE

Most of the significant facial injuries can be detected by gentle, symmetrical palpation and inspection. The presence of lost or loose teeth should be established, as well as the stability of the maxilla, by gently pulling the latter forward to see if the middle third of the face is stable. Middle-third fractures can be associated with both an airway obstruction and base of skull fractures. However, only those injuries co-existing with an airway obstruction need to be treated immediately. Mandibular fractures can also cause airway obstruction because of the loss of stability of the tongue.

THE NECK

If this has not already occurred during the log-roll, the neck should be carefully examined. While in-line manual stabilization is being maintained, the neck should be inspected for any deformity, bruising and lacerations. The cervical spinous processes and neck muscles can then be palpated for tenderness or deformity. The conscious patient can assist in this examination by indicating the site of any pain or tenderness.

Lacerations should *never* be probed, since torrential haemorrhage can occur if there is an underlying vascular injury. If the wound penetrates the platysma, definitive radiological or surgical management will be needed, the choice depending upon how stable the patient is.

THE THORAX

There are several potentially life-threatening conditions (Table 3.10) which need to be considered at this stage, as well as some minor thoracic injuries (for example, fractured ribs). The former will require further investigations to confirm their presence. Because this will usually mean taking the patient out of the resuscitation room, it is essential that it is done only when clinical suspicion is present and more serious conditions have been treated or excluded. Information regarding the mechanism of injury, as well as a detailed examination, is therefore particularly important.

Table 3.10 *Potentially life-threatening thoracic conditions*

- Pulmonary contusions
- Cardiac contusion
- Ruptured oesophagus
- Disruption of the thoracic aorta
- Diaphragmatic rupture
- Rupture of the trachea or main bronchi

Acceleration and deceleration forces can produce extensive thoracic injuries, including aortic disruption as well as pulmonary and cardiac contusions. However, these often leave marks on the chest wall which should lead the team to consider particular types of injury. For example, the diagonal seat belt bruise may overlap a fractured clavicle, a thoracic aortic tear, pulmonary contusion or pancreatic laceration. The rate, effort and symmetry of breathing should also be re-checked.

The presence of any crepitus, tenderness and subcutaneous emphysema must be noted when the sternum and ribs are palpated. Auscultation and percussion of the whole chest can then be carried out in order to check again if there is any asymmetry between the right and left sides of the chest.

THE ABDOMEN

The key objective of the abdominal examination is to decide if a laparotomy is required. This requires a thorough examination of the whole abdomen, including the pelvis and perineum. All bruising, abnormal movement and wounds must be noted, and any exposed bowel covered with warm saline-soaked swabs. As with the scalp, wounds should not be probed blindly as further damage can result. Furthermore, the actual depth of the wound cannot be determined if underlying muscle is penetrated. Consequently these cases will require further investigations (see Chapter 7).

Following inspection, palpation should be carried out in a systematic manner so that areas of tenderness can be detected. Percussion is an ideal way of locating these sites without distressing the patient.

The rate of urine output is an important indicator in assessing the shocked patient, and therefore it should be measured in all trauma patients. If this requires catheterization, a transurethral approach should be used if there is no evidence of urethral injury (Table 3.11). In contrast, when the patient is unable to urinate a suprapubic catheter may be necessary. The urine which is voided initially should be tested for blood and saved for microscopy and subsequent possible drug analysis.

Marked gastric distention is frequently found in crying children, adults with head or abdominal injuries, and patients who have been ventilated with a bag-and-mask technique. The insertion of a gastric tube facilitates the abdominal examination of these patients and reduces the risks of aspiration.

Table 3.11 *Signs of urethral injury in a male patient*

- Bruising around the scrotum
- Blood at the end of the urethral meatus
- High-riding prostate

> **An intra-abdominal bleed should be suspected if the patient is haemodynamically unstable for no apparent reason, especially if the lower six ribs are fractured or there are marks over the abdominal surface**

Abdominal examination is unreliable if there is a sensory defect due to neurological damage or drugs, or if there are fractures of the lower ribs or pelvis. In these cases further investigation will be required. The choice is dependent upon the resources available and the haemodynamic stability of the patient. Ultrasound and diagnostic peritoneal lavage can be done in the resuscitation room, but may not be diagnostic. Computed tomography (CT) provides greater information, particularly when contrast is used, but requires the patient to be moved.

EXTREMITIES

The limbs are examined in the traditional manner of inspection – palpation and active and passive movement. This will enable any bruising, wounds and deformities to be detected as well as crepitus, instability, neurovascular abnormalities, compartment syndrome or soft-tissue damage. Any wounds associated with open fractures must be swabbed and covered with a non-adherent dressing. Gross limb deformities should also be corrected, and the pulses and sensation re-checked, before any radiographs are taken.

All limb fractures need splintage to reduce fracture movement and hence reduce pain, bleeding, the formation of fat emboli and secondary soft-tissue swelling and damage. In the case of shaft of femur fractures, a traction splint should be used.

NEUROLOGICAL ASSESSMENT

A detailed neurological examination needs to be carried out at this stage to determine if there are any abnormalities in the peripheral and sympathetic nervous systems. Motor and sensory defects, and in male patients also, the presence of priaprism, can help to indicate the level and extent of the spinal injury.

SOFT-TISSUE INJURIES

The whole of the patient's skin must be examined to determine the number and extent of the soft-tissue injuries. Each wound needs to be inspected to determine its site, size, depth and the presence of any underlying structural damage. Once the clinical state of the patient stabilizes, superficial wounds can be cleaned, irrigated and dressed. Deeper wounds, and those involving vital structures, will require surgical repair.

THE BACK

Following the initial assessment of the back during the log-roll, this should be supplemented (if clinically indicated) by a more comprehensive assessment. The whole of the back, from occiput to heels, can then be checked and the back of the chest auscultated. The viability of the decubitus skin should be assessed.

Patients who cannot move due to neurological impairment, and also the elderly, have a high risk of developing pressure sores. Preventive steps must therefore be taken from the outset. The spinal board should be removed as soon as possible and the decubitus area moved every 30 min, using hip lifts for example.

Analgesia

Pain control is a fundamental aspect of the management of trauma patients. This is not only for humanitarian reasons, but also because pain can reduce the tolerance of the patient to hypovolaemia.[8,16] However, analgesia may mask important clinical signs and symptoms. For example, systemic analgesia can hide a fall in conscious level from a rise in intracranial pressure. Furthermore, in extremity injuries, systemic and regional analgesia can mask the symptoms of rising compartment pressure. Specialist teams involved in the patient's definitive care therefore need to know what analgesia has been given so that early signs are not missed. It is also important to maintain careful monitoring of the patient's status once the analgesia has been administered.

Good communication, explanation and gentle handling are important preliminaries to pain relief. Correct immobilization of injured limbs can also be very effective. In addition, the team should be proficient in providing the other common types of analgesia such as entonox, morphine and regional analgesia.[17]

Radiography

Over 90% of UK trauma victims will have been subjected to a blunt force. All these patients require chest and pelvic radiographs in the resuscitation room. Radiographs of the cervical spine should also be taken if clinically indicated. At the end of the secondary survey further radiographs will also need to be taken to help identify suspected skeletal and spinal abnormalities. The team leader needs to determine which investigations are required, and when. Radiographs of particular sites of injury can then be performed on stable patients along with other specialized investigations. The latter may involve transporting the patient to specialized areas where magnetic resonance imaging (MRI), CT or angiography can be carried out. This decision-making process can be helped greatly by discussing the case with the different specialists involved in the patient's care.

Medical history

There are five key pieces of information which need to be gathered on all trauma victims (Table 3.12). Often, this AMPLE history is acquired piece-meal while the patient is resuscitated. Nevertheless, time should be spent at the end of the secondary survey to ensure that it is complete.

Table 3.12 *An AMPLE history*

- A – Allergies
- M – Medicines
- P – Past medical history
- L – Last meal
- E – Events leading to the incident

Obtaining details about the patient's past medical history is particularly important in the UK because trauma victims here have a high incidence of illness.[18] The most common is cardiovascular disease, followed by psychiatric and respiratory problems. This information can be gained from the patient or his/her relatives, or by inspection of previous hospital records or communication with the patient's general practitioner.

> **Pre-existing disease in a trauma victim increases their chances of dying**

Assimilation of information

Because the condition of the patient can change quickly, repeated examinations and constant monitoring of the vital signs is essential. This enables the following questions to be answered:

1. Is the patient's respiratory function satisfactory? If it is not adequate, then the cause must be sought and corrected as a priority.

2. Is the patient's circulatory status satisfactory? It is essential that the trauma team recognizes shock early in its progress and intervenes promptly. It is equally important to evaluate the patient's response to the resuscitative measures.

If there has been less than 20% of the blood volume lost, the vital signs usually return to normal after less than 2 l of fluid. If the signs then remain stable, the patient is probably not actively bleeding. However, care and constant supervision is needed in these cases because such trauma victims may deteriorate later.

Transient responders are patients who are actively bleeding or recommence bleeding during the resuscitation. Therefore their vital signs initially improve but then deteriorate. They have usually lost over 30% of their blood volume, and require an infusion with typed blood. Control of the bleeding source invariably requires an operation.

Little or no response to fluid resuscitation by the shocked patient indicates either that the condition is not due to hypovolaemia, or the patient has lost over 40% of their blood volume and is bleeding faster than the infusion rate. The history, mechanism of injury and the physical findings will help to determine which is the most likely. The former requires invasive techniques to monitor the pulmonary and central venous pressures. In the case of major haemorrhage, an operation and a blood transfusion are urgently required. The source of the bleeding is usually in the chest, abdomen or pelvis.

3. What are the extent and priorities of the injuries? The ABC system is used to categorize injuries so that the most dangerous is treated first. For example, problems with the airway must be corrected before those of the circulation.

4. Have any injuries been overlooked?   The mechanism and pattern of injury must be considered in order to avoid overlooking sites of damage. Victims of blunt trauma have the injuring force dispersed over a wide area. As a result, trauma rarely 'skips' areas. For example, if an injury has been found in the thorax and femur, but not in the abdomen, then it has probably been missed. The patient must be re-examined.

5. Are tetanus toxoid, human antitetanus immunoglobulin or antibiotics required?   These will depend on both local and national policies, which should be known by the team leader.

Documentation and property

Comprehensive medical and nursing notes are required so that the specialist looking after the patient is fully aware of what injuries have been identified, and the treatment which has been provided. Many units have a purpose-designed single trauma sheet to help this process. If the patient is unconscious, his/her clothing and belongings should be searched. This may provide clues to the person's identity, as well as essential medical information.

Any possessions brought in with the patient must be logged and kept safe, along with the patient's clothing. This should be with their permission if they are conscious. Rings and other constrictive jewellery must also be removed as the fingers may swell. If a criminal case is suspected, all clothing, possessions, loose debris, bullets and shrapnel are required for forensic examination. These must be collected in labelled bags and signed for before releasing them to the police.

Relatives

Communication with the relatives usually carries on during the resuscitation, either directly or by the relatives' nurse. Nevertheless, once the secondary survey is completed it is useful for the team leader to appraise the relatives of the current findings and management plan. In doing this he/she should be accompanied by the relatives' nurse so that he/she is aware of what has been said.

TRANSITION TO DEFINITIVE CARE

Once the patient has been adequately assessed and resuscitated, definitive care can start. In many cases this will require either an operation(s) or intensive care management or, frequently, both. This requires the patient's injuries to be given their correct priority (Table 3.13).

Table 3.13 *Factors affecting the priority of an injury*

- Are the injuries immediately life-threatening?
- Are the injuries potentially life-threatening?
- Are the injuries limb-threatening?
- What is the physiological state of the patient?
- What resources are available in the hospital?
- Will the patient require intra-hospital transfer for further specialist care?

Because around 95% of UK trauma patients are victims of a blunt force, many have sustained multiple injuries.[19] A further consideration therefore is the logistics of carrying out several procedures on the patient, and how well he/she can physiologically cope. It may be appropriate in certain cases of significant multiple injuries to use a staged operative procedure, with the patient returning to the Intensive Care Unit between theatre sessions. This will enable the operations to be carried out when the patient is in their optimal physiological state.

Finally, the team leader should consider if there is any advantage in carrying out certain treatments in patients who require transfer to another hospital for some of their injuries. For example, it would be essential that a haemodynamically unstable head-injured patient is not transferred to a neurosurgical centre until the source of his/her bleeding has been identified and treated.

> **Optimum definitive care requires accurate information on the patient's injuries and physiological state, clinical experience, and a good liaison with all the specialists involved in the patient's care**

SUMMARY

Initial trauma care is best provided by a team of trained staff who are carrying out their tasks simultaneously under the direction of an experienced team leader. In this way, the immediately life-threatening conditions can be identified first and treated appropriately. Subsequently, a full history can be obtained while a detailed head-to-toe examination is carried out. The team leader can then list the patient's injuries, and their priorities for both further investigations and definitive treatment.

REFERENCES

1. Driscoll P, Monsell F, Duane L, Wardle T, Brown T. Optimal long bone fracture management. Part II – initial resuscitation and assessment in the accident and emergency department. *International Journal of Orthopaedic Trauma* 1995; **5**: 110–7.
2. Driscoll P, Vincent C. Organising an efficient trauma team. *Injury* 1992; **23**: 107–10.
3. Driscoll P, Vincent C. Variation in trauma resuscitation and its effect on patient outcome. *Injury* 1992; **23**: 111–15.
4. Burdett-Smith P. Airey G, Franks A. Improvement in trauma survival in Leeds. *Injury* 1995; **26**: 455–8.
5. Lecky F, Woodford M, Yates D. Trends in trauma care in England and Wales 1989–97. *Lancet* 2000; **355**: 1771–5.
6. Joint working party RCS England and British Orthopaedic Association. *Better Care for the Severely Injured*. Royal College of Surgeons (England), 2000.
7. Walker J, Driscoll P. Trauma team protection from infective contamination. In: Driscoll P, Gwinnutt C, Jimmerson C, Goodall O (eds). *Trauma Resection: The Team Approach*. London: Macmillan Press Ltd, 1993.
8. Rady M, Little R, Edwards D, Kirkman E, Faithful S. The effect of nociceptive stimulation on the changes in haemodynamics and oxygen transport induced by haemorrhage in anaesthetised pigs. *Journal of Trauma* 1991; **31**: 617–21.
9. Driscoll P. Changes in systolic blood pressure, heart rate, shock index, rate pressure product and tympanic temperature following blood loss and tissue damage in humans. Leeds University, MD Thesis, 1994.
10. Little R, Kirkman E, Driscoll P, Hanson J, Mackway-Jones K. Preventable deaths after injury: why are the traditional 'vital' signs poor indicators of blood loss. *Journal of Accident and Emergency Medicine* 1995; **12**: 1–14.
11. Scalea T, Simon H, Duncan A, *et al.* Geriatric blunt multiple trauma: increased survival with early invasive monitoring. *Journal of Trauma* 1990; **30**: 129–34.
12. Owens T, Watson W, Prough D, Kramer G. Limiting initial resuscitation of uncontrolled hemorrhage reduces internal bleeding and subsequent volume requirements. *Journal of Trauma* 1995; **39**: 200–9.
13. Bickell W, Wail M, Pepe P, *et al.* A comparison of immediate versus delayed fluid resuscitation for hypotensive patients with penetrating torso injury. *New England Journal of Medicine* 1994; **331**: 1105–9.

14. Kaweski S, Sise M, Virgillo R. The effect of prehospital fluids on survival in trauma patients. *Journal of Trauma* 1990; **30**: 1215–18.

15. Krausz M, Bar-Ziv M, Rabinovich R *et al*. 'Scoop and run' or stabilize hemorrhagic shock with normal saline or small-volume hypertonic saline? *Journal of Trauma* 1992; **23**: 6–10.

16. Kirkman E, Little R. Cardiovascular regulation during hypovolaemic shock: central integration. In: Secher N, Pawelczyk J, Ludbrook L (eds). *The Bradycardic Phase in Hypovolaemic Shock*. London: Edward Arnold, 1994.

17. Driscoll P, Gwinnutt C, Nancarrow J. Analgesia in the emergency department. *Pain Reviews* 1995; **2**: 187–202.

18. Wardle T, Driscoll P, Oxbey C, Woodford M, Campbell F. Pre-existing medical conditions in trauma patients. *40th Annual Proceedings of the Association for the Advancement of Automotive Medicine* 1996: **40**: 351–61.

19. Anderson I, Woodford M, Irving M. Preventability of death from penetrating injury in England and Wales. *Injury* 1989; **20**: 69–71.

4

Airway management

OBJECTIVES

- To understand the importance of airway maintenance, ventilation and oxygenation in the trauma patient
- To recognize airway obstruction
- To understand the principles of basic and advanced airway management techniques
- To recognize the importance of simultaneous cervical spine control

INTRODUCTION

The airway and breathing are the first priorities in trauma resuscitation. Airway obstruction is common in trauma victims, and may lead to *preventable* deaths – preventable often by simple and basic measures.[1] Trauma patients die from *tissue hypoxia*, either from poor oxygenation, inadequate circulation, or both.

> **The airway is the first priority in resuscitation**

In the 'A,B,C' of resuscitation, 'A' comes before 'B', and 'B' before 'C'! If a problem is found at any stage it must be corrected immediately, before moving on to the next step. An obstructed airway must be cleared immediately, or severe hypoxic brain damage and cardiac arrest will occur within minutes. Likewise, a clear airway does not guarantee adequate ventilation, and any further treatment is futile if hypoxia cannot be corrected. Therefore the airway, breathing and oxygenation are assessed and managed *first*, and must not be overlooked even if there are other, more dramatic injuries!

Cervical spine injuries may be exacerbated by airway management. In any trauma patient at risk, the cervical spine must be stabilized *simultaneously* with any necessary airway manoeuvre.

> **Airway and cervical spine control must occur simultaneously**

AIRWAY PROBLEMS IN TRAUMA

Airway problems in the trauma patient may be due to:

- soft-tissue obstruction. In the unconscious patient, muscle tone in the neck and pharynx is lost, and the tongue 'falls back'. In fact, the airway also obstructs at other sites including the soft palate and epiglottis, particularly if the patient is generating negative pressure by respiratory efforts.[2]
- oedema, haematoma or other swelling, due to trauma or burns of the head and neck. Airway burns in particular can cause very rapid and severe oedema, which may be fatal

without early intubation. Direct trauma to the larynx or trachea may also cause obstruction.[3]

- foreign bodies or foreign material – either intrinsic or extrinsic. Teeth, dentures, pieces of tissue, blood clots, semi-solid stomach contents or any other foreign matter may block the airway.
- displaced facial bones. A fractured maxilla may be displaced postero-inferiorly, obstructing the airway by the soft palate against the back of the pharynx. Similarly, a 'flail segment' of jaw from a bilateral mandibular fracture allows the tongue to fall backwards.[4]
- suspected cervical spine injuries. In such patients the head and neck must be immobilized in-line, to prevent further damage due to airway management. Immobilization will itself make airway management more difficult.
- aspiration of gastric contents. Many patients sustain trauma 'on a full stomach', and protective laryngeal reflexes are likely to be obtunded in those who are not fully conscious. Regurgitation may lead to potentially fatal aspiration pneumonia.

PATHOPHYSIOLOGY

Oxygen is essential for cellular metabolism, and therefore for organ function. In the presence of oxygen, cells metabolize biochemical fuels aerobically to generate energy and carbon dioxide. Under conditions of hypoxia, cells convert to anaerobic metabolism. This cannot be sustained: it is much less efficient in generating energy, and causes progressive metabolic acidosis due to lactic acid production. Cells cease to function, and eventually are permanently damaged: 'lack of oxygen stops the machine and then wrecks the machinery'.[5]

Hypoxia means reduced tissue oxygen availability. This can be due to inadequate circulation, and/or *hypoxaemia* (low oxygen content of arterial blood). It also occurs when cells are unable to utilize the delivered oxygen, as in carbon monoxide and cyanide poisoning.

As well as a clear airway, tissue oxygen supply depends on:

- *ventilation* – the mechanical process by which air is drawn into the lungs.
- *diffusion* – of oxygen across the alveolar–capillary membrane and of carbon dioxide in the reverse direction.
- *perfusion* – the circulation carries oxygenated blood to the tissue capillary beds, from which oxygen and carbon dioxide pass into and out of cells.

Ventilation is discussed in Chapter 5. Essentially, normal inspiration results from contraction of the diaphragm and the external intercostal muscles, although in respiratory difficulty the accessory muscles (scalene and sternomastoid) are also active. However, expiration is normally a passive process, resulting mainly from the elastic recoil of the lungs. During inspiration, muscle tone in the pharynx increases to counteract the negative airway pressure generated, and the vocal cords abduct. This increased tone is abolished in the unconscious patient, contributing to inspiratory 'collapse' of the pharynx and consequent airway obstruction.

Airway obstruction and hypoventilation lead to *hypoxaemia* and *hypercarbia*. Relief of airway obstruction may also lead to post-obstructive pulmonary oedema.[6]

Causes of hypoxaemia

The causes of hypoxaemia are given in Table 4.1.

A fall in cardiac output will lower mixed venous oxygen saturation, because the body continues to extract oxygen at the same rate from a slower circulation. If impaired alveolar–capillary diffusion is also present, hypoxaemia is exacerbated by systemic 'shunting' of this abnormally desaturated venous blood.

Table 4.1 *Causes of hypoxaemia*

- Low partial pressure of inspired oxygen – e.g. smoke inhalation
- Airway obstruction
- Apnoea or hypoventilation:
    central nervous system depression (head injury or drugs)
    spinal cord injury, affecting the diaphragm or intercostal
    muscles
- Mechanical interference with ventilation:
    flail chest
    tension pneumothorax
    haemothorax
- Impaired diffusion across alveolar–capillary membrane:
    pulmonary oedema
    lung contusion
    lung consolidation or collapse
    aspiration of blood, fluid or vomit
- Low cardiac output:
    hypovolaemia
    myocardial contusion
    cardiac tamponade
    tension pneumothorax

Effects of hypoxia

Different organs have different sensitivities to hypoxia, the heart and brain being the most sensitive. The main effects of hypoxia are:

- *metabolic*: anaerobic metabolism, metabolic acidosis, hyperkalaemia (although in practice *hypo*kalaemia commonly occurs due to the hormonal 'stress response').
- *neurological*: cerebral vasodilation and raised intracranial pressure leading to confusion, agitation, drowsiness, fits and coma.
- *cardiovascular*: impaired contractility, dysrhythmias (*severe* hypoxia leads to serious bradycardia and ultimately asystole).
- *respiratory*: increased respiratory drive (unless hypoxia is due to hypoventilation).
- *renal*: impaired renal function, acute renal failure.
- *gastrointestinal*: hypoxic liver dysfunction; increased gut mucosal permeability leading to systemic inflammatory response.

Effects of hypercarbia

The main effects of hypercarbia are:

- *metabolic*: respiratory acidosis, hyperkalaemia.
- *neurological*: cerebral vasodilation and raised intracranial pressure leading to drowsiness and unconsciousness.
- *cardiovascular*: sympathetic stimulation, causing hypertension, tachycardia and dysrhythmias.
- *respiratory*: increased respiratory drive (unless the hypercarbia is due to hypoventilation).

ASSESSMENT OF THE AIRWAY AND BREATHING

A thorough structured assessment of the airway is essential in order to:

- identify a *compromised* airway and breathing.
- identify the *potential for deterioration* of airway and breathing. Deterioration may occur as a result of:
  - a decreasing level of consciousness, leading to soft tissue obstruction

- increasing oedema (especially from burns or fractures) or haematoma
- an accumulation of blood, secretions or regurgitated matter.
- identify *potential risks* of airway management, for example:
  - cervical spine injury
  - laryngeal fracture or other airway trauma (which may be worsened by intubation).

Airway assessment and management take place simultaneously, but assessment is described here separately for clarity. Continual re-assessment is vital because of the risk of deterioration. If the patient deteriorates in any way, it is essential to return to the basic 'A,B,C' approach and to re-assess the airway. For example, an increased respiratory rate may be due to an obstructing airway, progression of a pneumothorax or deteriorating hypovolaemic shock.

Continual re-assessment is vital

The 15-second assessment

During this rapid first assessment (see Chapter 3), it is important to take a 'quick look' for obvious airway problems, such as cyanosis or respiratory distress. A patient who answers questions sensibly must have a clear airway, reasonable breathing and reasonable cerebral perfusion, as well as being grossly intact neurologically.

Detailed assessment

The detailed assessment of the airway can be divided into three phases: *Look*, *listen* and *feel*.

- *Look* at:
  - *the airway*: for visible obstruction, oedema, haematoma, foreign body, trauma or burns; and
  - *the neck and chest*: for breathing (rate, pattern and depth), use of accessory muscles, tracheal tug, tracheal deviation, abnormal movement, or visible trauma.
- *Listen* for:
  - breath sounds at the mouth;
  - snoring noises (possible soft-tissue obstruction);
  - gurgling noises (possible blood, vomit or saliva in the airway);
  - stridor (an inspiratory 'crowing' sound, signifying *partial* upper airway obstruction or laryngospasm); and
  - hoarseness (possible laryngeal obstruction or injury).
- *Feel* at:
  - the mouth, for air movement; and
  - the neck and chest: for signs of injury (tenderness, crepitus, subcutaneous emphysema).

Upper airway obstruction leads to paradoxical see-sawing movement, whereby the chest moves out and the abdomen moves in on inspiration, and the opposite on expiration. The accessory muscles will be active, and tracheal tug may occur. (In children, intercostal and subcostal recession are seen.)

Laryngeal injuries may not be obvious, but signs include swelling, voice change, laryngeal crepitus and subcutaneous emphysema.[3]

It should be noted that airway obstruction is only shown by most of the above signs *if the patient is breathing!* In the apnoeic, the only sign may be difficulty ventilating the patient.

Remember 'respiratory distress' may be due not only to an airway or breathing problem, but also to:
- **severe shock (respiratory centre activation)**
- **head injury (causing tachypnoea, bradypnoea or irregular breathing)**

AIRWAY MANAGEMENT SUMMARY

This section describes an overall plan of airway management in the trauma patient. Specific skills and equipment are described later.

Immediate actions

The important components of the initial management of the airway in the trauma victim include the following.

CERVICAL SPINE CONTROL

If the patient is not already immobilized, the cervical spine should be stabilized immediately if there is any suspicion of spinal injury. If there is any doubt, the neck should be immobilized, as this can always be discontinued later if it is found to be unnecessary.

If the patient is conscious and has a clear airway, after initial manual stabilization, immobilization should be achieved with a semi-rigid cervical collar, head blocks or sandbags, and forehead strapping. If the patient has a decreased conscious level or airway compromise, manual in-line stabilization (MILS) should be performed until the airway is secured.

OXYGEN

High-flow oxygen should be given as soon as possible in any patient with significant trauma. Again, it can always be removed later if found to be unnecessary.

> **Oxygen comes with the 'A' and 'B' of the primary survey**

CRICOID PRESSURE

Cricoid pressure can be used to prevent gastric regurgitation. If manpower allows, cricoid pressure should be applied as soon as possible in unconscious patients needing assisted ventilation or advanced airway management.

PULSE OXIMETRY

Monitoring the patient's pulse oximetry reading will provide useful information regarding tissue oxygenation; however, it does not provide information about levels of carbon dioxide and can be falsely reassuring in cases of respiratory insufficiency.

ANAESTHETIC HELP

If advanced airway techniques seem indicated, anaesthetic assistance should be sought sooner rather than later.

> **Always obtain early anaesthetic assistance**

The patient must be re-assessed after every intervention. It is important not to *assume* that an action has had its desired effect.

Basic airway management

A plan for basic airway management is given below.

1. Assess the airway and breathing.
   - If airway clear, go to '7' below.
   - If the patient is already intubated, check the tube position carefully and go to '12' below.

Otherwise:

2. Check the mouth for foreign matter.
    If it is present, it can be removed by suction (wide-bore Yankauer sucker) for liquids, or Magill's forceps for solids, under direct vision or laryngoscopy.
3. If obstruction persists and the patient is not fully conscious, try a jaw thrust or jaw lift. It is important to avoid head tilt as it may exacerbate cervical spine injury. However, the airway takes priority over the cervical spine (see below).
4. If obstruction persists, try either:
    –   An oropharyngeal airway in the unconscious patient without a gag reflex.
    –   A nasopharyngeal airway if a gag reflex is present, or an oral airway cannot be inserted (caution in suspected base of skull or maxillary fractures).
    If an oral airway causes gagging, coughing or laryngospasm, it should be removed and a nasopharyngeal airway considered.
5. If facial trauma is present, forward traction on a fractured maxilla, mandible or the tongue may relieve the obstruction.[4]
6. If obstruction persists despite the above manoeuvres, proceed to advanced airway control (below). However, it is important to consider the following first:
    –   Persistent soft-tissue obstruction: reposition for optimal jaw thrust.
    –   Foreign body: see '2' above.
    –   Wrong size of oral/nasal airway: consider changing size.
    –   Oral airway ineffective: try a nasal airway.
7. If the airway is clear, check the breathing.
    If there is spontaneous adequate breathing, 10–15 l/min oxygen should be administered via a non-rebreather reservoir mask. If the breathing is inadequate, the patient should be ventilated using a bag-and-mask, with oxygen at 10–15 l/min, while preparations are made to proceed with advanced airway management. Expert anaesthetic assistance should be sought if this has not already been obtained.

Advanced airway management

8. Use orotracheal intubation with MILS if:
    –   There is inadequate ventilation or apnoea.
    –   The patient is unconscious, and unable to maintain or protect their airway.
    –   There is actual or potential airway obstruction (airway swelling or burns).
    –   The patient has a head injury, with Glasgow Coma Score either ≤8 or deteriorating.
    –   There is hypoxaemia unrelieved by other measures.
    Anaesthetic drugs and expertise are needed if the patient is not deeply unconscious.
9. If intubation is difficult, temporary alternatives should be considered including:
    –   The laryngeal mask airway (LMA).
    –   The oesophageal–tracheal Combitube®.
10. In the conscious patient with impending airway obstruction, it may be necessary to consider, if expertise allows, one or more of the following manoeuvres:
    –   Awake fibreoptic intubation.
    –   Intubation after gaseous induction of anaesthesia.
    –   Surgical cricothyrotomy under local anaesthesia.
11. Perform immediate needle cricothyrotomy if complete airway obstruction cannot be relieved by intubation or any other method. This can be followed by specialist techniques for intubation, or by a formal surgical airway.
12. It is important to be alert for tube displacement and complications of ventilation such as tension pneumothorax.

Be alert for tube displacement

---

13. Early blood gas analysis will provide vital information. Arterial line insertion should be considered early, but only if it will not delay life-saving surgery. This allows:
    –   Continuous second-by-second monitoring of blood pressure.
    –   Frequent blood sampling for arterial blood gases and other tests.

CERVICAL SPINE STABILIZATION

Cervical spine injury (CSI) must be assumed in all patients with an appropriate mechanism of injury (see Chapters 2 and 9). However, CSI can only be excluded by a combination of radiological investigation and clinical examination in the *conscious patient*, or possibly by MRI scan in the unconscious. Plain X-radiography alone cannot 'clear' the spine[7-9] (although negative X-rays reduce the likelihood of the presence of CSI). Therefore:

- cervical spine X-rays must never be allowed to delay life-saving interventions; and
- CSI must still be assumed in patients with decreased levels of consciousness, even if X-rays are negative.

Adequate methods for cervical immobilization are:

- MILS;
- spinal board, cervical collar, head blocks and strapping; and
- cervical collar, sandbags or head blocks, and strapping.

If the patient has not already been immobilized before arrival, MILS must be applied immediately. A collar, sandbags and strapping can then be substituted if appropriate to 'free up' the person providing MILS. However, cervical collars make airway management and intubation more difficult, mainly by limiting mouth opening, and also limit access to the neck for cricoid pressure or cricothyrotomy. Therefore, the following plan is recommended.[7,10,11]

On arrival in the resuscitation room, the patient must be removed from a long spine board as soon as the primary survey is completed.

> **Intravenous fluid bags are not adequate substitutes for sandbags**

Sandbags or head blocks and tape should only be used if the patient is conscious, and the airway is not at risk; otherwise, MILS should be continued until the airway is secure. If the patient is already immobilized, this should be removed and carefully substituted by MILS if the airway is at risk. For intubation MILS should be used and the anterior portion of the cervical collar opened to allow adequate mouth opening. MILS does 'tie down' one person, but the importance of airway control dictates that it should be used when indicated.

> **Remove the anterior part of the collar and the sandbags and tape before attempting intubation**

Although cervical spine movement should be avoided if possible, the airway always takes priority. Advanced airway techniques will usually work if basic ones fail, but neck movement must be accepted if the airway cannot be cleared in any other way. Only a small percentage of unconscious trauma victims actually have a cervical spine injury, and even if one is present, neck movement may or may not make it worse. On the other hand, death is certain if the airway remains blocked.

> **The airway takes priority over the cervical spine**

Spinal immobilization is assumed in all the airway skills described in this chapter. However, if CSI can be excluded, then head extension should be used to facilitate all methods except nasotracheal intubation.

BASIC AIRWAY MANAGEMENT

Individual techniques are described below.

Both jaw thrust and chin lift relieve soft-tissue obstruction by pulling the tongue, anterior neck tissues and epiglottis forwards. The jaw thrust is preferable, as it can be performed by one person who can simultaneously stabilize the cervical spine. This person can also modify his/her grip to hold a facemask in position, if ventilation is needed. A chin lift needs a second person to stabilize the cervical spine, and prevents application of a tight-fitting facemask.

Oropharyngeal and nasopharyngeal airways are aids to, but not substitutes for, these methods. If using these airways, it is important not to be lulled into a false sense of security and to re-assess the patient, and continue the jaw thrust if necessary.

> **Without continued jaw thrust, an airway alone may not relieve obstruction**

Chin lift

The chin is gripped between the thumb and forefinger of one or both hands with the thumb(s) anterior to the symphysis menti and pulled forwards. Methods of chin lift which involve placing the thumb in the patient's mouth are potentially dangerous, and should be abandoned except in the case of patients with bilateral mandibular fractures where a gloved hand can be used to pull the anterior fragment forwards.

Jaw thrust

METHOD A

From above the patient's head both hands are positioned, and the head is stabilized by pressure between the palms of both hands. The mouth is then opened with both thumbs anterior to the symphysis menti and the jaw pushed anteriorly, with the fingers behind the angles of the jaw on each side.

METHOD B

From above the patient's head or beside his/her body, the thumbs are placed on the patient's zygomas at each side, while pushing the angles of the jaw forwards with the fingers.

Oropharyngeal (Guedel) airway

This is used in unconscious patients without a gag reflex.

INSERTION METHOD

The sizes of oropharyngeal airways used depend on the patient size: small adult, size 2; medium adult, size 3; and large adult, size 4.

Alternatively, the airway can be sized using the distance between the incisors and the angle of the jaw. The mouth is opened and the tip of the airway inserted with the airway inverted (convex downwards). The airway is then passed backwards over the tongue, rotating through 180° as it goes, until the flange lies anterior to the teeth. The patient is then re-assessed and jaw thrust maintained if needed.

If complications (see below) occur, the airway should be removed and a nasopharyngeal airway considered.

Complications
These include:

- trauma (to teeth, mucosa, etc.);
- worsening airway obstruction (the tongue may be pushed further backwards, or a large airway may lodge in the vallecula);
- gagging or coughing;
- laryngospasm; and
- vomiting and aspiration.

Nasopharyngeal airway

This may be better tolerated than an oropharyngeal airway in semi-conscious patients with a gag reflex, and is useful when trismus or facial swelling prevent the insertion of an oral airway.

CONTRAINDICATIONS

Suspected base of skull or maxillary fractures are relative contraindications due to the theoretical danger of the airway penetrating the cribriform plate into the cranial vault. However, careful insertion is justified if hypoxia cannot be relieved otherwise.

INSERTION METHOD

Nasopharyngeal airway sizes are as follows:

- Adult female: 6.0–7.0 mm (internal diameter);
- Adult male: 7.0–8.0 mm (internal diameter).

(or use one of similar diameter to patient's nostril).

The airway should be lubricated with water-soluble jelly before insertion, and a safety pin inserted through the flanged end to prevent the airway being inhaled. The airway can be inserted through either nostril, by directing it *posteriorly* along the floor of the nasopharynx. Gentle rotation between the thumb and finger will ease its passage. If resistance is felt on one side, the other nostril or a smaller airway can be tried. The airway is inserted until the flange lies at the nostril. If coughing, laryngospasm or airway obstruction occur, it should be withdrawn by 1–2 cm. The patient should then be re-assessed, and the jaw thrust maintained if necessary.

Complications
These include:

- trauma to turbinates and the nasal mucosa;
- bleeding from the nasal mucosa (potentially severe);
- gagging, vomiting, laryngospasm and airway obstruction if the airway is too long; and
- a theoretical possibility of penetration of the cribriform plate in the presence of basal skull fracture.

Cricoid pressure

Unconscious trauma patients must be assumed to have a full stomach, and to be at risk of aspiration. Cricoid pressure prevents regurgitation by occluding the oesophagus against the vertebral column. It also reduces gastric inflation during facemask ventilation, and (if applied correctly) improves the view at laryngoscopy.[12] Although usually taught as an advanced airway technique, cricoid pressure should ideally be applied *early*, as unconscious patients may aspirate at any time.

CONTRAINDICATIONS

Active vomiting (due to the risk of oesophageal rupture[13]) and laryngeal trauma are contraindications.

TECHNIQUE

Firm backwards pressure is applied to the cricoid cartilage with thumb and index finger, and must not be released until the airway is secured and instructed by the intubationist.

Bimanual cricoid pressure may be safer in suspected CSI, although evidence is lacking.[14,15] The back of the neck is supported with the other hand, unless support is already given by the posterior half of a rigid cervical collar.

Bag–valve–mask ventilation

This is discussed later under 'assisted ventilation'.

ADVANCED AIRWAY MANAGEMENT

Advanced airway management includes the following techniques:

- tracheal intubation;
- laryngeal mask airway;
- oesophageal–tracheal Combitube;
- needle cricothyrotomy; and
- surgical cricothyrotomy.

Tracheal intubation

Tracheal intubation is the definitive method of airway control. A cuffed tracheal tube allows: (i) a completely clear airway; (ii) adequate ventilation, without air leak or stomach distension; (iii) administration of 100% oxygen; (iv) protection of the lungs from aspiration (stomach contents, blood, secretions or foreign material); (v) bronchial suction; and (vi) delivery of drugs during cardiopulmonary resuscitation. However, the technique requires training and experience to perform, and its complications include hypoxia and death from unrecognized oesophageal intubation. Therefore, intubation should never be attempted by those who have not been properly trained.

Unrecognized oesophageal intubation is rapidly fatal

INDICATIONS

Indications include inadequate ventilation or apnoea; unconscious or semi-conscious patients who are unable to maintain or protect their airway, and are at risk of aspiration; actual or potential airway obstruction (unconsciousness, burns, haematoma or oedema); head injury, with Glasgow Coma Score either ≤8 or deteriorating (see Chapter 8); and hypoxaemia unrelieved by other measures.

CONTRAINDICATIONS

The main contraindication is the lack of training in intubation.

Complications

The most dangerous complication of intubation is oesophageal intubation. If unrecognized, this will cause hypoxia and death in the apnoeic patient. Hypoxia may also be due to:

- tube displacement following successful intubation;
- prolonged intubation attempts;
- intubation of a main bronchus (usually the right) if the tube is inserted too far; and
- exacerbation of prior trauma to the airway: following damage to the larynx or trachea, complete airway obstruction may result.[16]

Other immediate complications include: trauma to the teeth, pharynx, larynx or trachea; exacerbation of cervical spine injury; gagging, coughing, laryngospasm, regurgitation or vomiting in the semi-conscious patient; exacerbation of raised intracranial pressure, in patients with head injury; and cardiac dysrhythmias: tachycardia, bradycardia or extrasystoles (bradycardia is usually due to hypoxia).

Table 4.2 *Equipment required for adult orotracheal intubation*

- Laryngoscope (Macintosh, standard and large adult blades) – preferably two
- Suction equipment with wide-bore (Yankauer) catheter
- Cuffed tracheal tubes, sizes:
    Males: 8.0–9.0 mm internal diameter; 23–25 cm length
    Females: 7.0–8.0 mm internal diameter; 20–22 cm length
- Gum-elastic bougie, or intubating stylet
- Water-soluble lubricating jelly
- Magills forceps (to remove foreign bodies, or guide the tube through the cords)
- 10-ml syringe
- Ventilating bag (or mechanical ventilator), and oxygen
- Stethoscope, and other device (below) to confirm position
- Adhesive tape or tie
- Catheter mount (not essential)

> **Never attempt intubation without proper training**

TECHNIQUE FOR ADULT OROTRACHEAL INTUBATION

This is a step-wise procedure:

1. Check the intubation equipment and ensure that suction is available.
2. Monitor with a pulse oximeter, and preferably ECG, throughout intubation.
3. Position the patient as described above under 'cervical spine stabilization'.
4. Pre-oxygenate the patient for at least 30–60 s, using high-flow oxygen and a facemask, ventilating if necessary.
5. Apply cricoid pressure.
6. Insert the laryngoscope (held in the left hand) into the right-hand corner of the mouth, sliding the blade down over the curve of the tongue towards the larynx, so that the tongue is displaced to the left.
7. As the epiglottis comes into view, lift along the line of the laryngoscope handle (do not lever on the teeth) to show the vocal cords beneath. The tip of the curved blade should be in the vallecula, between the epiglottis and base of the tongue.
8. If the vocal cords are visible, insert the tracheal tube via the right-hand side of the mouth, making sure that you see it pass through the cords. Do not attempt intubation blindly. If laryngoscopy is difficult, use a gum-elastic bougie or other aid if experience allows; otherwise, use an alternative technique.
9. Attach the ventilation bag to the 15-mm connector on the end of the tube, either directly or via a catheter mount. Ventilate the lungs with oxygen and inflate the cuff with air until a leak is no longer heard at the mouth.
10. Check the tube position carefully as described below. Have a high index of suspicion for misplacement: *if in doubt, take it out*. Cricoid pressure is released only when tube position and ventilation are confirmed and the cuff is inflated (in an adult).
11. Secure the tube with adhesive tape or a tie. An oropharyngeal airway may be inserted to prevent biting on the tube if consciousness returns.
12. Continue ventilation: keep a constant watch to ensure the tube does not become displaced, and ventilation remains adequate.

It is vital not to let the patient become hypoxic during intubation. If pulse oximetry is not possible, no longer than 30 s should be allowed for the attempt. If unsuccessful, re-oxygenation by facemask ventilation for another 30–60 s will be necessary before a further attempt can be made. Mark the time by either: (i) asking someone to count time during the intubation attempt; or (ii) holding your breath as you start to intubate: when you need to breathe again, so does the patient!

Recognition of tube placement

Confirmation of tracheal tube placement is vital in order to avoid death from oesophageal intubation. The following routine should become second nature. Methods include:

- *Seeing* the tube pass through the cords at intubation.
- *Feeling* the ventilating bag as you inflate. (The lungs normally feel elastic and 'springy': after oesophageal intubation it is usually either impossible to inflate, or the bag deflates with a 'squelch'.)
- *Watching* the chest rise and fall with ventilation (both sides equally), and see that the abdomen does not distend.
- *Listening* to:
  - both lungs – for breath sounds. (Listen in the axillae, otherwise transmitted tracheal sounds may be heard, and intubation of one main bronchus may be missed.)
  - the stomach – for lack of breath sounds.
- Using a device as described below, ideally a capnograph, to confirm tracheal intubation.

Clinical tests for tube placement can mislead, especially in the obese patient.[17] The most reliable clinical sign is to see the tube pass through the cords (although the inexperienced may mistake the oesophagus for the trachea). Assessing movement and breath sounds over the chest and abdomen is not completely accurate, and condensation inside the tube is *not* a reliable sign. Oesophageal intubation will eventually cause cyanosis, but this may be delayed for several minutes after pre-oxygenation, by which time the cause may be overlooked. In any case, by the time cyanosis occurs it is almost too late!

$$\boxed{\textbf{If in doubt, take the tube out!}}$$

At least one of the following devices should be available (and used) to confirm tracheal placement:

Capnograph   This device measures concentrations of carbon dioxide (CO_2) in expired air. Detection of CO_2 is an almost foolproof way of confirming tracheal intubation, but there are pitfalls:[17]

- False positives: after oesophageal intubation, CO_2 may be detected *for a few breaths only*, if:
  - prior facemask ventilation has forced expired air into the stomach; or
  - the patient has recently consumed carbonated drinks (the 'cola complication'!).
- False negatives: in very low cardiac output states, CO_2 delivery to the lungs is reduced and expired concentrations may be very low.

Disposable CO_2 detector   When attached to the tracheal tube, this compact plastic device detects CO_2 during ventilation by an indicator colour change.[18] The same inaccuracies apply as for the capnograph, and the colour change is also caused by contamination with stomach acid.

Wee's oesophageal detector device   This device consists of a 50-ml syringe attached to a catheter mount, which fits over the 15-mm connector on the tracheal tube.[19] Easy aspiration of air from the syringe suggests tracheal placement; failure to aspirate air suggests oesophageal placement, as the walls of the oesophagus collapse around the tube. It is vital to check the device is airtight before use.

Difficult intubation

Intubation difficulties may be due to: (i) persistent muscle tone in the semi-conscious; (ii) swelling, haematoma or foreign material in the airway; (iii) the need for cervical spine stabilization; and (iv) anatomical variations.

In the first case, anaesthetic expertise is needed. Otherwise, invaluable aids to intubation (for those appropriately trained) are:

- The gum-elastic bougie[20] (a long, flexible guide which can be passed blindly through the cords when laryngoscopy is difficult, and the tube railroaded over it). This should always be available in any resuscitation room, and should be used the moment any difficulty in intubation is encountered.

- The McCoy laryngoscope[21] (a laryngoscope with the standard curved blade adapted to lever at the tip, improving the view of the cords).

Other techniques (given appropriate experience) include: (i) intubation via a laryngeal mask;[22–24] (ii) using a fibreoptic laryngoscope; (iii) blind nasotracheal intubation (see below); and (iv) using an alternative technique, e.g. laryngeal mask or Combitube.

Blind nasotracheal intubation

Nasotracheal intubation (NTI) can be performed without laryngoscopy and with minimal neck movement. Unlike oral intubation, it may be possible in semi-conscious patients with a gag reflex. Although once thought preferable to oral intubation in suspected cervical spine injury, evidence suggests that it is no safer.[11,25–27] It also has the following drawbacks:

- the patient must be breathing spontaneously;
- gagging, vomiting, laryngospasm, hypoxia and raised intracranial pressure may still occur;
- a smaller-diameter tube is needed than with oral intubation;
- oesophageal intubation is a significant risk; and
- basal skull fracture or middle-third facial fractures are relative contraindications, as intracranial passage of the tube through the cribriform plate is possible,[28,29] and meningitis is also a risk. (However, NTI is justifiable if hypoxia cannot be relieved otherwise,[30] provided that care is taken to direct the tube posteriorly.)

NTI is an alternative to oral intubation only for those who are skilled in its use. It can be used if oral intubation is not possible.

> **Blind nasal intubation should only be attempted by those who are specifically trained and skilled in its use**

Anaesthesia for intubation

Patients can only be intubated orally without anaesthesia if they are deeply unconscious. However, many trauma patients needing intubation (for example, after head injury) have a preserved gag reflex, muscle tone or clenched teeth. Attempted intubation of such patients without proper anaesthesia may lead to gagging, laryngospasm, regurgitation, hypoxia, bradycardia and (in the head-injured) raised intracranial pressure.

Oral intubation using a 'rapid sequence induction' (RSI) is normally used in these circumstances. This involves pre-oxygenation and cricoid pressure, after which an intravenous anaesthetic induction agent and a neuromuscular blocker ('muscle relaxant') are given. Intubation is performed with cervical spine stabilization as described earlier.

Anaesthetic drugs should only be given by those who are properly trained in their use, and who are skilled at intubation. Their greatest dangers are:

- loss of muscle tone, possibly leading to complete airway obstruction as well as apnoea. If both intubation and ventilation then prove impossible, catastrophic hypoxia will follow. RSI is therefore contraindicated if a 'difficult airway' is expected, and safer alternatives are awake fibreoptic intubation or cricothyrotomy under local anaesthesia.[7,31,32]
- hypotension, as induction agents generally cause vasodilation and sometimes cardiac depression. Hypotension may be severe in the hypovolaemic patient, who relies on vasoconstriction to maintain his/her blood pressure. Therefore before RSI, large-bore venous access should be established and hypovolaemia corrected.

The laryngeal mask airway

The laryngeal mask airway (LMA) is a wide-bore tube with a large, spoon-shaped inflatable cuff at the distal end. When inserted blindly into the mouth the cuff sits above the laryngeal inlet, maintaining the airway and allowing spontaneous or controlled ventilation. Insertion is usually easy, although less so with cervical spine immobilization.[33] Sizes and cuff inflation volumes are listed in Table 4.3.

Table 4.3 *Laryngeal mask airway (LMA) sizes and cuff inflation volumes*

Size of LMA	Patient size	Cuff inflation volume (ml)
3	30 kg – small adult	15–20
4	Small – medium adult	25–30
5	Medium – large adult	35–40

INDICATIONS

The laryngeal mask airway may be used: (i) as a *temporary* alternative to tracheal intubation in unconscious patients, when intubation is precluded by a 'difficult airway' or lack of expertise; (ii) as an alternative to bag-and-mask ventilation (the LMA may allow better ventilation than the latter method[34]); and (iii) by the experienced intubationist as an aid to difficult tracheal intubation.[22–24]

CONTRAINDICATIONS

Contraindications to use of the LMA include: (i) lack of training in the technique; (ii) patients with active gag reflexes; (iii) foreign-body airway obstruction (may impact the object further down in the pharynx); and (iv) severe oropharyngeal trauma.

DISADVANTAGES

Disadvantages of the LMA include the following:

- it may stimulate gagging, coughing and vomiting in the semi-conscious patient;
- it is easily displaced following insertion;
- it does *not* guarantee a clear airway or adequate ventilation if incorrectly placed;
- it does *not* protect against aspiration of stomach contents;
- ventilation with too-high pressures may lead to gastric distension, regurgitation and aspiration; and
- cricoid pressure may impede insertion.[35]

The laryngeal mask does not guarantee ventilation or prevent aspiration

---

The LMA therefore functions as a mask and not a tube (although when *in situ* it appears misleadingly like the latter!), and is an imperfect substitute for intubation in the trauma patient. However, the risks of poor ventilation, stomach distension and aspiration apply equally to facemask ventilation, and the LMA may be life-saving if ventilation is otherwise impossible.[36]

The oesophageal–tracheal Combitube

The Combitube is a double-lumen airway, which allows airway maintenance, ventilation, and protection from aspiration. When inserted blindly into the pharynx, the tube usually enters the oesophagus, or sometimes the trachea. In either case, ventilation should be possible through the appropriate lumen, and this is confirmed in the same way as for tracheal intubation. Laryngoscopy and intubation are possible past the Combitube by deflating the pharyngeal balloon. As with the LMA, it is potentially life-saving in emergency situations[37,38]

INDICATION

The Combitube may be used as a temporary alternative to tracheal intubation in unconscious patients when intubation is precluded by a 'difficult airway' or lack of expertise.

CONTRAINDICATIONS

These are similar to those for the LMA.

DISADVANTAGES

Disadvantages of the Combitube include its being unsuitable for use in children and its insertion being more traumatic than with the LMA. Moreover, gastric inflation may occur if the tube position is not checked carefully, while the pharyngeal balloon may be damaged by sharp teeth on insertion.

Cricothyrotomy

A *surgical airway* is created by either of two approaches. First, cricothyrotomy; which exists in two forms, namely 'needle' (using a cannula), and 'surgical' (by incision). The second approach is by tracheostomy.

Tracheostomy is unsuitable in emergency situations as it is technically difficult, time-consuming, and has serious complications from injury to adjacent neurovascular structures or the pleura. The cricothyroid membrane lies superficially in the notch between the thyroid and cricoid cartilages, and is relatively clear of major vessels and nerves. Therefore cricothyrotomy is the only option if life-threatening hypoxia is imminent, and only cricothyrotomy is discussed here.

Needle cricothyrotomy is a temporary life-saving measure, and must be replaced as soon as possible by intubation or tracheostomy. **Surgical cricothyrotomy** allows continued adequate ventilation, but is not intended for prolonged use.

INDICATIONS

Cricothyrotomy (needle or surgical) is indicated immediately when the airway and ventilation cannot be maintained in any other way, for example severe facial injury, haematoma, oedema, or foreign bodies.[39] Surgical cricothyrotomy may also be considered in the following situations, where it may be quicker and safer than tracheostomy:

- in patients at risk of impending airway obstruction (from burns, oedema or haematoma), including:
  - unconscious patients, if intubation is otherwise impossible.
  - conscious patients (under local anaesthesia), when general anaesthesia may precipitate irreversible airway obstruction, and awake fibreoptic intubation is not possible.
- when intubation is otherwise indicated, and although ventilation is possible, a definitive airway cannot be obtained in any other way.

RELATIVE CONTRAINDICATIONS

These include laryngeal trauma,[16] while surgical cricothyrotomy is contraindicated in children, as it may cause upper-airway collapse.

TECHNIQUE

With either technique, speed is essential to prevent hypoxic brain damage if the airway is completely obstructed.

Needle cricothyrotomy

The procedure is carried out in step-wise fashion:

1. Prepare the equipment: 14 G intravenous cannula, syringe, oxygen source, delivery system and connectors (see below), stethoscope.
2. Position the patient, identify the cricothyroid membrane (Figure 4.1) and stabilize the larynx as above.
3. Puncture the skin in the midline over the cricothyroid membrane, using the cannula with syringe attached.
4. Aiming 30–45° caudally, and keeping to the midline, advance the cannula towards the *lower* cricothyroid membrane while aspirating on the syringe.

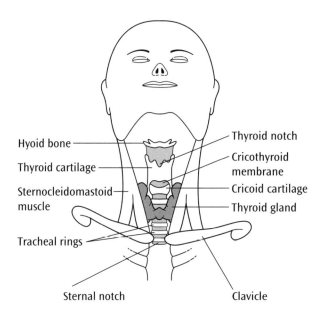

Figure 4.1 *Anatomy of the airway, showing the cricothyroid membrane.*

Hyoid bone

Thyroid cartilage

Sternocleidomastoid muscle

Tracheal rings

Thyroid notch

Cricothyroid membrane

Cricoid cartilage

Thyroid gland

Sternal notch

Clavicle

5. When air is aspirated, advance the cannula over the needle into the trachea.
6. Withdraw the needle and *aspirate again*, to confirm tracheal placement.
7. Attach the ventilating system (see below) to the cannula hub.
8. Ventilate as appropriate, checking for adequate inflation and oxygenation.
9. Secure the cannula in place (the safest way is to hold it continually!).

Surgical cricothyrotomy

As for needle cricothyrotomy, this is best performed in stages:

1. Prepare the equipment: Spencer-Wells forceps, scalpel blade, swab, tube (ideally size 6.0 tracheostomy tube, otherwise tracheal tube), self-inflating bag and oxygen source, 10-ml syringe, stethoscope, tape or bandage.
2. Ensure that an assistant stabilizes the head in the midline, and extend the neck if spinal injury is excluded.
3. Palpate the cricothyroid membrane between the thyroid and cricoid cartilages, and stabilize the larynx between thumb and fingers of the non-dominant hand.
4. Infiltrate local anaesthetic with adrenaline along the borders of the sternomastoids lateral to the cricothyroid membrane if appropriate.
5. Make a horizontal midline skin incision over the *lower* half of the membrane. (The small cricothyroid artery runs transversely across the upper third.)
6. Incise the membrane horizontally, and dilate the opening by inserting the scalpel handle and rotating it through 90° (or using forceps if available).
7. Insert a suitable lubricated tube as above.
8. Inflate the cuff, and ventilate if needed by attaching a self-inflating bag to the tube connector (directly, or via a catheter mount).
9. Check for adequate ventilation, as for tracheal intubation.
10. Fix the tube *securely* with a tape or a suture.

CRICOTHYROTOMY SETS

Purpose-designed cricothyrotomy sets are available, such as the Nu-Trach® or Patil®. Many of these are inserted through a cricothyroid puncture, but allow dilation to accommodate a larger tube with a 15-mm connector. This allows connection to a self-inflating bag or ventilator.

Complications

Complications may be identified as 'early' or 'late' in nature.

Early complications   These include:

*   Hypoxia and hypercarbia:
    *   prolonged insertion
    *   failed insertion

- misplacement
- inadequate ventilation
- air trapping
- Haemorrhage:
  - external
  - into the neck tissues
  - into the airway (potentially causing hypoxic respiratory arrest)
- Oesophageal perforation
- Surgical emphysema (from misplacement of cannula in needle cricothyrotomy)
- Air trapping due to inadequate exhalation in needle cricothyrotomy, leading to:
  - pneumothorax, pneumomediastinum
  - surgical emphysema
  - reduced venous return, reduced cardiac output and hypotension.

Late complications These include:

- Infection
- Subglottic stenosis, especially in children
- Voice dysfunction, due to vocal cord or cricothyroid muscle damage.

Although needle cricothyrotomy appears simple, serious complications arise from CO_2 and air trapping.[39,40] If the upper airway is not patent, exhalation through the relatively narrow cannula will be inadequate. This compromises ventilation further, and causes the complications of air trapping and high intrathoracic pressures described above. Although surgical cricothyrotomy seems more traumatic, it should give adequate ventilation and oxygenation. Therefore, needle cricothyrotomy should be converted to the surgical route *urgently* if exhalation is inadequate. In addition, needle cricothyrotomy does not prevent aspiration, or allow spontaneous breathing.

Oxygen delivery and ventilation systems

Needle cricothyrotomy   Ventilation systems are difficult to make up 'on the spot', and a suitable system should always be available.[39]

The ideal system is a jet injector system, powered by high-pressure (50–60 psi) oxygen from the wall outlet. This should give good oxygenation *and* ventilation.

Alternative systems are driven by high-flow (10–15 l/min) oxygen from the wall flowmeter and are of three types:

1. A length of green 'bubble' oxygen tubing: an expansion at one end is pushed firmly into the barrel of a 2-ml syringe, and a hole is cut across the side of the tubing just before the syringe. The syringe is pushed into the cannula hub, and the hole occluded intermittently ('one second on, four seconds off').
2. An IV-giving set cut off just below the drip chamber: the cut end is attached to the flowmeter, and the distal end connected to the cannula hub via a three-way tap. The open side-port on the three-way tap is occluded intermittently as above.
3. Two lengths of bubble oxygen tube separated by a Y-connector, with the base of the Y pointing towards the patient. The open end of the Y can then be occluded intermittently, as above. The 'patient end' of the tubing can be inserted into a syringe for connection as above.

These systems are driven by a lower pressure, which means that while oxygenation may be adequate, CO_2 may accumulate:[41] these methods provide only 20–40 min grace until replaced by intubation or tracheostomy.

However, if none of these is available, then ventilate with a self-inflating bag, attached to either:

- a 3-mm tracheal tube connector, the smaller end of which is pushed into the cannula hub;
- a 7-mm tracheal tube connector, the smaller end of which is pushed into the barrel of a 2-ml syringe, which is then attached to the cannula hub; or
- an adult-sized cuffed tracheal tube, inserted into the barrel of a large syringe and the cuff then inflated: the syringe is then attached to the cannula hub.

These can be assembled quickly, but may give very poor ventilation because of lower pressures and the large compressible volume of gas:[39] CO_2 may accumulate rapidly, and even oxygenation may not be adequate.

> **Always replace a needle cricothyrotomy with a definitive airway as soon as possible**

Surgical cricothyrotomy The 15-mm connector on a tracheostomy or endotracheal tube allows spontaneous or controlled ventilation, as with conventional intubation.

OXYGEN THERAPY AND VENTILATION

Oxygen therapy

The vital importance of oxygen was described earlier in Chapter 4. In major trauma it is essential to give as much oxygen as possible, and as soon as possible! There are very few medical contraindications to high-percentage oxygen, and the risk of CO_2 retention in certain patients with chronic obstructive pulmonary disease (COPD) is often overstated.[42] **Correction of hypoxia takes priority:** if in any doubt oxygen must be given and ventilation assisted if necessary.

Oxygen delivery

In the spontaneously breathing patient, oxygen is given by:

- Non-rebreather reservoir mask (NRRM): this is the best mask for giving high concentrations of oxygen. At flow rates of 10–15 l/min it gives at least 85% oxygen.
- Standard Hudson-type mask: this is second best, but can be can be used if a NRRM is not available. Even high flow rates will give at best 60–70% oxygen.

Nasal cannulae give relatively low and unpredictable concentrations of oxygen, and should not be used.

> **The non-rebreather reservoir mask gives close to 100% oxygen**

MONITORING OF OXYGENATION

Oxygenation may be monitored in three ways:

1. Clinically (although mild hypoxaemia is hard to detect).
2. By pulse oximetry (although this method does not detect hypoventilation if the patient is receiving oxygen, it may not 'pick up' due to poor peripheral perfusion, and may over-read if carboxyhaemoglobin is present).
3. By arterial blood gas measurement, if necessary.

ASSISTED VENTILATION

Facemask ventilation

If breathing is inadequate, then ventilation is initially given via a facemask, using either:

- a self-inflating bag–valve–mask (BVM) device (Ambu-type bag). This gives at least 85% oxygen, with flow rates of 10–15 l/min and a reservoir bag attached (although hyperventilation reduces the delivered percentage[43]). CO_2 rebreathing is eliminated by the one-way valve. However achieving a good seal with the facemask is difficult with one hand, therefore a two-person technique should be used by the inexperienced operator (one holds the mask and the other squeezes the bag).

- an anaesthetic reservoir bag ('black bag', or 'Waters circuit'). Although this delivers close to 100% oxygen at high flow rates, the adjustable valve makes it difficult to use, and rebreathing of CO_2 can occur. It is therefore best avoided by those not practised in its use.

TECHNIQUE

Whichever device is used,[44] it is imperative to: (i) use an airway if needed; (ii) hold the mask over the mouth and nose, using the thumb and index finger over the hard part of the mask, with one or preferably both hands; (iii) hook the remaining fingers under the jaw, with the little finger if possible behind the angle of the jaw, so the mask is held by a combined pincer grip and jaw thrust; and (iv) ventilate with oxygen at 12–16 breaths/min, enough to cause visible chest expansion.

COMPLICATIONS

Complications of facemask ventilation include:

- poor mask seal, with inadequate ventilation;
- gastric inflation, leading to diaphragmatic splinting and regurgitation;
- aspiration of regurgitated stomach contents, or matter from the pharynx;
- neck movement, and exacerbation of cervical spine injury; and
- pneumocephalus and meningitis in patients with basal skull fracture.[45]

Advanced ventilation methods

Once the airway is controlled by intubation, LMA, Combitube or surgical cricothyrotomy, ventilation is given by either: (i) self-inflating bag; (ii) an anaesthetic reservoir bag; or (iii) a mechanical ventilator.

> **If a ventilated patient deteriorates in any way, think first of oesophageal intubation**

Care of the ventilated patient

The ventilated patient must be treated with caution, and in step-wise manner:

- Set the ventilator appropriately, e.g.
  - tidal volume 8–10 ml/kg
  - rate 12–16 per minute.
- Sedate and paralyse the patient if necessary (anaesthetic expertise is essential here).
- Watch constantly to ensure that the tracheal tube is not displaced, either:
  - out of the trachea
  - into one main bronchus.
- Ensure that ventilation remains adequate, by:
  - clinical observation
  - pulse oximetry
  - capnography
  - airway pressure monitoring
  - frequent arterial blood gases (all ventilated trauma patients should have an 'arterial line')
  - ventilator disconnect alarm.
- Use a tracheal suction catheter if airway secretions accumulate.
- Be alert for complications of positive-pressure ventilation:
  - ventilator disconnection (potentially fatal in the apnoeic)

- hypotension, due to raised mean intrathoracic pressure and reduced venous return (may be severe in hypovolaemia or cardiac tamponade)
- tension pneumothorax (which develops easily from a 'simple' pneumothorax during ventilation)
- inadequate ventilation due to traumatic bronchopleural fistula
- dynamic hyperinflation[46] (air trapping due to inadequate exhalation, which 'tamponades' the heart in a similar way to tension pneumothorax)
- air embolism, following chest trauma.[47,48]

SUMMARY

Provision of a patent-protected airway is key to the management of any trauma patient. Many patients will not require any airway intervention, while a majority of the remainder will respond rapidly to simple manoeuvres expertly performed. Carrying out the steps defined in this chapter in a logical sequence of increasing complexity will ensure that preventable deaths from airway obstruction are avoided.

REFERENCES

1. Hussain LM, Redmond AD. Are pre-hospital deaths from accidental injury preventable? *British Medical Journal* 1994; **308**: 1077–80.
2. Nandi PR, Charlesworth CH, Taylor SJ, Nunn JF, Dore CJ. Effect of general anaesthesia on the pharynx. *British Journal of Anaesthesia* 1991; **66**: 157–62.
3. Wilson RF, Arden RL. Laryngotracheal trauma. In: Wilson RF, Walt AJ (eds). *Management of Trauma – Pitfalls and Practice*. Baltimore: Williams & Wilkins, 1996; pp. 288–313.
4. Parkins DRJ. Maxillofacial injuries in immediate care. *Journal of the British Association for Immediate Care* 1996; **19**: 34–6.
5. Nunn JF. *Nunn's Applied Respiratory Physiology*. Oxford: Butterworth-Heinemann, 1993; pp. 529–36.
6. Willms D, Shure D. Pulmonary oedema due to upper airway obstruction in adults. *Chest* 1988; **94**: 1090–2.
7. Hastings RH, Marks JD. Airway management for trauma patients with potential cervical spine injuries. *Anesthesia and Analgesia* 1991; **73**: 471–82.
8. Roberge RJ, Wears RC, Kelly M, *et al*. Selective application of cervical spine radiography in alert victims of blunt trauma: a prospective study. *Journal of Trauma* 1988; **28**: 784–8.
9. Woodring JH, Lee C. Limitations of cervical radiography in the evaluation of acute cervical trauma. *Journal of Trauma* 1993; **34**: 32–9.
10. Heath KJ. The effect on laryngoscopy of different cervical spine immobilization techniques. *Anaesthesia* 1994; **49**: 843–5.
11. Criswell JC, Parr MJA, Nolan JP. Emergency airway management in patients with cervical spine injuries. *Anaesthesia* 1994; **49**: 900–3.
12. Sellick BA. Cricoid pressure to control regurgitation of stomach contents during induction of anaesthesia. *Lancet* 1961; **ii**: 404–6.
13. Ralph SJ, Wareham CA. Rupture of the oesophagus during cricoid pressure. *Anaesthesia* 1991; **46**: 40–1.
14. Gabbott DA. The effect of single-handed cricoid pressure on neck movement after applying manual in-line stabilization. *Anaesthesia* 1997; **52**: 586–8.
15. Nolan JP, Parr MJA. Tracheal intubation in trauma. *British Journal of Anaesthesia* 1998; **80**: 270.
16. Gussak GS, Jurkovich GJ. Treatment dilemmas in laryngotracheal trauma. *Journal of Trauma* 1988; **28**: 1439–44.
17. Clyburn P, Rosen M. Accidental oesophageal intubation. *British Journal of Anaesthesia* 1994; **73**: 55–63.
18. Denman WT, Hayes M, Higgins D, Wilkinson DJ. The Fenem CO_2 detector device. *Anaesthesia* 1990; **45**: 465–7.

19. Wee MYK. The oesophageal detector device. *Anaesthesia* 1988; **43**: 27–9.

20. Nolan JP, Wilson ME. Orotracheal intubation in patients with potential cervical spine injuries. An indication for the gum elastic bougie. *Anaesthesia* 1993; **48**: 630–3.

21. Gabbott DA. Laryngoscopy using the McCoy laryngoscope after application of a cervical collar. *Anaesthesia* 1996; **51**: 812–14.

22. Chadd GD, Ackers JWL, Bailey PM. Difficult intubation aided by the laryngeal mask airway. *Anaesthesia* 1989; **44**: 1015.

23. Heath ML, Allagain J. Intubation through the laryngeal mask. *Anaesthesia* 1991; **46**: 545–8.

24. Baskett PJF, Parr MJ, Nolan JP. The intubating laryngeal mask. Results of a multicentre trial with experience of 500 cases. *Anaesthesia* 1998; **53**; 1174–9.

25. Crosby ET. Tracheal intubation in the cervical spine-injured patient. *Canadian Journal of Anaesthesia* 1992; **39**: 105–9.

26. Wood PR, Lawler PGP. Managing the airway in cervical spine injury. *Anaesthesia* 1992; **47**: 792–7.

27. Holley J, Jorden R. Airway management in patients with unstable cervical spine fractures. *Annals of Emergency Medicine* 1989; **18**: 1237–9.

28. Horellou MF, Mathe D, Feiss P. A hazard of nasotracheal intubation. *Anaesthesia* 1978; **33**: 73–4.

29. Patrick MR. Airway manipulations. In: Taylor TH, Major E (eds). *Hazards and Complications of Anaesthesia*. Edinburgh: Churchill Livingstone, 1987.

30. Rhee KJ, Muntz CB, Donald PJ, Yamada JM. Does nasotracheal intubation increase complications in patients with skull base fractures? *Annals of Emergency Medicine* 1993; **22**: 1145–7.

31. Gwinnutt CL, McCluskey A. Management of the upper airway. In: Driscoll PA, Skinner DV (eds). *Trauma care. Beyond the Resuscitation Room*. London: BMJ Books, 1998; pp. 19–33.

32. Benumof JL. Management of the difficult adult airway. *Anesthesiology* 1991; **75**: 1087–110.

33. Asai T, Neil J, Stacey M. Ease of placement of the laryngeal mask during manual in-line neck stabilization. *British Journal of Anaesthesia* 1998; **80**: 617–20.

34. Alexander R, Hodgson P, Lomax D, Bullen C. A comparison of the laryngeal mask airway and Guedel airway, bag and facemask for manual ventilation following formal training. *Anaesthesia* 1993; **48**: 231–4.

35. Gabbott DA, Sasada MP. Laryngeal mask airway insertion using cricoid pressure and manual in-line neck stabilization. *Anaesthesia* 1995; **50**: 674–6.

36. Calder I, Ordman AJ, Jackowski A, Crockard HA. The Brain laryngeal mask airway. An alternative to emergency tracheal intubation. *Anaesthesia* 1990; **45**: 137–9.

37. Banyai M, Falger S, Roggla M, *et al*. Emergency intubation with the combitube in a grossly obese patient with bull neck. *Resuscitation* 1993; **26**: 271–6.

38. Eichinger S, Schreiber W, Heinz T, *et al*. Airway management in a case of neck impalement: use of the oesophageal tracheal combitube airway. *British Journal of Anaesthesia* 1992; **68**: 534–5.

39. Benumof JL, Scheller MS. The importance of transtracheal jet ventilation in the management of the difficult airway. *Anesthesiology* 1989; **71**: 769–78.

40. Jorden RC, Moore EE, Marx JA, Honigman B. A comparison of PTV and endotracheal ventilation in an acute trauma model. *Journal of Trauma* 1985; **25**: 978–83.

41. Ryder IG, Paoloni CCE, Harle CC. Emergency transtracheal ventilation: assessment of breathing systems chosen by anaesthetists. *Anaesthesia* 1996; **51**: 764–8.

42. Bateman NT, Leach RM. Acute oxygen therapy. *British Medical Journal* 1998; **317**: 798–801.

43. Davey A, Moyle JTB, Ward CS. *Ward's Anaesthetic Equipment*. London: WB Saunders, 1992; pp. 188–94.

44. Lawrence PJ, Sivaneswaran N. Ventilation during cardiopulmonary resuscitation: which method? *Medical Journal of Australia* 1985; **143**: 443–6.

45. Klopfenstein CE, Forster A, Suter PM. Pneumocephalus. A complication of continuous positive airway pressure after trauma. *Chest* 1980; **78**: 656–7.

46. Conacher ID. Dynamic hyperinflation – the anaesthetist applying a tourniquet to the right heart. *British Journal of Anaesthesia* 1998; **81**: 116–17.

47. Morris WP, Butler BD, Tonnesen AS, Allen SJ. Continuous venous air embolism in patients receiving positive end-expiratory pressure. *American Reviews of Respiratory Disease* 1993; **147**: 1034–7.

48. Gavalas M, Tekkis P. Air embolism. In: Greaves I, Ryan JM, Porter KP (eds). *Trauma*. London: Arnold, 1998; pp. 237–41.

5

Thoracic trauma

OBJECTIVES

- To understand the pathophysiology of thoracic trauma and its relationship to other organ systems
- To understand how to assess the patient with thoracic trauma and be able to recognize thoracic injuries
- To be able to plan and carry out the initial management of the patient with thoracic injuries

INTRODUCTION

Thoracic injuries are directly responsible for 25% of all trauma deaths and are a major contributory factor to mortality in a further 25%.[1] Although many of these deaths occur almost immediately, there is a significant group of patients that may be salvaged with early effective management.

The majority (approximately 90%) of all patients who sustain thoracic trauma can be managed conservatively, with no more than a chest drain, monitoring and analgesia. Few patients require surgery, and an emergency department thoracotomy is indicated in only a very small minority.

PATHOPHYSIOLOGY OF CHEST TRAUMA

The main consequences of chest trauma occur as a result of its combined effects on respiratory and haemodynamic function.[2] The commonest manifestation of thoracic trauma is hypoxia, the causes of which include:

- haemorrhage;
- lung collapse and compression;
- ventilatory or cardiac failure;
- pulmonary contusion;
- changes in intrathoracic pressure; and
- mediastinal displacement.

The aim of early intervention is to restore adequate delivery of oxygen to the tissues. This includes the maintenance of an open airway, administration of a high concentration of inspired oxygen, and re-expansion of the lung by insertion of a chest drain. Successful management of thoracic trauma is dependent, therefore, on effective resuscitation and the rapid treatment of immediately life-threatening injuries.

Profound hypovolaemia in chest trauma is most often seen with great vessel damage, pulmonary hilar injury and cardiac or pericardial laceration without tamponade. Hypovolaemia produces a low cardiac output state, which further contributes to the pathophysiological consequences of chest injury.

Pulmonary contusion is one of the main factors responsible for the increased morbidity and mortality associated with chest trauma. It is a progressive condition, with initial alveolar haemorrhage and oedema, followed by interstitial fluid accumulation and decreased alveolar membrane diffusion. These changes produce relative hypoxaemia, increased pulmonary vascular resistance, decreased pulmonary vascular flow and reduced lung compliance. Importantly, there is a 'ventilation–perfusion mismatch' (alveoli are perfused, but are unavailable for gas exchange because they are full of blood) that can lead to an intrapulmonary shunt, often in excess of 30%. This contributes significantly to the hypoxaemia, especially in the early stages following trauma. Later, hypoxia-induced pulmonary vasoconstriction will divert the blood away from the non-ventilated alveoli, leading to a reduction of the intrapulmonary shunt to about 5%.

A loss of mechanical function of the chest wall will also result in hypoxia. If the chest wall is sufficiently disrupted, the patient may be unable spontaneously to generate sufficient movement of air to allow adequate gas transfer.

Cardiac output may be directly reduced by decreased myocardial contractility (e.g. myocardial contusion), cardiac disruption (e.g. a tear in a cardiac valve), reduced venous filling (e.g. in cardiac tamponade), or with changes in intrathoracic pressure such as occurs with the development of tension pneumothorax.

ASSESSMENT

On arrival in the emergency department, decisions and action need to be taken without delay. Important information may be obtained from the ambulance service relating to the patient's history and mechanism of injury. Actions taken before arrival need to be established; for example, a tension pneumothorax may have been decompressed. The sequence of questions in the hand-over to hospital care can be remembered as 'MIST':

- **M**echanism of injury
- **I**njuries found and suspected
- **S**igns (respiratory rate, SpO_2, pulse, blood pressure)
- **T**reatment given pre-hospital.

In every case, the system of a primary survey with simultaneous resuscitation is followed. In the stable patient, once this has been completed, a secondary survey can be performed.

Certain wounds or bruising patterns highlight the likelihood of underlying injury, for example a seat-belt mark on the chest wall may arouse suspicion of fractured ribs, lung contusion, or solid organ injury in the abdomen, whereas a penetrating wound medial to the nipple or the scapula suggests possible damage to the heart (with potential cardiac tamponade), the great vessels, or the hilar structures. However, major intrathoracic injuries may occur without obvious external damage. Additionally, some injuries point to possible associated more serious pathology; for example, fractures of the first and second ribs are associated with major vessel injury.

Primary survey

AIRWAY

The first priority is the patency of the airway, and the protocols described in Chapter 4 should be followed.

BREATHING

Before examining the chest, the neck should be carefully examined for wounds, bleeding, tracheal deviation, laryngeal crepitus, surgical emphysema and elevated jugular venous pressure. If a cervical collar is already in place, it should ideally be removed temporarily to allow examination, while maintaining manual in-line stabilization.

> **Do not forget to examine the neck**

The chest must be completely exposed so that respiratory movement and quality of ventilation can be assessed. The mechanics of breathing can be disrupted by major airway obstruction, haemothorax or pneumothorax, pain or pulmonary contusion. Impending hypoxia is sometimes indicated by subtle changes in the breathing pattern, which may become shallow and rapid.

Measure and record the respiratory rate

Visual inspection and palpation of the chest wall may reveal deformity, contusion, abrasion, penetrating injury, paradoxical breathing, tenderness, instability or crepitus. All are markers suggestive of underlying injury.

A systematic examination of the chest should now be carried out, including percussion and auscultation. The back of the chest should not be forgotten, and in particular there should be a search for blood on a gloved hand drawn behind the supine patient, from shoulder to buttocks. A more formal assessment of the back of the chest can be completed as part of the log-roll. This must be done expeditiously in penetrating trauma, so that life-threatening wounds are detected early.

Individual thoracic injuries are discussed below.

CIRCULATION

The pulse should be assessed for quality, rate and regularity. The peripheral circulation is assessed by skin colour, temperature and capillary return. Venous distension in the neck may not always be present in a patient with cardiac tamponade who has hypovolaemia. ECG monitoring is an important adjuvant.

DISABILITY

The hypoxic patient will initially be confused and may become combative. Primary head injury will also cause an altered mental state, which will be compounded by hypoxia or hypercarbia. It is essential that airway and ventilation are optimized in the presumed head-injured patient, as the confusion of hypoxia may be reversed and harmful secondary brain injury prevented.

Secondary survey

Once the immediately life-threatening conditions have been diagnosed and treated or excluded, the patient can be assessed thoroughly. This assessment includes a detailed history and full examination, and is described in more detail in Chapter 3.

CHEST INJURIES

Immediately life-threatening injuries

There are six specific thoracic injuries which will be fatal if they are not recognized and treated immediately:[3]

- **a**irway obstruction
- **t**ension pneumothorax
- **o**pen pneumothorax
- **m**assive haemothorax
- flail chest
- cardiac tamponade.

They can be usefully remembered by the mnemonic **atomic**. All of these injuries require high-flow oxygen as the first step in their treatment.

AIRWAY OBSTRUCTION

Complete obstruction of the pharynx or trachea will result in death within minutes if it is not immediately relieved, and should be eliminated as the first priority.

Treatment
This is described in Chapter 4.

TENSION PNEUMOTHORAX

A tension pneumothorax develops when air enters the pleural space secondary to a laceration of the lung, bronchus or chest wall. Unlike a simple pneumothorax, in a tension pneumothorax the airflow is unidirectional. Air flows into the pleural space on inspiration, but cannot escape during expiration due to the effective formation of a flap valve. This causes a progressive accumulation of air in the pleura with collapse of the ipsilateral lung, producing hypoxia and eventually shift of the mediastinum to the opposite side. The consequent reduced venous return will result in a low cardiac output. In advanced cases, hypoxia-induced myocardial failure may further reduce cardiac output.

Tension pneumothorax is a clinical diagnosis, and is recognized by:

- respiratory distress;
- over-inflated hemithorax, ± visibly splayed ribs;
- hyper-resonant percussion note (ipsilateral);
- reduced or absent breath sounds (ipsilateral);
- tracheal deviation; and
- distended neck veins.

Tracheal deviation away from the side of the lesion is a late sign and treatment should not be delayed until it is present if there is an otherwise high index of suspicion of the diagnosis. Distended neck veins may not be visible if the patient is hypovolaemic from an associated injury.

Treatment
The treatment of tension pneumothorax is immediate needle decompression, which should not be delayed to perform a chest radiograph (see Practical procedures, p.66).

If needle decompression fails to demonstrate tension pneumothorax, the needle should be left in place. The needle serves as a reminder that a simple pneumothorax may be present, and should be secured in place using tape; it must not be capped. If the decompression fails but the clinical suspicion remains strong, the chest wall may be thicker than the length of the needle: a second needle should be placed laterally.

> **Needle decompression, 2nd intercostal space, midclavicular line.**
> **If this fails and the diagnosis is still suspect:**
> **needle decompression, 4th intercostal space anterior to midaxillary line**

Following this, intravenous access is obtained and a formal intercostal drain should be placed through the fifth intercostal space anterior to the midaxillary line (see Practical procedures, p.65).

OPEN PNEUMOTHORAX

When a penetrating chest wall injury creates a direct communication between the thoracic cavity and the external environment, an open pneumothorax results. This communication between the thoracic cavity and atmospheric air may lead to preferential influx of air through the chest wall defect (the path of least resistance) if the diameter of the chest wall defect is bigger than two-thirds of the diameter of the trachea. Although most penetrating injuries usually seal off, larger defects may remain open, causing a 'sucking chest wound' with immediate equilibration between atmospheric and intrathoracic pressures. This quickly causes collapse of the lung on the affected side, and potential failure adequately to ventilate the uninjured lung. The clinical signs are those of a pneumothorax: namely, reduced breath sounds, a resonant percussion note and decreased expansion, together with a penetrating chest wall injury.

Treatment

The defect should be covered either with an Ashermann chest seal or initially, as a less sophisticated first-aid measure, with a sterile waterproof dressing secured on three sides to act as a flutter valve. An intercostal drain should be placed away from the open wound. Surgical débridement and closure of the wound will be necessary later. Antitetanus protection (for the non-immune) and antibiotics will be necessary.

MASSIVE HAEMOTHORAX

Massive haemothorax is usually caused by penetrating injury, but it can also result from blunt trauma. A life-threatening haemothorax may result from major lung parenchymal laceration, injury to the pulmonary hilum, or from direct cardiac laceration. A massive haemothorax is usually defined as the presence of more than 1500 ml of blood in the hemithorax, or 200 ml per hour (3 ml/kg/h) from the chest drain.

As well as causing hypotension due to blood loss, a massive haemothorax will also occupy space in the thoracic cavity normally occupied by lung, and the subsequent lung collapse will cause hypoxia. The signs of massive haemothorax are those of hypovolaemic shock together with:

- dullness to percussion (ipsilateral);
- absent or reduced breath sounds (ipsilateral); and
- decreased chest movement (ipsilateral).

Treatment

Infusion of fluids through large-calibre intravenous lines must be started before any attempt is made to drain a massive haemothorax, otherwise sudden decompression may result in haemodynamic decompensation from further hypovolaemia as the tamponade effect is released.

Blood should be given as soon as it is can be typed. A large-bore intercostal drain (28 French gauge or larger) is required for adults (see Practical procedures, p.65). Until a cardiac or vascular injury has been ruled out, the systemic pressure should not be allowed to rise uncontrollably, as this may precipitate further bleeding and cause death (see Chapter 6). Continuing blood loss of greater than 3 ml/kg body weight per hour indicates the need for surgical exploration. The patient should ideally have a central venous line placed in order to monitor right-sided cardiac filling pressure.

> **Always gain intravenous access before draining a massive haemothorax**

FLAIL CHEST

Severe direct chest wall injury may cause extensive disruption, with multiple rib and sternal fractures. When a segment of chest wall loses bony continuity with the thoracic cage (in other words, two or more adjacent ribs are broken in two or more places), it becomes flail and will move paradoxically on respiration, reducing tidal volume and compromising ventilation. The principal cause of hypoxia with flail chest, however, is the inevitable accompanying pulmonary contusion. Associated rib fractures may be accompanied by significant blood loss.

The diagnosis is usually clinical, by observation of abnormal chest wall movement and the palpation of crepitus. Splinting from chest wall muscular spasm may mask the paradoxical movement, and the diagnosis is not uncommonly delayed until these muscles relax (due to exhaustion, or when paralysing drugs are given). The chest radiograph will not always reveal rib fractures or costochondral separation. An anterior flail chest can be particularly difficult to diagnose, as paradoxical movement (although present) is hard to detect when movement appears symmetrical. Careful inspection from a low level, looking along the chest, is likely to be helpful. The possibility of a central flail should be particularly considered in patients who have sustained steering-wheel injuries.

Treatment

If respiratory compromise is present, this may be initially managed by stabilization of the chest wall by direct pressure. Pain reduces the patient's tidal volume with inadequate ventilation of the basal segments, resulting in atelectasis. Pain also inhibits coughing, allowing secretions to obstruct bronchi and cause acute respiratory failure. Effective pain relief is therefore essential.

The injured lung is sensitive to inadequate perfusion subsequent to shock, and also to fluid overload (there is already capillary leakage); therefore, careful fluid management is essential. The degree of respiratory distress and hypoxia determines the need for ventilation, and it is important to be aware that pulmonary contusion may develop insidiously. Functional, not physical integrity is the principal aim. Adequate analgesia, careful fluid management and ventilatory support for severe underlying contusion are the cornerstones of management. Operative stabilization of fractures is very rarely indicated.

CARDIAC TAMPONADE

Although penetrating injuries are usually responsible for cardiac tamponade, blunt trauma may damage the heart or great vessels, causing bleeding into the pericardium. It only requires a small amount of blood within the fixed, fibrous pericardium to severely restrict cardiac function. The characteristic features are those of Beck's triad (although all these signs may be difficult to illicit in a noisy resuscitation room):

- Elevated central venous pressure
- Hypotension
- Muffled heart sounds.

The neck veins in a hypovolaemic patient can be empty. Kussmaul's sign of paradoxical elevated venous pressure on inspiration associated with tamponade may also be seen. Low-amplitude complexes may be seen on the ECG. Cardiac tamponade is usually a diagnosis of exclusion unless there are clear signs, such as an anterior stab wound medial to the nipple.

Treatment
The ideal management of cardiac tamponade is surgical decompression and exploration. Pericardiocentesis (see Practical procedures, p.67) may be life-saving and can be performed while the patient is awaiting surgery.

Potentially life-threatening injuries

The primary or secondary survey may reveal one of eight potentially life-threatening thoracic injuries:

- Cardiac contusion
- Aortic disruption
- Diaphragmatic rupture
- Major airway injury
- Oesophageal injury
- Pulmonary contusion
- Simple pneumothorax
- Haemothorax.

CARDIAC CONTUSION

Cardiac contusion is the most commonly missed fatal thoracic injury. It occurs when there is direct compression of the heart, or as a result of rapid deceleration. It is often associated with sternal fractures, and in such cases the right ventricle is more commonly damaged. The associated chest pain is usually assumed to be due to chest wall contusion or rib fractures. The diagnosis is established from the mechanism of injury, serial cardiac enzyme measurements, electrocardiographic changes and two-dimensional echocardiographic evidence of ventricular wall dysfunction and pericardial effusion.

Approximately 20% of patients with myocardial contusion suffer from dysrhythmias, including sinus tachycardia, supraventricular tachycardia and ventricular extrasystoles. It is also possible to develop conduction defects ranging from bundle branch block to complete heart block. Conduction defects may rarely require pacemaker insertion. Myocardial contusion following blunt injury can lead to decreased cardiac contractility and decreased compliance of the ventricle, resulting in a low cardiac output state due to myocardial failure. Associated coronary artery injury or injury to smaller vessels within the contused area can lead to tissue necrosis and infarction. Non-specific ST-segment and T-wave changes, and conduction abnormalities such as right bundle branch block may all be seen on the ECG.

Treatment

Conduction defects may rarely require anti-arrhythmic agents or pacemaker insertion. Cardiogenic shock is rare, but when it occurs conventional protocols should be followed. Urgent surgical repair using cardiopulmonary bypass is sometimes necessary for valvular trauma or ventricular septal rupture. These injuries may go unnoticed in the presence of more obvious associated injuries, but can be diagnosed using echocardiography.

TRAUMATIC AORTIC DISRUPTION

Tears of the aorta are immediately fatal in approximately 90% of cases. They occur as a result of blunt or deceleration injuries, typically in a road traffic accident or fall from a height. The aorta may be completely or partially transected, or may have a spiral tear.

The aorta is firmly fixed at three points: the aortic valve; the ligamentum arteriosum; and the hiatus of the diaphragm. Sudden deceleration will allow the mobile parts of the aorta to continue moving relative to the fixed parts. The commonest site of rupture is at the attachment of the ligamentum arteriosum, at which point the aorta remains tethered to the main pulmonary artery.

The immediate survival of the patient depends on the development of a contained haematoma, maintained by the intact adventitia. The survival of patients after reaching hospital depends on early diagnosis followed by urgent surgical repair. The diagnosis should be suspected in any high-energy chest trauma with a suggestive examination and radiographic findings, although there is no pattern of skeletal injuries that accurately predicts this condition.[4] No single radiographic sign absolutely predicts aortic rupture, but a widened mediastinum is the most consistent finding (Table 5.1).

Any suspicion of traumatic aortic disruption should prompt further investigation (see Investigations, p.64).

Table 5.1 *Radiographic signs of aortic disruption*

• Widened mediastinum
• Apical haematoma (cap)
• Fractured first or second rib
• Elevation of the right main bronchus
• Depressed left main bronchus
• Loss of definition of the aortic knuckle
• Tracheal deviation to the right
• Left haemothorax*
• Deviation of a nasogastric tube in the oesophagus to the right
• Obliteration of the aortic window

* Without any other obvious cause.

Treatment

The survival of patients after reaching hospital depends on early diagnosis, followed by urgent surgical repair.

If transfer is necessary the patient should be mechanically ventilated and the systolic blood pressure kept below 100 mmHg, using infusions of propanolol or sodium nitroprusside, or both. This is to prevent elevations of systemic blood pressure that may rupture the flimsy adventitial layer, causing fatal haemorrhage. Particular caution should, however, be taken in the use of these drugs in patients with myocardial contusion. A policy of 'hypotensive' fluid resuscitation is essential in this condition. The cardiothoracic surgeons should be contacted immediately for both advice and management of the patient.

There are special circumstances under which surgery for a diagnosed aortic disruption may be delayed. The usual scenario is in the presence of multiple trauma, where a condition such as a severe operable head injury may take priority. In such a case, all measures should be taken to maintain a lower blood pressure while the other injuries are being treated, although it must be accepted that this will involve some compromise with regard to cerebral perfusion pressure.

DIAPHRAGMATIC RUPTURE

Penetrating injuries cause small diaphragmatic perforations that are rarely of immediate significance. By contrast, blunt trauma produces large radial tears of the diaphragm and easy herniation of abdominal viscera. The right hemidiaphragm is relatively protected by the liver, and left-sided ruptures are therefore more common, although if right-sided rupture does occur it has a substantially higher mortality.[5] Left-sided ruptures are more easily diagnosed because of the appearance of gut in the chest. Bilateral rupture is rare. Pulmonary complications are common in patients undergoing surgery.

The chest radiograph can be misinterpreted as showing a raised hemidiaphragm, acute gastric dilatation or a loculated pneumothorax. Contrast radiography, or locating an abnormal position of the stomach (by identifying the tip of a nasogastric tube) on plain radiography confirms the diagnosis. Computed tomography (CT) scanning may also be of value. In some centres thoracoscopy is successfully employed, with up to 98% accuracy for diagnosis of diaphragmatic rupture.[6]

Treatment

Unless intracranial injuries or potentially fatal haemorrhage require immediate surgery, repair of the diaphragm should not be delayed. This is often performed through a laparotomy for associated abdominal injuries, but may equally be performed through a thoracotomy or thoracoscopy. Preoperative insertion of a nasogastric tube is mandatory to prevent gastric distension and its sequelae.

MAJOR AIRWAY INJURY

Extensive free air in the neck, mediastinum or chest wall should always raise the suspicion of major airway damage. Laryngeal fractures are rare, but are indicated by hoarseness, subcutaneous emphysema and palpable fracture crepitus. Transection of the trachea or a bronchus proximal to the pleural reflection causes extensive deep cervical or mediastinal emphysema, which rapidly spreads to the subcutaneous tissues. Injuries distal to the pleural sheath result in pneumothorax.

Blunt tracheal injuries may not be obvious, particularly if the conscious level of the patient is depressed. Penetrating injuries are usually apparent, and all require surgical repair. They may be associated with injury of adjacent structures, most commonly the oesophagus, carotid artery or jugular vein. Laboured breathing may be the only indication that there is airway obstruction.

Injury to a major bronchus is usually the result of blunt trauma. There are often severe associated injuries, and most victims die at the site of the accident. For those who reach hospital, there is at least a 30% mortality rate.

Signs of bronchial injury may include:

- haemoptysis;
- subcutaneous emphysema;
- tension pneumothorax; and
- pneumothorax with a large and persisting air-leak.

Most bronchial injuries occur within 2.5 cm of the carina, and the diagnosis is again confirmed by bronchoscopy. Mucosal oedema and debris can obscure the extent of a bronchial injury, so the site should be carefully inspected.

Treatment

Attempted intubation is warranted if the airway is completely obstructed or there is severe respiratory distress, but should be performed by a senior clinician. The airway may be hazardous to secure and may require either rigid bronchoscopy or immediate tracheostomy followed by surgical repair. Bronchial tears must be repaired on an urgent basis in the operating theatre, through a formal thoracotomy.

OESOPHAGEAL TRAUMA

Damage to the oesophagus is usually caused by penetrating injury. Blunt oesophageal injury is rare, except with sudden compression causing a 'burst' type of defect. This occurs after a severe blow to the upper abdomen when gastric contents are forced up into the oesophagus, producing a linear tear through which the contents are then able to leak. Mediastinitis, with or without rupture into the pleural space with empyema formation, follows.

The clinical picture may be identical to that of spontaneous rupture of the oesophagus, but the diagnosis is often delayed. The diagnosis is confirmed by cautious contrast study of the oesophagus, or by endoscopy.

Treatment

Treatment is by formal surgical repair in the operating theatre, with drainage of the pleural space and/or mediastinum. In selected patients (usually the severely debilitated), a conservative approach may be taken. Aggressive, broad-spectrum intravenous antibiotic therapy should be employed immediately in all patients with oesophageal rupture.

PULMONARY CONTUSION

All patients with significant chest wall trauma are likely to have underlying pulmonary contusion. Contusion usually develops clinically and radiographically over the first 1–3 days, but in severe trauma there may be ventilatory failure and chest X-radiographic signs on presentation.

Spiral CT is more sensitive than chest X-radiography for detecting early pulmonary contusions, and in one series[7] the presence of a normal early CT correlated with failure to develop evidence of pulmonary contusion.

Treatment

Treatment involves high-flow oxygen therapy, serial blood gas analysis, appropriate analgesia, judicious fluid replacement and physiotherapy. In some patients a period of mechanical ventilation is required.

SIMPLE PNEUMOTHORAX

The presence of air in the pleural cavity without either penetration from the outside, or the presence of tensioning, constitutes a simple pneumothorax. Signs include reduced chest expansion on the affected side, decreased air entry, increased resonance to percussion, and visible air on the chest X-radiography. This may not be visible on a supine film, particularly if the pneumothorax is small.

Treatment

A chest drain should be inserted in the fifth intercostal space, just anterior to the mid-axillary line (see Practical procedures, p.65).

HAEMOTHORAX

Blood in the thoracic cavity may come from lung laceration or injury to any of the vessels supplying the hemithorax. Signs include reduced chest expansion, dull percussion note, and decreased air entry on the affected side. These signs may be not be detectable early on in the patient's chest X-radiography in a noisy resuscitation room, especially if supine. Likewise, a supine chest X-radiography may fail to identify small or moderate blood in the hemithorax for the observer who expects to see a fluid level, as it will appear as diffuse shadowing. An erect or semi-erect film should reveal blunting of the costophrenic angle.

Treatment
A large-bore chest drain should be inserted on the affected side (see Practical procedures, p.65).

FLUID RESUSCITATION

A policy of controlled resuscitation has already been described, and this is particularly important in thoracic trauma

Over-vigorous infusion is undoubtedly hazardous to certain patients, and improved strategies have been sought.[8,9] Overenthusiastic infusion is particularly dangerous in patients with cardiac tamponade, traumatic aortic disruption, and pulmonary contusion.[10,11]

Traumatic disruption of the aorta (TDA) and pulmonary contusion merit special mention. Patients who have a TDA are often clinically very stable and well, but the adventitial layer of the aorta is the only thing preventing rupture and massive exsanguination, the medial and intimal layers having torn. This is a precarious situation, and a rise in blood pressure beyond a certain point may cause this to disrupt, resulting in sudden death.

Pulmonary contusion is characterized by increased capillary permeability, and leakage of tissue fluid into the alveoli, creating pulmonary oedema. Indiscriminate infusion of intravenous fluid in these patients will exacerbate the injury in much the same way as fluid will in cases of cardiogenic pulmonary oedema. Great caution is therefore necessary when there is a possibility that pulmonary contusion is present.

The priority in treating continued significant haemorrhage remains control of the bleeding at source.

Base deficit is a sensitive indicator of oxygen debt and changes in oxygen delivery, and will therefore reflect the adequacy of tissue perfusion and resuscitation. Low cardiac output states may additionally benefit from the administration of intravenous calcium or inotropes, but it is important to recognize that these are of no use in the absence of an adequate circulating volume. Haemorrhage from cardiac or vascular laceration that has stopped following tamponade may re-bleed fatally if such injuries are not identified before resuscitation raises the arterial and intracardiac pressures.

INVESTIGATIONS

Imaging is essential in the accurate diagnosis of many of the conditions mentioned in this chapter. Considerable advances have been made in the application of imaging techniques to the trauma situation.

Chest radiography

A plain chest radiograph is the most important investigation in a patient with thoracic trauma, and should be performed with the patient as erect as possible. An erect film enables best assessment of lung expansion and free air or blood in the chest cavity. Widening and shift of the mediastinum may be evident. Serious injuries such as cardiac tamponade, transection of the aorta, ruptured diaphragm and major airway injury can usually be diagnosed from the chest radiograph.

In practice, however, the radiograph is often performed with a seriously injured patient in a supine (or at best partially erect) position. Interpretation of a supine film has many pitfalls: small pneumo- and haemothoraces may be missed due to the air or blood being evenly distributed throughout the hemithorax; the mediastinum usually appears widened, leading to false-positive diagnoses of traumatic aortic disruption; and air under the diaphragm pointing to hollow viscus perforation may not be evident. Additionally, subcutaneous emphysema further complicates radiograph interpretation.

Multiple rib fractures, fractures of the first or second ribs, or scapular fractures indicate that severe force has been delivered to the chest and its internal organs, and highlight the need for careful assessment for further unsuspected injuries. Pneumomediastinum, pneumopericardium or air beneath the deep cervical fascia suggest tracheobronchial disruption. Surgical emphysema of the chest wall and haemopneumothorax are generally indicative of pulmonary laceration following rib fractures.

Ultrasound/echocardiography

In order to diagnose or eliminate the majority of the conditions presenting potential threats to life, various imaging modalities are now available. Portable ultrasound is increasingly being used, and although operator-dependent, may be of considerable use in the diagnosis of pericardial and pleural fluid collections.[12–14] The most benefit has been seen with blunt thoracic trauma, particularly in suspected aortic injury, but it can also evaluate intracardiac shunts, valvular injury and pericardial effusions (tamponade).[15]

Transoesophageal echocardiography (TOE) is an ultrasound technique which is useful for eliminating the very high false-positive rate for traumatic disruption of the aorta in cases of a widened mediastinum on plain chest radiograph.[16] There is supporting evidence for its use in patients with a high likelihood of aortic disruption based on mechanism of injury and clinical findings, in the presence of a normal chest X-radiography.[17] Again, it is dependent on a skilled operator, and there still remain some 'blind spots' (aortic arch branches and distal ascending aorta), which may be missed areas that account for up to 20% of lesions.[18] There is little experience with its use in trauma in the UK.

Computed tomography

Computed tomography (CT) is particularly useful in aiding the diagnosis of aortic injuries.[19,20] It is recommended as the first-line investigation of stable patients with low or moderate probability of aortic disruption, as it has a high sensitivity (92–100%) and specificity (81.7–100%).[21,22] It also allows accurate detection of other thoracic injuries, and it is now common practice for most patients who have sustained significant thoracic trauma to undergo a CT scan of the chest at an early stage of their management, the urgency being dictated by clinical condition. The newer generation of machines are rapid in operation (one breath-hold time), and can accurately detect pulmonary parenchymal changes, such as pneumatocysts, haematomas, haemorrhage and acute respiratory distress syndrome (ARDS).[15]

The risks associated with the transfer of a potentially unstable patient to the CT scanner should never be underestimated. Monitoring and resuscitative procedures are difficult, and there is increased risk of critical infusions, drips and drains becoming disconnected.

Angiography

Angiography is the 'gold standard' for the diagnosis of aortic disruption and injury to major thoracic arteries. Angiographic equipment is constantly improving, and almost all imaging is now by digital subtraction. This allows multiple projections of computer reconstructions of the vessel.[15] However, it is invasive, takes a long time, and needs the patient to be relatively stable. It should be used for investigation of patients with a high likelihood of traumatic aortic disruption, and for those with CT-confirmed diagnosis who need further localization before surgery[23] (at the request of the cardiothoracic surgeon).

Thoracoscopy

Thoracoscopy, whether video-assisted (VATS) or direct, has a definite place in the management of thoracic trauma. The commonest indications are for diagnosis of point of origin of bleeding to form a haemothorax, and drainage of a haemothorax.[6] It also has a delayed use in the evacuation of retained haemothoraces. More recently, its role in the evaluation of mediastinal injuries has been under scrutiny. Only certain patients are suitable, and haemodynamic stability is necessary. Contraindications include suspected injuries to the heart and great vessels, blunt trauma causing contusion, widened mediastinum on radiography, massive haemothorax or continued bleeding, and inability to tolerate single-lung ventilation.[24]

Laboratory tests

There remains no specific blood test for myocardial injury following trauma. Many of the recognized cardiac enzymes have been tried, such as creatine phosphokinase (CPK) and its myocardial band isoenzyme (CK-MB), but they may also rise in the presence of other confounding variables such as skeletal trauma and other pre-morbid conditions.[25] More recent markers such as troponin I and troponin T have also yet to be shown to be specific indicators of myocardial contusion.[26,27]

PRACTICAL PROCEDURES

Intercostal chest drain insertion

Insertion of an intercostal chest drain is the single commonest intervention in patients who have sustained significant thoracic trauma. It may be life-saving or simply prophylactic, but the procedure carries a significant morbidity and must be performed correctly.

The fifth intercostal space, just anterior to the mid-axillary line is chosen because:

- the chest wall is usually thin at this location due to absence of muscle cover;
- the patient can subsequently lie on their front or back;
- the cosmetic effect is limited; and
- key structures are unlikely to be damaged.

PROCEDURE

The procedure is carried out in step-wise fashion:

- High-flow oxygen is administered.
- The fifth intercostal space on the affected side, just anterior to the mid-axillary line is identified.
- The skin is cleaned and draped.
- Local anaesthetic is infiltrated under the skin and down to the pleura if the patient is conscious.
- A 3-cm incision is made along the line of the rib.
- A track is dissected bluntly through the subcutaneous tissues, staying above the rib.
- The parietal pleura is punctured with the closed end of a clamp.
- A gloved finger is inserted through the pleura, and a finger sweep performed to determine the presence of adhesions (beware the presence of bony spicules from rib fractures).

One of the two options detailed below should then be followed, depending on the available equipment.

Whether a chest drain is being inserted for a haemothorax or a pneumothorax, it should always be directed towards the lung apex. A measure of the correct amount of drain which needs to be inserted can be gained by comparing the drain to the size of the patient's chest. If too much is inserted the drain will kink with loss of function; if too little, it is possible that one of the drain side holes will lie outside the chest – resulting in an air leak, or within the chest wall – resulting in surgical emphysema.

Option 1
- A primed chest drain bag apparatus is attached to the intercostal catheter.
- The flexible introducer is inserted through a distal eye in the catheter.
- The catheter and introducer are inserted into the chest, after which the introducer is withdrawn.

- Misting of the inside of the drain, or blood in the drain, are sought to confirm placement.

Option 2

- The distal end of the chest drain is clamped (after removal of the trocar).
- The tip of the drain is held in a clamp, and inserted through the pleura, after which the clamp is removed.
- Misting of the inside of the drain, or blood in the drain, are sought to confirm placement.
- The tube is connected to an underwater seal, and checked for swinging.
- The underwater seal must remain below the level of the patient's chest at all times.

Then in either case:

- The tube is firmly sutured in place and the incision closed.
- The area is dressed.
- A check chest X-ray is performed.

The wound is best closed with mattress sutures. A suture on either side of the drain (centrally placed within the wound) can be tied to close the wound, and a central suture can be inserted but left untied until removal of the drain. This produces a neat, linear scar. So-called purse-string sutures should not be used. The drain should be sutured in place using a gaiter-type suture or other similar method.

The wound should be dressed with a number of 10×10-cm swabs, each with a slit cut in one side, placed around the wound before adhesive tape is applied. This reduces kinking of the drain.

COMPLICATIONS

Complications of the procedure include:

- misplacement (usually extrapleural);
- damage to chest or abdominal organs by instruments;
- damage to intercostal neurovascular bundle;
- infection (local, or empyema); and/or
- subcutaneous emphysema.

Needle thoracocentesis

This is a life-saving procedure that should be undertaken on clinical suspicion of tension pneumothorax. It is a safe procedure, and is simple to perform. The much-quoted rush of air on puncturing the pleura is often absent or missed.

Failure to improve after this procedure may be due to an incorrect diagnosis, or possibly due to the cannula being too short: 50% of patients in a series had chest walls greater than 3 cm thick, but only 5% were thicker than 4.5 cm.[28] Therefore, the needle used should be a minimum of 4.5 cm long.

PROCEDURE

Again, the procedure is performed step-wise:

- High-flow oxygen is administered.
- The second intercostal space in the mid-clavicular line is identified.
- The skin is rapidly cleaned (an alcohol swab is adequate).
- Using a large-bore cannula, the skin is punctured just above the third rib aiming directly down, at 90° to the skin.

A rush of air may confirm placement, though this may not occur until the trochar is removed due to blockage with tissue and may, on occasion even be missed. The cannula is then taped in place. A chest drain should be inserted as soon as is practical and a chest radiograph obtained.

COMPLICATIONS

The two main complications include: (i) failure to puncture the pleura; and (ii) creation of pneumothorax.

Pericardiocentesis

Pericardiocentesis is a procedure used to buy time in a patient with cardiac tamponade. The removal of only 15 ml of blood can be life-saving while preparations are made for cardiothoracic surgery.

PROCEDURE

The procedure used is as follows:

- High-flow oxygen is administered.
- The patient's ECG rhythm is monitored.
- The site of puncture is cleaned.
- Local anaesthetic is infiltrated if the patient is conscious.
- A large cannula is attached to a 50-ml syringe.
- The needle is introduced one finger's breadth inferior to, and just left of, the xiphisternum.
- The needle is aimed towards the tip of the left scapula.
- The ECG is monitored at all times while advancing: QRS and ST changes indicate myocardial stimulation, and the needle should be partially withdrawn.
- As much blood as possible is withdrawn from the pericardium – it will probably not clot, and there should be less than 50 ml.
- The appearance of the ECG changes during aspiration indicate that the needle should be partially withdrawn.
- Once the procedure is completed, the capped-off cannula should be secured in place.
- Thoracotomy should be arranged – note, further aspiration may be needed in the interim.

COMPLICATIONS

Complications of the procedure include: (i) misplacement (into the ventricle); (ii) myocardial injury; (iii) dysrhythmia; (iv) pneumothorax; and (v) puncture of the great vessels.

EMERGENCY THORACOTOMY

Emergency thoracotomy is associated with a high mortality, and has the best chance of success if performed by an experienced surgeon. It is a controversial procedure, and history has recorded its practice in hopeless situations.[29–31] There are very few indications for its application, which are specific and evidence-based, and attempting this major undertaking outside established guidelines will almost inevitably end in failure.[32–38]

Definite **indications** are few: only those patients who have sustained certain injuries and who fulfil specific criteria should be considered for this procedure (Table 5.2). A thoracotomy should be performed wherever possible in theatre by a cardiothoracic surgeon. Only if urgency absolutely dictates should the procedure be performed elsewhere. Definite **contraindications** to performing an emergency thoracotomy are listed in Table 5.3. However, it is important to remember that this issue is a perpetual controversy, and the application of firm rules is not always appropriate.

There is an extremely high mortality associated with all thoracotomies performed anywhere outside the operating theatre, particularly by non-cardiothoracic surgeons. Patients requiring thoracotomy in the emergency room, even in established trauma centres, for anything other than isolated penetrating heart injury rarely survive.[39] Outcome is even worse for those having this procedure performed in the field. Salvage thoracotomies for blunt trauma are almost always hopeless. In the majority of blunt chest trauma cases *in extremis*, the injuries discovered will not be repairable, the continued blood loss is enormous, and the outcome fatal.[40] There is commonly much venous bleeding, particularly from lacerated pulmonary veins, and posterior intercostal and lumbar vessels. Control of such large-volume haemorrhage under suboptimal conditions is usually impossible. There may be pressure on the attending surgeon to 'open the chest' as a last resort, but it seldom has a beneficial outcome.

Table 5.2 *Indications for emergency thoracotomy*

- Penetrating trauma (cardiac tamponade diagnosed), with definite signs of life at scene
- Uncontrollable life-threatening haemorrhage into the airways (hilar clamping required)
- Requirement for aortic cross-clamping (uncontrollable subdiaphragmatic haemorrhage)
- Open cardiac massage (rarely required)

Table 5.3 *Contraindications to emergency thoracotomy*

- Blunt trauma with no signs of life at scene
- CPR for more than 5 min without endotracheal intubation
- Asystolic or pulseless electrical activity (PEA) arrest for over 10 min

When indicated, thoracotomy enables relief of tamponade, internal cardiac massage, and cross-clamping of the aorta which will help to restore the perfusion pressure to the brain and the coronary arteries while reducing intra-abdominal haemorrhage. This emergency surgery may take the form of median sternotomy, anterolateral thoracotomy or lateral thoracotomy depending upon the nature of the injury, the surgeon's experience and the facilities available.

Urgent thoracotomy

The indications for urgent thoracotomy rather than immediate emergency thoracotomy are shown in Table 5.4.

Table 5.4 *Indications for urgent thoracotomy*

- Ruptured aorta
- Open pneumothorax
- Ruptured diaphragm
- Massive haemothorax
- Oesophageal trauma
- Major airway injury
- Penetrating cardiac injury

ANALGESIA

As already stated, chest injuries can cause hypoxaemia directly through lung damage, but also indirectly through reduced chest excursion secondary to pain. Therefore, adequate analgesia is essential. The mainstay of analgesia in trauma is the use of opiates, and these should be used as required in thoracic trauma, although it is important to remember that they can reduce ventilation and decrease the clearance of secretions.

Local anaesthetic infiltration, such as intercostal bupivacaine, can be invaluable for extensive rib fractures, effectively blocking the neurovascular bundles in the spaces above and below the fracture sites. An injection of 3–5 ml of 0.5% bupivacaine (with or without adrenaline) is ideal. Intercostal blocks should be placed at the level of injury and two levels above and below.[41] They should be placed 7–9 cm lateral to the posterior midline, where the angle of the rib is palpable. This ensures blocking of the lateral intercostal branch (sensory innervation of the anterior and posterior thorax).

In the longer term, admitted patients gain excellent pain relief from epidural infusions of local anaesthetic.

COMMON ERRORS AND PITFALLS

Common errors and pitfalls of thoracic trauma include the following:

- Victims of blunt chest trauma who appear outwardly well without external signs or symptoms may be concealing life-threatening injuries.
- Pulmonary contusion may have an insidious onset, and may present as respiratory failure requiring ventilation several days after the initial injury.
- Injudicious administration of clear fluids in victims of chest trauma is associated with a worse outcome than in those patients who have cautious fluid resuscitation.
- Isolated minor chest wall trauma only usually requires analgesia. It is of most importance to exclude underlying organ damage. Rib fractures only require operative stabilization in exceptional circumstances. Sternal fractures, again, rarely need operative stabilization. As with fractured ribs, pain is often a major factor in prevention of adequate respiratory mechanics.

SUMMARY

Thoracic injuries are common and make a major contribution to potentially avoidable mortality. A logical, systematic approach to examination, assessment and treatment is essential. Failure to achieve this will result in injuries being missed and in avoidable morbidity and mortality.

REFERENCES

1. Mansour KA. *Trauma of the Chest*. Philadelphia: WB Saunders, 1997.
2. Rooney SJ, Hyde JAJ, Graham TR. Chest Injuries. In: Driscoll P, Skinner D, Earlham R (eds). *ABC of Major Trauma* (3rd edn). London: BMJ Books, 2000, pp. 16–26.
3. The American College of Surgeons Committee on Trauma. *Advanced Trauma Life Support for Doctors: Instructor Course Manual*. Chicago: American College of Surgeons, 1997.
4. Lee J, Harris JH, Duke JH, Williams JS. Non correlation between thoracic skeletal injuries and acute traumatic aortic tear. *Journal of Trauma* 1997; **43**: 400–4.
5. Epstein LL, Lempke RE. Rupture of the right hemidiaphragm due to blunt trauma. *Journal of Trauma* 1968; **8**: 19.
6. Villavicencio RT, Aucar JA, Wall MJ. Analysis of thoracoscopy in trauma. *Surgical Endoscopy* 1999; **13**: 3–9.
7. Schild HH, Strunk H, Weber W, *et al*. Pulmonary contusion: CT vs plain radiograms. *Journal of Computer-Assisted Tomography* 1989; **13**: 417–20.
8. Westaby S. Resuscitation in thoracic trauma. *British Journal of Surgery* 1994; **81**: 929–31.
9. Bickell W, Pepe PE, Mattox KL. Complications of resuscitation. In: Mattox KL (ed). *Complications of Trauma*. New York: Churchill Livingstone, 1994, pp. 126–31.
10. Hyde JAJ, Rooney SJ, Graham TR. Fluid management in thoracic trauma. *Hospital Update* 1996; **22**: 448–52.
11. Hyde JAJ, Rooney SJ, Graham TR. Hypotensive resuscitation. In: Greaves I, Porter KM, Ryan JM (eds). *Trauma*. London: Edward Arnold, 1997.
12. Catoire P, Orliaguet G, Liu N, *et al*. Systematic transoesophageal echocardiography for detection of mediastinal lesions in patients with multiple injuries. *Journal of Trauma* 1995; **38**: 96–102.
13. Freshman SP, Wisner DH, Weber CJ. 2-D echocardiography: emergent use in the evaluation of penetrating precordial trauma. *Journal of Trauma* 1991; **31**: 902.

14. Karalis DE, Victor MF, Davis GA, *et al*. The role of echocardiography in blunt chest trauma: a transthoracic and transoesophageal echocardiographic study. *Journal of Trauma* 1994; **36**: 585–93.

15. Mattox K, Wall M. Newer diagnostic measures and emergency management. *Chest Surgical Clinics of North America* 1997; **7**: 213–26.

16. Saletta S, Lederman E, Fein S, *et al*. Transoesophageal echocardiography for the initial evaluation of the widened mediastinum in trauma patients. *Journal of Trauma* 1995; **39**: 137–142.

17. Vignon P, Lagrange P, Boncooeur MP, *et al*. Routine transoesophageal echocardiography for the diagnosis of aortic disruption in patients without enlarged mediastinum. *Journal of Trauma* 1997; **42**: 969–72.

18. Ahrar K, Smith DC, Bansal RC, Razzouk A, Catalano RD. Angiography in blunt thoracic aortic injury. *Journal of Trauma* 1997; **42**: 665–9.

19. Brasel KJ, Weigelt JA. Blunt thoracic aortic trauma: a cost-utility approach for injury detection. *Archives of Surgery* 1996; **131**: 619–26.

20. Durham RM, Zuckerman D, Wolverson M, *et al*. Computed tomography as a screening exam in patients with suspected blunt aortic injury. *Annals of Surgery* 1994; **220**: 699–704.

21. Biquet JF, Dondelinger RF, Roland D. Computed tomography of thoracic aortic trauma. *European Radiology* 1996; **6**: 25–9.

22. Gavant ML, Menke PG, Fabian T, *et al*. Blunt traumatic aortic rupture: detection with helical CT of the chest. *Radiology* 1995; **197**: 125–33.

23. Savastano S, Feltrin GP, Miotto D, *et al*. Aortography in the diagnosis of traumatic aortic rupture due to blunt chest trauma. Report of thirty six patients. *Annales de Radiologie* 1991; **34**: 371–5.

24. Graeber GM. Thoracoscopy and chest trauma: its role. In: Westaby S, Odell J (eds) *Cardiothoracic Trauma*. London: Arnold, 1999; pp. 110–18.

25. Jones JW, Hewitt RL, Drapanas T. Cardiac contusion: a capricious syndrome. *Annals of Surgery* 1975; **181**: 567.

26. Hamm CW, Katus HA. New biochemical markers for myocardial cell injury. *Current Opinion in Cardiology* 1995; **10**: 355–60.

27. Mair P, Mair J, Koller J, *et al*. Cardiac troponin T release in multiply injured patients. *Injury* 1995; **26**: 439–43.

28. Britten S, Palmer SH, Snow TM. Needle thoracocentesis in tension pneumothorax: insufficient cannula length and potential failure. *Injury* 1996; **27**: 321–2.

29. Baxter BT, Moore EE, Moore JB, Cleveland HC, McCroskey BL, Moore FA. Emergency department thoracotomy following injury: critical determinants for patient salvage. *World Journal of Surgery* 1988; **12**: 671–5.

30. Bleetman A, Kasem H, Crawford R. Review of emergency thoracotomy for chest injuries in patients attending a UK Accident and Emergency department. *Injury* 1996; **27**: 129–32.

31. Jahangiri M, Hyde J, Griffin S, *et al*. Emergency thoracotomy for thoracic trauma in the accident and emergency department: indications and outcome. *Annals of the Royal College of Surgeons of England* 1996; **78**(3 [Pt 1]): 221–4.

32. Mattox KL, Pickard LR, Allen MK. Emergency thoracotomy for injury. *Injury* 1986; **17**: 327–31.

33. Baker CC, Thomas AN, Trunkey DD. The role of emergency room thoracotomy in trauma. *Journal of Trauma* 1980; **20**: 848–55.

34. Bodai BI, Smith JP, Ward RE, O'Neill MB, Auborg R. Emergency thoracotomy in the management of trauma. *Journal of the American Medical Association* 1983; **249**: 1891–6.

35. Mattox KL. Indications for thoracotomy: deciding to operate. *Surgical Clinics of North America* 1989; **69**: 47–58.

36. Boyd M, Vanek VW, Bourguet CC. Emergency room resuscitative thoracotomy: when is it indicated? *Journal of Trauma* 1992; **33**: 714–21.

37. Ivatury RR, Rohman M. Emergency department thoracotomy for trauma: a collective review. *Resuscitation* 1987; **15**: 23–35.

38. Velmahos GC, Degiannis E, Souter I, Allwood AC, Saadia R. Outcome of a strict policy on emergency department thoracotomies. *Archives of Surgery* 1995; **130**: 774–7.

39. Lewis G, Knottenbelt JD. Should emergency room thoracotomy be reserved for cases of cardiac tamponade? *Injury* 1991; **22**: 5–6.

40. Bodai BI, Smith JP, Blaisdell FW. The role of emergency thoracotomy in blunt trauma. *Journal of Trauma* 1982; **22**: 487–91.

41. Fouche Y, Tarantino DP. Anaesthetic considerations in chest trauma. *Chest Surgical Clinics of North America* 1997; **7**: 227–38.

6

Shock

OBJECTIVES

- To understand the physiological mechanisms responsible for tissue oxygen delivery
- To understand the mechanisms of shock following trauma
- To understand the body's compensatory mechanisms during shock
- To recognize and assess the shocked patient
- To demonstrate a structured approach in the management of the shocked trauma patient

INTRODUCTION

Shock is defined as a clinical state of under-delivery of oxygen and essential nutrients to the cells and tissues of the body. Inadequate supply or utilization of these vital substrates leads to anaerobic glycolysis, the activation of complex cellular and immune-mediated pathways, and cellular damage.[1]

PATHOPHYSIOLOGY OF OXYGEN DELIVERY

Interruption of the perfusion of tissues with oxygenated blood is a fundamental process in the pathophysiology of shock. It is therefore important to understand the mechanisms that maintain its integrity, in the healthy state, before considering how it can be impaired. The following factors affect tissue oxygen delivery (DO_2):

- The ability of the lungs to take up oxygen (see Chapter 4).
- The oxygen-carrying capacity of blood.
- Haemoglobin concentration.
- Blood flow.

Oxygen-carrying capacity of blood

Haemoglobin is a protein comprising of four subunits, each of which contains a haem molecule attached to a polypeptide chain. The haem molecule contains iron, which reversibly binds with oxygen, and each haemoglobin molecule can carry up to four oxygen molecules. Blood has a haemoglobin concentration of approximately 15 g/100 ml, and normally each gram of haemoglobin can carry 1.34 ml of oxygen if it is fully saturated. Therefore, the **oxygen-carrying capacity** of fully saturated blood is:

Hb (15) $\times$ 1.34 $\times$ Saturation of Hb (1) = 20.1 ml O_2/100 ml of blood

The relationship between the partial pressure of oxygen available (PaO_2) and oxygen uptake by haemoglobin is not linear, because the addition of each O_2 molecule to the haem complex facilitates the uptake of the next O_2 molecule. This produces a sigmoid-shaped oxyhaemoglobin dissociation curve (Figure 6.1).[1] In the normal healthy state haemoglobin

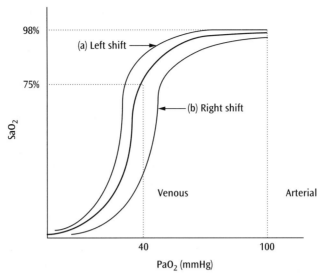

Figure 6.1 *The oxyhaemoglobin dissociation curve (thick line). Normal values of haemoglobin oxygen saturation (SaO₂; %) and partial pressure of oxygen in arterial blood (PaO₂; mmHg) are given for arterial and venous blood. The effects of a left shift (a) and a right shift (b) in the dissociation curve are represented by the thinner lines.*

is 97.5% saturated at a PaO_2 of 100 mmHg (13.4 kPa). It follows from this curve that increasing the PaO_2 further has little effect on the oxygen-carrying capacity.

An increase in the affinity of haemoglobin for oxygen at a particular PaO_2 means that oxygen is more actively retained, resulting in the oxygen disassociation curve being shifted to the left (Figure 6.1(a)). This is caused by:

- a decrease in hydrogen ion concentration (rise in pH);
- a decrease in $PaCO_2$;
- a decrease in concentrations of red cell 2,3-diphosphoglycerate (2,3-DPG); and
- a decrease in temperature.

At the tissue level, the partial pressure gradient of oxygen is opposite to that found at the alveolar–capillary interface. The capillary PO_2 is approximately 20 mmHg (2.6 kPa) and cellular PO_2 only 2–3 mmHg (<0.4 kPa). Furthermore, local factors reduce the affinity of haemoglobin for oxygen (shifting the curve to the right), allowing O_2 to be released more readily (Figure 6.1(b)).

Haemoglobin concentration

The normal haemoglobin concentration (as measured by haematocrit) is usually just above the point at which the oxygen transportation is optimal (approximately 10 g/dl). Consequently, a slight fall in haemoglobin concentration will actually increase oxygen transportation by decreasing blood viscosity. Approximately 60 times less oxygen is dissolved in plasma than is combined with haemoglobin. This amount is directly proportional to the PaO_2 and is approximately 0.003 ml/100 ml blood/mmHg of PaO_2. Consequently, the total content of oxygen in blood is equal to the oxygen associated with haemoglobin plus that dissolved in plasma.

Blood flow

VEINS

The venous system acts as a reservoir for over 50% of the circulating blood volume and is therefore often referred to as a *capacitance system*. The amount of blood stored at any one time is dependent on the size of the vessel lumen. This is controlled by sympathetic innervation and local factors, which can alter the tone of the vessel walls. If the veins dilate, more blood remains in the venous system and less returns to the heart. Should there be a requirement to increase venous return, then sympathetic stimulation increases, reducing the diameter of the veins and the capacity of the venous system. A change from minimal to maximal tone can decrease the venous capacitance by approximately 1 litre in an adult.

Conversely, a total loss of the tone causes so much dilatation that the normal blood volume is insufficient to fill it (see Neurogenic shock, p.75).

ARTERIES

The walls of the aorta and other large arteries contain relatively large amounts of elastic tissues that stretch during systole and recoil during diastole. The walls of arterioles contain relatively more smooth muscle. This is innervated by the sympathetic nervous system that maintains, to a large extent, vasomotor tone by stimulation of alpha adrenoreceptors. The arterial system is under constant control by sympathetic innervation and local factors to ensure that blood goes where it is needed most. This is exemplified in the shocked patient where differential vasoconstriction maintains supply to the vital organs (brain, heart, kidneys) at the expense of others (skin).

Cardiac output

This is defined as the volume of blood ejected by each ventricle per minute. Thus, the cardiac output equates to the volume of blood ejected with each beat (stroke volume) multiplied by the heart rate (beats per minute):

Cardiac output = Stroke volume × Heart rate = 4–6 l/min (normal adult)

To allow a comparison between patients of different sizes, the cardiac index (CI) is sometimes used, this being the cardiac output divided by the body surface area of the person.

Cardiac output can be affected by several factors, including:

- preload;
- myocardial contractility;
- afterload;
- heart rate; and
- systemic blood pressure.

PRELOAD

Preload is the volume of blood in the ventricle at the end of diastole. The left ventricular end-diastolic volume (LVEDV) is about 140 ml and the stroke volume (SV) 90 ml. Therefore, the end-systolic volume is approximately 50 ml and the left ventricular ejection fraction (SV/EDV) ranges from 50% to 70%. The greater the preload, the greater the consequent stroke volume (Starling's law). A clinical estimate of this volume, or force, is the end-diastolic pressure (EDP). As the left ventricular EDP (LVEDP) increases, so does the stroke volume. If the EDP exceeds a critical level, then the force of contraction declines and eventually ventricular failure ensues.

MYOCARDIAL CONTRACTILITY

Substances affecting myocardial contraction are termed inotropes. A positive inotrope produces a greater contraction for a given length (or EDP clinically). Adrenaline, noradrenaline and dopamine are naturally produced substances that have this effect. Dobutamine and isoprenaline are synthetic catecholamines with positive inotropic activity. Negative inotropes result in a reduced contractility for a given muscle length; these substances are often drugs such as anti-arrhythmics and anaesthetic agents. Many of the physiological states produced by shock will also depress contractility for example hypoxia, acidosis and sepsis. Myocardial injury has a similar effect.

AFTERLOAD

Afterload is the resistance faced by the ventricular myocardium during contraction. In the left ventricle this is mainly due to the resistance offered by the aortic valve and the compliance (stiffness) of the arterial blood vessels. Usually this latter component is the most important and is estimated by measuring the *systemic vascular resistance* (SVR).

HEART RATE

This is mediated via β_1 adrenoreceptors. These can be stimulated directly, by the sympathetic nervous system (SNS), or indirectly by the release of catecholamines from the adrenal medulla. This is termed a *positive chronotropic effect*.

Stimulation of the parasympathetic nervous system (PNS), which supplies the sinoatrial node and atrioventricular node via the vagus nerve, decreases heart rate and thus has a *negative chronotropic effect*. Beta-blockers and other drugs that inhibit the SNS can produce a similar effect. An increased heart rate may follow inhibition of the PNS M receptors. Usually faster heart rates enhance cardiac output; however, ventricular filling occurs during diastole, and it is this phase of the cardiac cycle that is predominantly shortened as the heart rate increases. A sinus tachycardia above 160 beats/minute in the young adult drastically reduces the time for ventricular filling. This leads to a progressively smaller stroke volume and a fall in cardiac output. The critical heart rate when this occurs is also dependent on the age of the patient and the condition of the heart. For example, rates over 120 beats/minute may be sufficient to cause inadequate filling in the elderly.

SYSTEMIC BLOOD PRESSURE

The systemic blood pressure can be defined as the pressure exerted on the walls of the arterial blood vessels, and is the maximal pressure generated in the large arteries during each cardiac cycle, while diastolic pressure is the minimum. The difference between them is the pulse pressure. The *mean arterial pressure* is the average pressure during the cardiac cycle and is approximately equal to the diastolic pressure plus one-third of the pulse pressure. As the mean arterial pressure is the product of the cardiac output and the systemic vascular resistance, it is affected by all the factors already discussed.

Tissue oxygen consumption

The total consumption of oxygen per minute (VO_2) for a resting healthy male is 100–160 ml/min/m^2. As the DO_2 is 500–720 ml/min/m^2, the tissues use only 20–25% of the oxygen that is available. Thus body tissues have a tremendous potential to extract more oxygen from the circulating blood. In a healthy subject, the VO_2 is constant throughout a wide range of oxygen delivery. Under normal circumstances an increase in oxygen demand is met by increasing the oxygen delivery, usually from a rise in the cardiac output. However, should this not be possible, or inadequate, then VO_2 can be maintained to a limited extent by increasing the oxygen extraction ratio. Should this also fail, then VO_2 will begin to fall because it is now directly dependent on DO_2.

MECHANISMS OF SHOCK IN TRAUMA

The causes of shock are conventionally divided into:

- Hypovolaemic
- Cardiogenic
- Neurogenic
- Septicaemic
- Anaphylactic.

Anaphylaxis and septicaemic shock will not be discussed in great detail as they are rare in the initial trauma patient contact:[2-5] nevertheless, septicaemic shock can occasionally occur if patients are found sometime after their initial trauma, and anaphylaxis can complicate the clinical picture as a consequence of the administration of drugs such as antibiotics or morphine.

Hypovolaemic shock

In trauma there are three pathophysiological entities which will result in shock: reduced venous return, impaired cardiac function, and reduced vascular tone. Hypovolaemic shock causes reduced venous return. Causes of hypovolaemic shock include haemorrhage, burns and crush injury.

Cardiogenic shock

Cardiogenic shock results from impaired cardiac function, and causes include:

- cardiac contusion or tamponade;
- ischaemic heart disease (which may have been the cause of the initial trauma);
- anti-arrhythmic drugs; and
- underlying cardiomyopathy.

In addition, tension pneumothorax, cardiac tamponade pulmonary embolism and high airway pressure in positive-pressure ventilation cause impedance to venous return, further exacerbating the shock state.

Neurogenic shock

Neurogenic shock results from reduced vascular tone. A spinal lesion above T6 can impair the sympathetic nervous system outflow from the cord below this level sufficiently to result in generalized vasodilatation, bradycardia and loss of temperature control. As it leads to a reduction in blood supply to the spinal column, it gives rise to additional nervous tissue damage. In the presence of other injuries both the reflex tachycardia and vasoconstriction responses to hypovolaemia are eliminated. Shock does not occur as a result of head injuries. In the patient with a cervical cord injury and hypotension, it is essential that it is not assumed that the hypotension is due simply to neurogenic shock. Any injury of sufficient energy to result in a cervical cord injury is likely to be sufficient to produce significant injuries and haemorrhage elsewhere.

Septicaemic shock

As a result of established systemic infection, release of inflammatory mediators causes a loss of venous tone, with blood pooling and an initially hyperdynamic circulation, before venous return and cardiac output fall and clinical shock becomes established. Causes of septicaemic shock in trauma include translocation of bacteria across the gut wall, infection of wounds, aspiration and gastrointestinal perforation.

Anaphylactic shock

In anaphylaxis, antigen-induced IgE-mediated release of vasoactive substances (including histamine) from mast cells causes generalized vasodilatation. In addition there is an increase in vascular permeability that causes fluid to leak into the extravascular space. As a consequence of these mechanisms both venous return and venous tone fall.

COMPENSATORY MECHANISMS IN SHOCK

Patients cannot remain permanently in a state of shock – they either improve or die – and shock could be looked upon as a momentary pause on the way to death. To help stop the fatal decline, the body has several compensatory mechanisms that attempt to maintain adequate oxygen delivery to the essential organs.

Oxygen uptake

Sympathetically induced tachypnoea occurs in shocked patients. Unfortunately, this does not produce any sizeable increase in the amount of oxygen uptake per 100 ml of blood because the haemoglobin in blood passing ventilated alveoli is already 97.5% saturated. The slight rise in PaO_2 due to the hypocapnia from hyperventilation only increases this value by around 1%. However, the clinician can help to prevent any decline in saturation by increasing the inspired concentration of oxygen and ensuring that there is adequate ventilation.

Blood flow

There are pressure receptors in the heart and baroreceptors in the carotid sinus and aortic arch. These trigger a reflex sympathetic response via control centres in the brainstem in response to hypovolaemia. The sympathetic discharge stimulates many tissues in the body, including the adrenal medulla. This leads to a further release of systemic catecholamines, enhancing the effects of direct sympathetic discharge, particularly on the heart. This response prevents, or limits, the fall in cardiac output by positive inotropic and chronotropic effects on the heart and by increasing venous return secondary to venoconstriction.

Furthermore, selective arteriolar and pre-capillary sphincter constriction of non-essential organs (for example, skin and gut) maintains perfusion of vital organs (for example, the brain and heart). Selective perfusion also leads to a lowering of the hydrostatic pressure in those capillaries serving non-essential organs. This reduces the diffusion of fluid across the capillary membrane into the interstitial space, thereby decreasing any further loss of intravascular volume. It also has the effect of increasing the diastolic pressure and thereby reducing the pulse pressure. Increased sympathetic activity is therefore responsible for many of the clinical signs associated with shock:

- tachypnoea;
- tachycardia – direct sympathetic stimulation;
- reduced pulse pressure;
- pallor, sweating and coolness of the skin due to reduced perfusion; and
- ileus due to reduced gut perfusion.

A further source of circulatory control is found in the kidney. The juxtaglomerular apparatus detects any reduction in renal blood flow and causes renin release. This leads to the formation of angiotensin II and aldosterone. These, together with antidiuretic hormone (ADH) released from the pituitary, increase the reabsorption of sodium and water by the kidney and reduce urine volume. In addition, the thirst centre of the hypothalamus is also stimulated. The overall result is that the circulating volume is increased. Renin, angiotensin II and ADH can also produce generalized vasoconstriction and so help to reduce venous capacitance. In addition, the body attempts to enhance the circulating volume by releasing osmotically active substances from the liver. These increase plasma osmotic pressure and so cause interstitial fluid to be drawn into the intravascular space.

MANAGEMENT OF THE SHOCKED PATIENT

The detection of shock is dependent on certain physical signs that are produced as a result of poor oxygen delivery.[6,7] Similarly, the treatment of shock consists of restoration of an adequate delivery of oxygen. The A,B,C approach to diagnosis and management of patient problems and injuries is paramount, and any information gained from pre-hospital personnel and/or family members is vital as a part of this process.

Airway and breathing

The first priority in any shocked patient is to clear and secure the airway and administer high-flow oxygen. The immediately life-threatening thoracic conditions should then be looked for, and treated when found.

Circulation

Following trauma, hypovolaemia is the sole or main contributor cause in most cases. An essential component of the initial assessment of the shocked patient is the identification of the location of the blood loss. Potential sites for haemorrhage are:

- external ('on the floor');
- chest;
- abdomen and retroperitoneum;
- pelvis; and
- long-bone fractures.

```
'Blood on the floor and four more'
```

External blood loss should be apparent, although a careful examination of the back is essential in order not to miss a posterior injury. External bleeding into the confines of a splint must be sought and excluded. Major bleeding into the chest should already have been identified during the 'breathing' assessment, but continued observation will be necessary to exclude lesser degrees of haemorrhage.

Palpation of the abdomen in the conscious patient or visible distension may indicate the possibility of abdominal haemorrhage and indicate the need for further investigation. However, abdominal examination is not sensitive and a high index of suspicion should be maintained dependent on the mechanism of injury, physical signs and specialized investigation.

A single attempt to spring the pelvis may provide evidence of disruption pending the completion of appropriate radiographs. This procedure assesses lateral compression and anteroposterior movement and should not be repeated (absence of positive findings does not rule out pelvic fractures, hence the need for definitive X-rays).

Significant long-bone fractures should become apparent during the 'exposure' component if they are not already obvious. Early splintage of such fractures will significantly reduce blood loss, and also help with the patient's pain relief. Traction splintage of femoral fractures (when there is not a pelvic fracture at the point of proximal purchase) decreases the space and volume for potential blood loss. Realignment also makes patient analgesia and subsequent handling easier.

Retroperitoneal haemorrhage is invariably occult, and may only become apparent when all other sites of bleeding have been excluded or controlled.

```
Beware retroperitoneal haemorrhage
```

INITIAL HAEMOSTASIS

It is easy to underestimate the extent of blood loss from external sources. A large amount of the evidence may be left at the scene and bleeding – especially from head wounds – can be insidious. Manual pressure applied to bleeding points will normally control venous bleeding, particularly when combined with elevation of the wound above the level of the heart. This is therefore best achieved with the patient laying supine. When dealing with arterial bleeding however, tourniquets are often necessary. Limb arterial bleeding is best controlled by using a sphygmomanometer cuff inflated above systolic pressure. Where this is not possible, a triangular bandage should be applied over the dressing covering the wound such that its knot lies above the bleeding point. If a rigid bar is then incorporated under the knot, and twisted, increased pressure can be exerted.

```
The time a tourniquet is applied should be clearly marked in the patient's
notes so that inappropriately long-limb ischaemia is avoided
```

Controlling external haemorrhage

This is carried out by:
- applying direct pressure over the bleeding site;
- elevation of the bleeding site above the level of the heart; or
- applying a tourniquet.

Traditional methods of recognizing shock utilize assessment of the physiological response to hypoxia such as heart rate (HR), blood pressure (BP) and respiratory rate (RR). These have the advantages of requiring little equipment, of permitting rapid and repeated measurement by numerous people with minimal training, and of being easily understood. The response to blood loss is, however, not uniform (see below).

RECOGNITION

In established shock, the patient will be pale,[8] sweating and distressed, and the neck veins may be seen to be flat or distended. Nevertheless, in the early stages of the shock process, all these abnormalities may be absent and the patient may look completely normal. In established shock, the capillary refill time will be prolonged beyond its normal value of 2 s. This is estimated by pressing on the nail bed for 5 s and counting how long it takes for the normal pink colour to return after the compression is released. This sign is not reliable in the cold patient, and if there is a proximal injury on the tested limb may only give an indication of local rather than general perfusion.

The pulse should be assessed for the presence of either a brady- or a tachycardia. Vasodilatation with a bounding pulse is suggestive of septic shock. The presence of a radial pulse implies a systolic blood pressure of at least 80 mmHg, a femoral pulse implies a systolic blood pressure of 70 mmHg. If only the carotid is palpable, the systolic blood pressure will be approximately 60 mmHg.

Radial pulse	systolic BP 80mmHg
Femoral pulse	systolic BP 70 mmHg
Carotid pulse	systolic BP 60 mmHg

A blood pressure of 80 mmHg (the presence of a palpable radial pulse) is usually adequate to maintain essential central organ perfusion.

Accessory information can be gained from pulse oximetry and ECG and blood pressure monitoring, and these must be routinely applied.

Estimating volume loss and grading shock

The compensatory mechanisms evoked by 'shock' are related to the decline in function of various organs. It is possible to divide the physiological changes of hypovolaemic shock into four categories depending on the percentage blood loss (Table 6.2).

Tachypnoea can indicate shock as well as underlying respiratory or metabolic pathology. A tachycardia often occurs early due to the sympathetic response. In Grade 2 shock the diastolic blood pressure rises, without any fall in the systolic component, leading to a narrowed pulse pressure. This is due to the compensatory sympathetic nervous system-mediated vasoconstriction. Consequently, a narrow pulse pressure with a normal systolic blood pressure is an early sign of shock. Hypotension indicates a loss of approximately 30% of the circulating volume.

> **A fall in blood pressure will only take place when no further compensation is possible. It is therefore a LATE sign in shock**

Table 6.2 *Clinical presentation of an adult with hypovolaemic shock*[6]

Category of hypovolaemic shock Parameter	I	II	III	IV
Blood loss (litres)	<0.75	0.75–1.5	1.5–2.0	>2.0
Blood volume loss (%)	<15	15–30	30–40	>40
Respiratory rate (per minute)	14–20	20–30	30–40	>35 or low
Heart rate (per minute)	<100	100–120	120–140	>140 or low
Capillary refill time	Normal	Delayed	Delayed	Delayed
Diastolic blood pressure	Normal	Raised	Low	Very low
Systolic blood pressure	Normal	Normal	Low	Very low
Pulse pressure	Normal	Low	Low	Low
Urine output (ml/h)	>30	20–30	5–15	Negligible
Mental state	Normal	Anxious	Anxious/ confused	Confused/ drowsy

Limitations to estimations of hypovolaemia

For some patient groups, undue reliance on the clinical signs alone might lead to a gross over- or underestimation of the blood loss. It is therefore important that management is based on the overall condition of the patient and not on isolated physiological parameters.

The *elderly patient*[9] is less able to compensate for acute hypovolaemia as their sympathetic drive is reduced. Consequently, the loss of smaller volumes can produce a fall in blood pressure.

A variety of commonly prescribed *drugs* can alter the physiological response to blood loss. For example, beta-blockers will prevent tachycardia and also inhibit the normal sympathetic positive inotropic response. Therefore a beta-blocked patient is unlikely to become tachycardic after a 15% blood volume loss. However, they will become hypotensive at relatively low levels of haemorrhage.

Table 6.3 *Pitfalls in assessing blood loss*

- The elderly patient
- Drugs
- Pacemakers
- The athlete
- Pregnancy
- Hypothermia
- Tissue damage

An increasing number of patients have *pacemakers* fitted each year. Some types only allow the heart to beat at a particular rate irrespective of the volume loss. Therefore they will give rise to the same errors in estimation as beta-blockers.

The physiological response to training will mean that the serious *athlete* will have a larger blood volume and a resting bradycardia (about 50 beats/min). A pulse of 100 beats/min may represent compensatory tachycardia in these patients.

During *pregnancy*,[10-12] the heart rate progressively increases so that by the third trimester it is 15–20 beats faster than normal. Blood pressure falls by 5–15 mmHg in the second trimester, and returns to normal during the third trimester as the blood volume has increased by 40–50%. Supine hypotension due to compression of the inferior vena cava may exacerbate shock, and must be prevented by positioning or insertion of a wedge as part of the primary survey (see Chapter 14).

Hypothermia[13] will reduce the blood pressure, pulse and respiratory rate irrespective of any other cause of shock (see Chapter 15). Hypothermic patients are often resistant to cardiovascular drugs, defibrillation or fluid replacement. Estimation of the fluid requirements of these patients can therefore be very difficult, and invasive monitoring is often required.

TREATMENT

Treatment of shock is subdivisible into the followng components:

- Control of external haemorrhage.
- Intravenous access.
- Fluid resuscitation.
- Investigations.
- Surgical intervention.

Control of external haemorrhage

Control of external haemorrhage has already been discussed, and forms an essential part of the primary survey. In cases where the external haemorrhage is associated with compound fractures, appropriate splintage must be applied, although the timing of this must be judged according to clinical priority.

PERIPHERAL INTRAVENOUS ACCESS

The largest cannula possible (ideally a 14 or 16 G) should be inserted, the antecubital fossa being the site of choice. The use of an elbow splint will improve flow and decrease the risk of complications such as loss of the venflon or clotting of the line. Short, wide cannulae should be used because the flow of a liquid in a tube is inversely proportional to cannula length and directly related to the fourth power of its radius. However, in the shocked patient this can be difficult. Ideally, a second cannula should also be placed, although other life-saving interventions should not be delayed while struggling to achieve this. Once intravenous access is achieved, the cannula must be firmly secured; in the case of femoral or other central lines, this means stitching it in place. Once intravenous access has been achieved, 20 ml of blood should be taken for laboratory tests (FBC, U&E, cross-match and, if clinically appropriate, glucose, blood cultures, clotting and toxicology).

All fluids given to patients need to be warmed before administration, in order to prevent iatrogenically-induced hypothermia. A simple way of achieving this is to store a supply of colloids and crystalloids in a warming cupboard. This eliminates the need for warming coils during this phase of resuscitation. These increase the resistance to flow and thereby slow the rate of fluid administration.

If peripheral intravenous access cannot be effectively achieved (and multiple, increasingly fruitless attempts to cannulate ever smaller veins should be avoided), access should be achieved via the femoral vein. The insertion of small-bore neck lines for the purpose of intravenous infusion should be avoided. Access to the neck is likely to be difficult due to the need for neck immobilization following blunt trauma; moreover, the volumes of fluid which can be infused are small and the procedure is technically difficult. In addition, infraclavicular approaches are associated with a high incidence of complications such as pneumothorax, which can be potentially catastrophic in the trauma victim. A useful site is therefore the femoral vein.

INSERTION OF FEMORAL VENOUS LINE

The groin is exposed and quickly cleaned. Aseptic technique for line insertion is ideal. The anatomical markings are the anterior superior iliac spine (ASIS) laterally, and the pubic symphysis in the midline. Half-way along a line drawn between these landmarks is the surface marking of the femoral artery. The femoral vein lies medial to the artery in a direction pointing towards the umbilicus. The femoral nerve lies lateral to the artery (necessary for local anaesthetic infiltration in femoral fractures) (Figure 6.2).

In the severely compromised patient there is a degree of urgency in obtaining vascular access, and therefore local anaesthetic infiltration over the puncture site should be omitted.

The technique described briefly below is called the Seldinger method. There are various

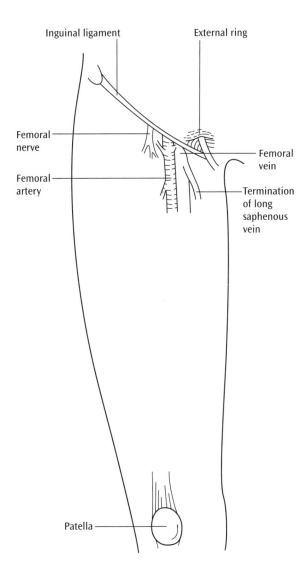

Inguinal ligament

External ring

Femoral nerve

Femoral artery

Femoral vein

Termination of long saphenous vein

Patella

Figure 6.2 *Anatomical landmarks for an insertion of a femoral line.*

proprietary kits available for central venous access, and they have differing numbers and calibres of lumen.

- A wide-bore needle attached to a syringe is inserted over the landmark described and the syringe aspirated until a constant flash-back of venous blood is obtained.
- The syringe is removed from the needle and a guidewire inserted down the needle into the vein. There should be no resistance to the passage of the wire.
- The needle is then removed, leaving the wire in place. The dilator is then passed over the wire and a small nick in the skin is made with a knife to allow easier passage. The dilator is then removed, the definitive venous line is inserted over the wire, and the wire is then removed. The wire can be used for blood collection and infusion. It is important to keep hold of the wire at all stages so as not to lose it!

In extremis, the insertion of a large-gauge cannula into the femoral vein provides a stopgap until a more definitive line can be placed. The presence of either a pelvic or femoral fracture is not a contraindication to the insertion of a femoral line if this is the only practical option for the rapid infusion of life-saving fluids.

COMPLICATIONS OF FEMORAL AND PERIPHERAL VENOUS ACCESS

These include:

- failed cannulation;
- haematoma;
- extravasation of fluid or drugs;

- damage to adjacent structures;
- air embolism; and
- damage to the cannula (usually due to attempts to re-insert the trochar into the cannula).

VENOUS CUT-DOWN

This procedure requires time, surgical skill and anatomical knowledge of the position of suitably placed vessels (antecubital veins, femoral vein, long saphenous vein). It is therefore a technique for experienced personnel in patients who have difficult vascular access when other techniques are used.

- The long saphenous vein is found 2 cm above and anterior to the medial malleolus of the ankle.
- The site should be prepared with aqueous antiseptic solution and towelled to give the operator a sterile area. Local anaesthetic should be infiltrated along the line of proposed incision in the conscious patient.
- A transverse incision is made over the landmark through the skin.
- The vessel is located and isolated from adjacent adventitia, taking care to avoid the saphenous nerve.
- Using a haemostat, two ligature ties are passed beneath the vessel. The distal one is tied, after which a clip is placed on the tie to allow manipulation of the vessel.
- A tranverse venotomy is made and a large-bore intravenous catheter is inserted proximally.
- The proximal tie is then secured around the vessel and catheter, and the overlying cut-down wound is cleaned and dressed with a sterile water-proof dressing.

The complications of intravenous cut-down are similar to those of peripheral venous access.

INTRA-OSSEOUS ACCESS AND INFUSION[14-16]

This procedure should be used early in the approach to attaining vascular access in the child. It is fast, without the anatomical variations that can complicate direct intravenous access, relatively easy, and fluids and drugs may be administered via this route. There are various anatomical sites, but the most common is the anterior surface of the tibia 2 cm below and medial to the tibial tuberosity or insertion of the patellar tendon. Potential complications of insertion include infection, fracture and growth plate damage.

- The site should be prepared with aqueous antiseptic and a small amount of local anaesthetic should be infiltrated into the skin and down to the periosteum of the conscious patient.
- A small incision is made in the skin and, using the intra-osseous needle in a twisting and downwards motion, the device is inserted perpendicular to the skin. A loss of resistance is found on entry into the marrow cavity.
- The central trochar is then removed and a three-way tap can be attached to the needle and blood withdrawn for haematology and biochemistry. Fluid can be injected via a syringe three-way tap and giving set. Gravity flow alone does not produce adequate flow rates, and syringe-administered aliquots are therefore necessary.
- The intra-osseous needle is a bulky device and needs to be protected with suitable dressings to avoid displacement.

SUBCLAVIAN AND JUGULAR LINES

Insertion of internal jugular and subclavian lines is a difficult technique with a relatively high incidence of complications that occur more frequently in inexperienced hands. In addition, if not performed by someone with considerable experience, unnecessary time can be wasted in the attempt. The narrow-bore lines conventionally used for this approach are not suitable for the rapid administration of fluids and are more appropriately reserved for subsequent patient monitoring. For this reason, insertion of these lines is only recommended as a last resort, and only then by experienced clinicians.

Insertion of a low-approach internal jugular venous line
- The Seldinger technique is used.
- The patient's cervical collar is removed and the patient's head and neck is held in neutral alignment. Some head-down tilt of the patient is helpful, but not mandatory.
- The landmark for insertion is the posterior border of the sternocleidomastoid muscle 2–3 cm above the clavicle.
- The needle is advanced just behind the muscle in a direction towards the suprasternal notch. The vein can be reached within the length of a green needle. The needle should be advanced in a straight direction, and if blood is not aspirated then a second pass is made. The advantage of this approach is that arterial puncture can be controlled by direct pressure, unlike the subclavian route.
- Once the definitive line has been inserted and secured, the head blocks and straps may be replaced. Due to the low placement of the line this does not interfere with the head blocks.
- A portable chest X-ray should be obtained before the infusion of large quantities of fluid.
- Whichever approach is chosen, it should be performed by experienced staff because of the potential for damaging the vein and neighbouring structures.

Insertion of a subclavian line
- The Seldinger technique is used after removal of the cervical collar and establishment of manual in-line stabilization.
- The area is cleaned and surgical drapes applied.
- The junction of the middle and outer thirds of the clavicle and the suprasternal notch are identified.
- The needle is inserted 1 cm below the clavicle, at the junction of the middle and outer thirds, and advanced towards the suprasternal notch, passing under the clavicle.
- The vein is usually located at a depth of 4–6 cm.

Complications of jugular and subclavian lines
These include: (i) arterial puncture; (ii) haematoma; (iii) haemothorax; (iv) pneumothorax; (v) air embolism; (vi) loss of the guidewire; and (vii) cardiac arrythmias.

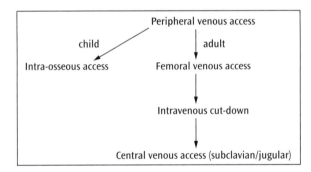

Figure 6.3 *A flow diagram for intravenous access.*

Fluid resuscitation

TYPES OF RESPONSE

Patients will either respond to fluid infusion by the return of cardiovascular stability, or will fail to respond and continue to progress through the stages of shock. In some cases, transient stability will be achieved but the patient will continue to bleed.

Thus, cases can be divided into: responders; transient responders; and non-responders.

Initial fluid resuscitation should begin with the administration of warmed crystalloid, usually Hartman's solution in general. In a fit adult, 2 l of Hartman's solution is an appropriate initial volume.

Responders
In these cases no more than maintenance fluids are usually required once the initial deficit has been replaced. Examples of such cases include those with external bleeding which has been controlled or a closed fractured shaft of femur following application of a traction splint.

Transient responders

Transient responders will mount an initial response to intravenous fluids with some stabilization of their vital signs, but will subsequently deteriorate due to continued haemorrhage. In these cases, following initial administration of crystalloid, administration of blood will be necessary as well as an urgent surgical opinion. Group-specific blood should be available, although on occasion administration of O-negative blood may be necessary. Examples of injuries of this type include the patient with a ruptured spleen.

Non-responders

Non-responders fail to mount any haemodynamic improvement following the administration of intravenous fluids, due to ongoing haemorrhage at a greater rate. These patients need an urgent surgical opinion. In addition, they will require the vigorous administration of intravenous fluids in order to maintain systolic blood pressure at a level consistent with essential organ perfusion. After initial administration of crystalloid, blood (usually type-specific or O-negative initially, followed by fully cross-matched blood) will be required.

Transient and non-responders invariably require an urgent senior surgical opinion

---

In administering intravenous fluids to the patient with ongoing haemorrhage, it is necessary to determine the accepted systolic blood pressure which is to be maintained pending surgical control of haemorrhage. Current evidence suggests that the best course of action is to administer sufficient fluids to maintain perfusion of essential organs. In practice, this means maintaining a systolic blood pressure in the region of 80 mmHg in the previously normotensive, which is equivalent to the presence of a palpable radial pulse.[17,18] A significantly higher pressure may be needed in those with a history of significant hypertension.

Resuscitation end point = presence of a radial pulse (systolic BP of 80 mmHg)

Currently, the evidence for this approach is patchy, although the theoretical basis for it (and the evidence from animal studies[19,20]) is strong. The technique of limited resuscitation or permissive hypotension is designed to avoid the acceleration of ongoing haemorrhage, disruption of established thrombus and dilution of clotting factors which can result from over-vigorous fluid administration.

The management of hypovolaemic shock is summarized as follows:

- The fluid of choice for immediate resuscitation in hypovolaemic shock is warmed crystalloid.
- Urgent surgical assessment is required for all patients who are shocked, or who have an obvious source on ongoing haemorrhage.
- Vigorous fluid resuscitation in hypotensive patients where there is a definite bleeding source that has not been controlled will lead to further bleeding, and a worse prognosis.
- Until the source of the bleeding is controlled, hypovolaemic patients require controlled resuscitation to maintain a blood pressure at 80 mmHg.

Turning the tap off!

The only appropriate end-point in the management of ongoing haemorrhage is surgery. No procedure should be performed in the resuscitation room which might increase mortality and morbidity by delaying urgent transfer to theatre. Nevertheless, in some cases procedures such as placement of an external fixator on an open-book pelvic fracture,[21–23] or (rarely) thoracotomy and cross-clamping of the aorta,[24,25] may be life-saving in the moribund patient.

ASSESSMENT AND MONITORING

The shocked patient's vital signs should be continuously monitored (Table 6.4).

Table 6.4 *Monitored vital signs in hypovolaemic patients*

- Respiratory rate
- Peripheral oxygen saturation
- Heart rate
- Blood pressure
- Pulse pressure
- Cardiac monitoring
- Temperature
- Urinary output
- Glasgow Coma Scale

Regular blood gas analysis is an essential component of the management of the shocked patient, and will allow the monitoring of the haematocrit as well as the base excess and lactate which are indicators of response or deterioration in the shock state.

Accurate measurement of urinary volume will obviously require the insertion of a urinary catheter. This should be connected to a system permitting accurate volume measurement that can be recorded whenever the other vital signs are measured.

COAGULATION ABNORMALITIES AFTER MASSIVE BLOOD LOSS

Coagulation abnormalities may occur in the resuscitation room as a result of the initial management of shock, due to dilution of clotting factors by administered fluids. This will be exacerbated by release of tissue factors which inhibit clotting and the low concentration of clotting factors in stored blood. Treatment of any type of coagulation disorder has to be guided by the results of the clotting studies and liaison with the haematologist. In cases of massive blood loss, consideration should be given to the administration of fresh-frozen plasma.

SUMMARY

The commonest cause of shock in trauma is haemorrhage. Establishment of the presence and location of haemorrhage is the cornerstone of effective management of shock. Appropriate intravenous fluids should be administered, but in many cases the only effective management of bleeding is surgery. If surgery is necessary, patient management should seek to expedite this without increasing morbidity and mortality due to excessive delays while unnecessary procedures are performed. In the patient with ongoing haemorrhage, a blood pressure of approximately 80 mmHg – which is sufficient to maintain vital organ perfusion – should be used as an end-point pending surgical control of haemorrhage. Initial fluid replacement should be with warmed crystalloid, with blood being administered as the second fluid if necessary.

REFERENCES

1. William F Ganong. *Review of Medical Physiology*. Prentice-Hall, 1999.
2. American College of Chest Physicians/Society of Critical Care Medicine Consensus Conference: definitions for sepsis and organ failure and guidelines for the use of innovative therapies in sepsis [see comments]. *Critical Care Medicine* 1992; **20**: 864–74.

3. Shoemaker WC. Circulatory mechanisms of shock and their mediators. *Critical Care Medicine* 1987; **15**: 787–94.

4. Shoemaker WC. Pathophysiology of shock as a basis for monitoring and therapy for the critically ill patient. In: Shoemaker WC, Tavares BM (eds), *Current Topics in Critical Care Medicine*. Basel: Karger, pp. 23–40.

5. Shoemaker WC, Appel PL, Kram HB, Bishop M, Abraham E. Hemodynamic and oxygen transport monitoring to titrate therapy in septic shock. *New Horizons* 1993; **1**: 145–59.

6. American College of Surgeons Committee on Trauma. Advanced life support course for physicians. Chicago, 1997.

7. Baskett PJ. ABC of major trauma. Management of hypovolaemic shock [see comments]. *British Medical Journal* 1990; **300**: 1453–7.

8. Redmond AD, Redmond CA, Jones JM, Hillier V. The significance of patient appearance in predicting severity of injury. *Injury* 1994; **25**: 81–2.

9. Wardle TD. Co-morbid factors in trauma patients. *British Medical Bulletin* 1999; **55**: 744–56.

10. Marx GF. Clinical management of the patient in shock. Shock in the obstetric patient. *Clinical Anesthesia* 1965; **2**: 151–65.

11. Esposito TJ, Gens DR, Smith LG, Scorpio R, Buchman T. Trauma during pregnancy. A review of 79 cases. *Archives of Surgery* 1991; **126**: 1073–8.

12. Mighty H. Trauma in pregnancy. *Critical Care Clinics* 1994; **10**: 623–34.

13. Mizushima Y, Wang P, Cioffi WG, Bland KI, Chaudry IH. Should normothermia be restored and maintained during resuscitation after trauma and hemorrhage? *Journal of Trauma* 2000; **48**: 58–65.

14. Guy J, Haley K, Zuspan SJ. Use of intraosseous infusion in the pediatric trauma patient. *Journal of Pediatric Surgery* 1993; **28**: 158–61.

15. Neal CJ, McKinley DF. Intraosseous infusion in pediatric patients. *Journal of the American Osteopathic Association* 1994; **94**: 63–6.

16. Hodge D, III. Intraosseous infusions: a review. *Pediatric Emergency Care* 1985; **1**: 215–18.

17. Deakin CD. Early fluid resuscitation in haemorrhagic shock. *European Journal of Emergency Medicine* 1994; **1**: 83–5.

18. Bickell WH, Wall MJ Jr, Pepe PE, *et al.* Immediate versus delayed fluid resuscitation for hypotensive patients with penetrating torso injuries [see comments]. *New England Journal of Medicine* 1994; **331**: 1105–9.

19. Kowalenko T, Stern S, Dronen S, Wang X. Improved outcome with hypotensive resuscitation of uncontrolled hemorrhagic shock in a swine model. *Journal of Trauma* 1992; **33**: 349–53.

20. Cutress R. Fluid resuscitation in traumatic haemorrhage [see comments]. *Journal of Accident and Emergency Medicine* 1995; **12**: 165–72.

21. Yang AP, Iannacone WM. External fixation for pelvic ring disruptions. *Orthopedic Clinics of North America* 1997; **28**: 331–44.

22. Ghanayem AJ, Stover MD, Goldstein JA, Bellon E, Wilber JH. Emergent treatment of pelvic fractures. Comparison of methods for stabilization. *Clinical Orthopedics* 1995; 75–80.

23. Bassam D, Cephas GA, Ferguson KA, Beard LN, Young JS. A protocol for the initial management of unstable pelvic fractures. *American Surgeon* 1998; **64**: 862–7.

24. Brown SE, Gomez GA, Jacobson LE, Scherer T III, McMillan RA. Penetrating chest trauma: should indications for emergency room thoracotomy be limited? *American Surgery* 1996; **62**: 530–3.

25. Demetriades D. Penetrating injuries to the thoracic great vessels. *Journal of Cardiac Surgery* 1997; **12**: 173–9.

Abdominal trauma

INTRODUCTION

Abdominal injury is a contributing factor in 20% of trauma deaths, either early from exsanguinating haemorrhage or late from bowel injury, subsequent sepsis or multiple organ failure. Advances in technology and an increased appreciation of the significance of the physiological derangement associated with severe abdominal injury has led to changes in the resuscitation, investigation and surgical management of abdominal trauma.

Abdominal injury frequently occurs as part of the picture of multiple injury, and therefore prioritization issues become paramount in its management.

ANATOMY

External anatomy

The surface markings of the abdominal cavity extend from the level of the fifth interspace (nipple level in the male) on full expiration, to the inguinal ligaments and pubic symphysis inferiorly. It is vital that abdominal evaluation includes the flanks and back, since wounds can classically be concealed in these regions. The flank encompasses the area between the anterior and posterior axillary lines. The back lies posterior to this, and may benefit from some partial protection to penetrating stab wounds due to its thick musculature.

Internal anatomy

The abdomen is divided into the peritoneal cavity, retroperitoneum and the pelvis.

PERITONEAL CAVITY

The peritoneal cavity contains the majority of the abdominal organs including the liver, spleen, stomach, small bowel, parts of the duodenum and parts of the large bowel. On full expiration it extends up to the level of the fifth interspace, and the ribs provide some protection to the upper abdominal organs. Therefore abdominal injury should be suspected in all cases of lower chest trauma.

RETROPERITONEUM

The retroperitoneum is divided into zones that have relevance at operation, where the mechanism and location of injury will determine whether surgical exploration or conservative management is applied. The central zone (zone I) contains the major vessels, and haematomas should be explored surgically in both blunt and penetrating trauma. The lateral zones (zone II) containing the kidneys, ureters and colon are only explored in blunt injury when the haematoma is expanding; however, they should be explored with care in cases of penetrating injury. The pelvis comprises zone III, and while penetrating trauma in this zone should be explored, haematoma from blunt trauma should not: observation, packing and interventional radiology techniques are more appropriate.

PELVIC CAVITY

The pelvic cavity is surrounded by the pelvic bones and contains the bladder, rectum and the internal genitalia in females.

MECHANISM OF INJURY

Blunt trauma

Blunt trauma remains the commonest cause of abdominal injury in the UK. Blunt abdominal injury is frequently associated with multi-system injury, making abdominal evaluation difficult and presenting problems in the prioritization of investigation and management. Injuries may be produced by direct impact or by deceleration and rotational forces that impinge on the intra-abdominal organs, especially at the interface between mobile and fixed structures. The solid organs – especially the liver and spleen – are the most commonly injured in blunt trauma, and this can lead to devastating haemorrhage. Bowel injury occurs either through an acute increase in intra-luminal pressure on impact or by shearing at points of transition from retroperitoneal to mobile bowel on a mesentery.

Penetrating trauma

Stab wounds are more common in the UK than gunshot injuries. The injury is confined to the tract of the implement at wounding (investigation and management are discussed later). Injuries from gunshot wounds vary depending on the energy transferred by the missile. Handgun rounds typically produce a low-energy transfer that inflicts injury along the path of the bullet, but little collateral damage, while high-energy transfer wounds from military rifles are associated with a cavitation effect resulting in widespread destruction of surrounding tissue and gross contamination.

Blast injury

This is discussed in Chapter 16.

CLINICAL PRESENTATION

The clinical presentation of abdominal trauma varies widely, as abdominal injury may be an isolated injury or part of multi-system trauma. The presentation will also be complicated by the patient's level of consciousness and the presence of other distracting injuries. The patient's haemodynamic status and the initial response to fluid must also be assessed, and will obviously affect investigation and management.

Abdominal signs in trauma vary from the acute abdomen with peritonitis or marked distension through the subtle seat belt sign which is frequently associated with intra-abdominal injury, to the minimal abdominal tenderness often found with early intraperitoneal bleeding, especially when other distracting injuries predominate. It is vital to have a high index of suspicion and a low threshold for appropriately directed investigation.

IMMEDIATE ASSESSMENT

Early surgical referral is essential in all cases where abdominal injury is suspected, and particularly in cases of multiple injury.

Wherever possible, a clear history should be taken from the patient or paramedic personnel with regard to the incident and the mechanism of injury. This can provide vital information about the likelihood of an abdominal injury, and should include information on such features as speed, seat belts and weapons.

The initial priorities in the management of the trauma patient are Airway, Breathing, and Circulation. Assessment of the abdomen and pelvis takes place under *Circulation and haemarrhage control*. The abdomen is one of the five major sites of potential blood loss in the trauma patient, and as such it is evaluated initially as part of the assessment of circulation and needs to be excluded as a site of bleeding, especially in the presence of hypotension and multiple injuries. This early assessment will be clinical, but may include ultrasound as a screening tool, performed either by a radiologist or by trained surgical or emergency room personnel. The initial evaluation may lead to the unstable or hypotensive patient with abdominal signs being transferred directly to theatre.

The abdominal assessment comprises a full clinical examination, including inspection of the abdomen, flanks and back for bruising, penetrating wounds and distension. This is followed by palpation of the abdominal quadrants to elicit tenderness and/or peritonitis and percussion for subtle signs of tenderness. Auscultation in the busy emergency room may add little to the evaluation. Rectal (and vaginal where indicated) examinations are an essential component of this assessment. The rectal examination will elicit reduced tone from spinal cord injury, bleeding from lower gastrointestinal trauma, bony penetration in pelvic fracture and a high-riding prostate associated with pelvic fracture, which is also an indicator of potential urethral injury.

The abdomen must be formally re-assessed during the secondary survey, and clinical (and sometimes ultrasound) assessments need to be repeated at a later stage if they are initially negative. The assessment of the abdomen will direct the team towards immediate surgery, appropriate investigation or repeat clinical evaluation.

EARLY MANAGEMENT

Resuscitation

The best currently available evidence suggests that, especially in patients with penetrating injury, limiting fluid resuscitation to a systolic blood pressure of 80 mmHg may confer a survival advantage.[1] The theoretical basis for applying the principle to all trauma victims (with the exception of head injuries, where it may have a detrimental effect) is strong, and resuscitation to a blood pressure sufficient to maintain perfusion of vital organs, without disruption of established clot or precipitation of coagulation abnormalities, is recommended. Thus the most appropriate policy is judicious administration of warmed fluids in order to maintain perfusion of the vital organs. The administration of intravenous fluids is never an alternative to the rapid transfer of the patient to the operating theatre, laparotomy and the control of bleeding by a surgeon.

Adjuncts

Placement of a urinary catheter (only after rectal examination) and a nasogastric tube are integral parts of the clinical evaluation. The urinary catheter allows monitoring of the progress of resuscitation and may provide evidence of haematuria as a sign of urinary tract injury. Where there are indicators of urethral injury, consultation with a urologist followed by urethrography or a single gentle attempt at catheterization may be appropriate, the alternative being a suprapubic catheter inserted by an appropriately skilled practitioner.

The nasogastric tube decompresses the stomach, relieves acute gastric distension, and provides evidence of upper gastrointestinal bleeding from penetrating injury to the stomach or oesophagus. Oral insertion of a Ryles tube is sometimes necessary if there is significant facial or base of skull trauma, or if it is impossible to insert a tube via the nose. Both a nasogastric tube and urinary catheter are prerequisites to performance of diagnostic peritoneal lavage (DPL).

Indicators of urethral trauma

- **Blood at the urinary meatus**
- **High-riding prostate**
- **Scrotal or perineal haematoma**

INVESTIGATIONS

Abdominal trauma presents the surgeon with a diagnostic dilemma. The abdomen is often not the only injured area, raising questions about whether the abdomen or a remote injury should be managed first. Conventional physical examination of the abdomen may not be appropriate, as the result of neurological injury, paraplegia or intoxication and distracting pain at a nearby site may lead to confusion in the evaluation of the awake patient. These situations call for specific protocols in the approach to abdominal assessment.

Abdominal trauma is classically divided into 'blunt or penetrating' for the purposes of investigation and management. Numerous modalities have been used to aid in the diagnosis of abdominal injury, and each has its proponents and critics. However, what is apparent is that no single investigation is ideal in all circumstances and that often a combination of tests will be most appropriate and will allow an informed decision to be made whether to proceed to a laparotomy or to use conservative management. Possible investigative modalities include:

- DPL;
- Focused Abdominal Sonography for Trauma (FAST);
- computed tomography (CT) scanning; and
- laparoscopy.

The indications and contraindications of each of these procedures is discussed below.

Diagnostic peritoneal lavage (DPL)

DPL (Table 7.1) has been the 'gold standard' for the investigation of blunt abdominal injury for more than 30 years.[2] It has an accuracy in blunt abdominal injury of 97.3%, with false-positive and false-negative rates of only 1.4% and 1.3%, respectively.[3] In blunt abdominal trauma, lavage counts of 100 000 red cells per mm^3 (RCC) and 500 white cells per mm^3 have been accepted as providing the most appropriate level of sensitivity. The most frequent criticism of this technique is the rate of non-therapeutic laparotomy performed for positive cell counts. This is a consequence of the balance between false-negative results and oversensitivity, and is variously estimated at 10–15%. Unfortunately, DPL does not allow conservative management in the presence of blood in the abdominal cavity, but computed tomography (CT) may be used as an adjunct in the stable patient. The value of DPL in penetrating trauma remains controversial; lavage cell counts of between 1000 and 10 000 red cells per mm^3 have been used to attain an appropriate sensitivity.

The presence of scarring from previous abdominal surgery, especially from a lower midline incision, will make DPL more technically difficult and reduce the chances of a diagnostic result. In this situation, an urgent surgical consultation is usually more appropriate than attempts at alternative sites for catheterization in inexperienced hands. Complications of DPL include gut penetration, haemorrhage and infection.

Despite more recent investigative advances, DPL remains widely used and many institutions have switched to a percutaneous Seldinger technique that has been shown to be

Table 7.1 *Diagnostic peritoneal lavage (DPL)*

(catheterization and nasogastric tube are prerequisites)

Open technique
- Full surgical aseptic technique used
- Subumbilical midline infiltration with local anaesthetic with 1:100 000 adrenaline is performed
- A skin incision is made with dissection to the peritoneum
- The dialysis cannula is inserted under direct vision and directed down into the pelvis
- 1 litre of warmed saline is instilled and allowed to redistribute
- The fluid bag is positioned below the patient to allow drainage of lavage fluid
- One sample is sent to the laboratory for analysis (a second sample is retained with the patient in case the first sample is lost)

Closed technique
- After preparation as before, a small skin incision is made
- The introducing needle is inserted angled toward the pelvis
- Using a Seldinger wire technique, the needle is replaced by a lavage catheter into the pelvis
- Fluid infiltration and collection are carried out as before

of equal sensitivity, faster and associated with fewer complications than its open counterpart.[4]

Focused Abdominal Sonography for Trauma (FAST)

Kristensen *et al.* first reported the use of ultrasound in the investigation of abdominal trauma in 1971.[5] Since then this technique has become widely accepted in Europe and more recently in America. Rozycki and colleagues have developed the FAST technique – a standard approach to abdominal trauma ultrasound which involves imaging a limited number of ultrasound windows to detect fluid:

- right upper quadrant;
- left upper quadrant;
- pelvis; and
- pericardial window to assess for pericardial effusion.

A collected review of nearly 5000 patients[6] (whose FAST was performed by a surgeon rather than a radiologist) demonstrated a sensitivity of 93.4%, specificity of 98.7% and an accuracy of 97.5% for haemoperitoneum and visceral injury. FAST is a technique that can be successfully performed by radiologists, accident and emergency staff or surgeons as long as they have been adequately trained and maintain a sufficient level of experience.

The application of ultrasound is more limited in penetrating trauma as the volume of blood that can be reliably detected – approximately 100 ml – restricts the sensitivity. However, high-frequency probes have been used in an attempt to visualize wound tracts and determine peritoneal penetration.

Ultrasound can be used as a screening tool in the resuscitation room and, if positive, can be followed in the stable patient by CT scanning to determine organ specificity. Rapid trauma ultrasound screening of the abdomen has also been shown to have a major role in multiple casualty incidents.

Ultrasound is fast, non-invasive and, with the advent of hand-held machines, portable. It is, however, operator-dependent and limited by factors such as surgical emphysema and obesity.

Computed Tomography (CT)

The CT scanner is strictly off-limits to unstable trauma patients. However, in the patient that is cardiovascularly normal following resuscitation, CT is the investigation of choice in many institutions. The standard trauma CT scan with a modern spiral scanner can be completed in 3–5 min, and should include intravenous contrast. The scans should image from the top of the diaphragm, to visualize haemothorax and pneumothorax, to the pubic symphysis and pelvis to aid orthopaedic assessment of suspected pelvic fracture.

The organ specificity and ability to grade injuries offered by CT has advanced the cause of conservative management; nevertheless, this decision should be made only on clinical parameters. In addition, CT has the advantage of visualizing the retroperitoneal structures.

Laparoscopy

Diagnostic laparoscopy (DL) in trauma is a relatively new investigation, the role of which is evolving. Studies have shown DL to be 97% accurate[7] in blunt abdominal trauma, but there is little evidence to support its use in this scenario as its application is limited by time and cost, and hampered by the presence of peritoneal blood. However, there is a niche for DL within the investigation of penetrating trauma in stable patients. DL has a sensitivity of 100% for the identification of peritoneal penetration,[8] and therefore is valuable for evaluating penetration in abdominal stab wounds. Some centres have even used this approach to provide evidence of peritoneal penetration in gunshot wounds where the course of the bullet appears tangential.[9] Laparoscopy is also the most effective investigation for diagnosing ruptured diaphragm, and a number of cases have been reported of laparoscopic repair of these injuries. Time, the requirement for a general anaesthetic, and the difficulty in excluding hollow viscus perforation precludes the procedure being more widely applied.

Wound exploration

Wound exploration is not an alternative to a laparotomy, since if the patient has generalized abdominal signs then a laparotomy is indicated. Wound exploration is an imprecise technique and has been associated with an accuracy of only 55% and with 88% false-positive results.[10] When performed, it must be carried out in the operating theatre, by a surgeon, as a formal procedure with either local anaesthesia and a cooperative patient or general anaesthesia. The patient must consent to undergo a laparotomy (or consent must be acquired). The wound should be extended surgically if necessary and penetration of the peritoneum identified or excluded. Haemostasis can then be obtained and laparotomy carried out or the wound closed in an appropriate manner. This procedure is not recommended as a routine.

Choice of investigation of blunt abdominal trauma (Table 7.2)

There needs to be a high index of suspicion for abdominal injury in all cases of multiple trauma. The key issue in the choice of investigation for blunt abdominal trauma is the cardiovascular stability of the patient. Patients who are unstable with unequivocal abdominal signs require a laparotomy, and not investigation or imaging. The dilemma arises in multi-system injury where the abdomen is only one of the potential sources for the cardiovascular instability. In this situation a rapid bedside test is required – local resources and experience will dictate whether DPL or ultrasound is the primary choice. In the haemodynamically-normalized patient the appropriate choice of study is CT scan, which provides organ specificity and allows the option of conservative management of solid organ injury where appropriate.

Table 7.2 *Indications for investigation of blunt abdominal injury*

- High index of suspicion from the mechanism of injury
- Injuries above and below the diaphragm
- Clinical signs of abdominal injury
- Seat belt sign, bruising of the abdominal wall
- Inability to perform unequivocal clinical examination – distracting injury, intoxication, paraplegia, obtunded patient

> **Investigation of blunt abdominal trauma**
>
> - Unstable patient with abdominal signs – THEATRE
> - Unstable patient with uncertain abdominal injury – DPL or ultrasound
> - Stable patient – CT scan

INVESTIGATION OF PENETRATING TRAUMA

In penetrating trauma the sensitivity of CT and ultrasound are far too low to exclude an abdominal injury.

Stab wounds

In peritoneal penetration laparotomy is compulsory; therefore laparoscopy or wound exploration should be employed in the operating theatre, with evidence of peritoneal penetration as the end-point.

Gunshot wounds

Most institutions employ a policy of obligatory laparotomy for abdominal gunshot wounds, as the incidence of organ injury following gunshot wounds is high. The only exception to this rule is the stable patient where either the track of the bullet appears tangential, and there is real doubt whether peritoneal penetration has occurred, or the injury is in the thoracoabdominal region and assessment is required to determine whether the injury is wholly thoracic. In these instances laparoscopy in theatre with the patient prepped for laparotomy may be appropriate in institutions with experience in the assessment of gunshot injuries.

AREAS OF DIAGNOSTIC DIFFICULTY IN STABLE PATIENTS (Table 7.3)

Diaphragm

The diagnosis of diaphragm injury remains elusive to non-invasive modalities. An initial chest X-ray with a nasogastric tube *in situ* may confirm the diagnosis. DL is the investigation of choice in the stable patient where there is index of suspicion clinically, or from an equivocal chest X-ray appearance.

Table 7.3 *Summary of investigations for suspected intra-abdominal injury*

- Haemodynamically unstable patients with signs of intra-abdominal bleeding require surgery
- Haemodynamically unstable patients with uncertainty about the abdomen require rapid abdominal evaluation (DPL or ultrasound)
- Haemodynamically stable patients with other severe injuries should have rapid evaluation (DPL or ultrasound)
- In the presence of minor associated injuries, a haemodynamically-normal patient with a clinically equivocal abdomen requires CT evaluation
- Haemodynamically stable patients with abdominal signs should have CT, allowing non-operative management if appropriate

Renal tract

CT has replaced the intravenous urogram (IVU) as the investigation of choice in renal injury. It allows an assessment to be made of both function and anatomical disruption of the kidneys. A one-shot IVU is still useful in resuscitation or theatre to determine the presence of renal injury and that there are two functioning kidneys. The cystogram remains the investigation of choice for suspected bladder disruption, and gentle urethrography may be performed where there is a suspicion of a urethral tear.

Pancreas

Serum amylase has no value in the initial evaluation of pancreatic injury as it has a positive predictive value of only 10% and a negative predictive value of 95%[11] for pancreatic injury. Contrast spiral CT is probably the best investigation, though CT scans early in the investigation can miss injuries to the pancreas.

Stab wounds to the flank and back

The evaluation of penetration is difficult in these injuries as the muscles of the back are thick and penetration of retroperitoneal organs may not present with abdominal signs. Contrast CT (including rectal contrast) is the most sensitive investigation.

Penetrating injuries to the buttocks

It must be assumed that injuries to the buttocks penetrate the abdominal cavity; therefore appropriate investigation of the abdomen should be carried out as well as digital rectal and sigmoidoscopic examination for blood.

CRITICAL DECISION-MAKING AND PRIORITIZATION IN MULTI-SYSTEM INJURY

Indications for laparotomy

The following are indications for laparotomy:

- unstable patients with signs of intra-abdominal trauma;
- positive findings on DPL or ultrasound in unstable patients;
- positive findings on CT in patients unsuitable for non-operative management;
- peritoneal penetration in stab wounds;
- gunshot wound to the abdomen; and
- evisceration and retained foreign bodies.

Although abdominal injury may at times present in isolation, in the UK – where blunt trauma (especially due to road traffic accidents) predominates – such injury is frequently found as part of the picture of multiple trauma. Prioritization of the investigations in this situation has already been discussed; however, it is clear that prioritization of management of the injuries must occur to provide the best outcome for the injured patient. Firm leadership of the resuscitation team is paramount in order to organize the competing surgical response in the multiple injury scenario. Contention may arise in patients with abdominal injuries and co-existing head injury, pelvic injury or multiple fractures.

Patients who have sustained both head and abdominal injury (as frequently occurs in road traffic accidents) may present resuscitation, investigation and management dilemmas. Clearly, the policy of hypotensive resuscitation is not appropriate in this scenario, as attention must be paid to maintaining the cerebral perfusion pressure. Prioritization of investigation and management is difficult and depends upon the severity of the injuries. An exsanguinating abdominal injury demands a laparotomy to control bleeding, before assessment of the head injury – obviously an unstable patient should not be placed in the CT scanner. When the patient is more stable, a trauma CT from head to symphysis pubis is the appropriate investigation, and treatment is directed toward the most life-threatening injury first. These decisions are judgements made from experience of trauma management.

As has been well described, the fractured, open-book pelvis is a major source of blood loss in the trauma patient.[12] Therefore, where there is concomitant abdominal and pelvic injury, prioritization of management must occur. Clearly laparotomy before stabilization of the pelvis will open the pelvic haematoma and allow free bleeding; thus, the rapid application of an external fixator to stabilize the pelvis either in the resuscitation room or in theatre immediately before laparotomy is the appropriate response. Laparotomy can occur relatively easily with the external fixator frame *in situ*.

Modern trauma orthopaedic management includes the early fixation of multiple long-bone fractures and open orthopaedic injuries. When the abdomen is also injured, laparotomy should take priority following rapid splinting of fractures in the resuscitation room. Occasionally the physiological state of the patient may demand that minimal surgical procedures are carried out, namely damage control. It may be possible to place external fixators concurrently to abdominal surgery, but this should not be done in the face of a deteriorating patient and fixation may have to be delayed until the patient is more stable.

SURGICAL STRATEGIES

Non-operative management of solid-organ injury (Table 7.4)

There is an increasing volume of data supporting the non-operative management of adult patients with solid-organ injury from blunt abdominal injury.[13] The widespread use of CT in stable patients has allowed both an accurate diagnosis and an estimate of the severity of the organ injury to be made. When the latest therapeutic techniques in interventional radiology[14] are incorporated, an increasing number of patients with isolated abdominal solid-organ injury are likely to be managed without surgical intervention. It is important that clinical and not CT criteria are used to determine surgical intervention; therefore, patients with minimal physical signs, cardiovascular stability and a requirement of less than 2 units of blood in the acute phase with appropriate findings on CT are candidates for this approach. Patients managed non-operatively have great potential for rapid deterioration and must be monitored for haemodynamic instability, fluid and transfusion requirements in a High-Dependency Unit or Intensive Care Unit where signs of early deterioration can be detected and surgical intervention rapidly undertaken if required. If a policy of conservative management is to be followed, this policy must be instigated or sanctioned at consultant level.

Table 7.4 *Indications for non-operative management of solid organ injury*

- Appropriate injuries to solid organs shown on CT
- Minimal physical signs
- Cardiovascular stability with a requirement of less than 2 units of blood acutely
- High-Dependency or Intensive Care facilities available
- Patient available for repeated examination, for example not in theatre undergoing long orthopaedic procedures

Non-operative management may be appropriate in up to 50% of isolated blunt liver injuries in adults, and have a 50–80% success rate.[15] It has also been shown to be successful in 93%[16] of less severe injuries in blunt splenic trauma. The majority of renal injuries can also be managed non-operatively unless there is injury to the renal pedicle or massive damage, as determined by CT scan, intravenous urogram or selective arteriogram.

Interventional radiology

Angiography is an important diagnostic adjunct in trauma as it allows the accurate diagnosis of bleeding and provides therapeutic options in both surgical and non-operative management. In abdominal trauma, interventional radiological techniques have been widely accepted in the diagnosis and management of haemorrhage from complex pelvic fractures. Where closure of an open-book pelvic fracture with an external fixator has failed to control bleeding, it is appropriate to proceed to angiography and embolization of the bleeding vessels. Surgical exploration of an expanding pelvic haematoma is fraught with difficulties, and pelvic packing followed by embolization is now the procedure of choice.

Interventional radiology techniques can also be successfully employed as an adjunct to non-operative management of solid organ injury[15] by demonstrating haemorrhage, followed by control using coil embolization of the bleeding vessels.

Damage control

The majority of patients who undergo laparotomy for abdominal injury can tolerate definitive vascular and organ repair at the initial operation. However, up to 10% of patients with multiple trauma are in a state of physiological extremis that will not permit both injury control and reconstruction to proceed together.[17] A survival advantage has been demonstrated in this group of patients using a limited 'damage control' procedure compared to a definitive primary operation.[18]

Damage control is founded on the concept that patients in physiological extremis – hypothermia (<34oC), acidosis (pH <7.2) and a coagulopathy – will tolerate only limited surgical procedures aimed at arresting haemorrhage and controlling peritoneal contamination, before the metabolic deterioration becomes irreversible. Therefore the initial surgery is limited: bleeding vessels are ligated or shunted, and bowel injuries stapled or tied off and returned to the abdomen which is packed to control bleeding from solid organs.[19] The abdomen is rapidly closed using either towel clips, suture of an intravenous fluid bag into the wound (Bogata bag), suture to the skin or alternatives. The patient is then transferred to the Intensive Care Unit, where aggressive resuscitation is directed at correcting the core temperature and coagulopathy, and reversing the acid–base imbalance.

> **Massive or multiple injury in the face of :**
>
> - **Hypothermia – 35oC despite attempts at warming**
> - **Acidosis pH – <7.2**
> - **Coagulopathy**

Definitive surgery is delayed for 24–48 h until resuscitation has corrected the physiological imbalance. At this stage the abdominal packs are removed, bowel continuity is restored, and the abdomen formally closed if this is possible without the development of an abdominal compartment syndrome.

Evisceration and foreign bodies or weapons *in situ*

Some institutions with vast experience of the management of penetrating injuries and evisceration have advocated that eviscerated bowel and omentum can be safely cleaned and returned to the abdomen, avoiding laparotomy. This is not a principle that should be followed in units with far less experience of these injuries, and a policy of laparotomy for injuries that penetrate the peritoneum should be adhered to.

There is no role for the removal of retained foreign bodies or weapons anywhere but in theatre at laparotomy, under direct vision and with control of potential haemorrhage or contamination.

SUMMARY

Abdominal injury presents in the emergency room in many different ways, and therefore a high index of suspicion for abdominal trauma must be maintained in all trauma patients. Prioritization issues in resuscitation, investigation and management are paramount in multiple trauma involving the abdomen and physiological factors. Surgical factors should also be taken into consideration in the management plan. Investigations should be tailored toward the individual patient, haemodynamic stability and the mechanism of injury, and more than one modality when used in conjunction may improve the accuracy of diagnosis. Recent advances include the acceptance of technology to aid in diagnosis and management, a greater understanding of the importance of physiological exhaustion, and an increased approval for non-operative strategies.

REFERENCES

1. Bickell WH, Wall MJ, Pepe PE, Martin RR, Ginger VF, Allen MK, Mattox KL. Immediate versus delayed fluid resuscitation for hypotensive patients with penetrating torso injuries. *New England Journal of Medicine* 1994; **331**: 1105–9.
2. Root HD, Hauser CW, McKinley CR, Lafave JW, Mendiola RP. Diagnostic peritoneal lavage. *Surgery* 1965; **57**: 633–7.
3. Powell DC, Bivins BA, Bell RM. Diagnostic peritoneal lavage. *Surgery, Gynecology and Obstetrics* 1982; **155**: 257–64.
4. Velmahos GC, Demetriades D, Stewart M, *et al.* Open versus closed diagnostic peritoneal lavage: a comparison on safety, rapidity, efficacy. *Journal of the Royal College of Surgeons, Edinburgh* 1998; **43**: 235–8.
5. Kristensen JK, Buemann B, Kuehl E. Ultrasonic scanning in the diagnosis of splenic haematomas. *Acta Chemica Scandinavica* 1971; **137**: 653.
6. Rozycki GS, Shackford SR. Ultrasound, what every trauma surgeon should know. *Journal of Trauma* 1996; **640**: 1–4.
7. Leppaniemi AK, Elliot DC. The role of laparoscopy in blunt abdominal trauma. *Annals of Medicine* 1996; **28**: 483–9.
8. Zantut LF, Ivatury RR, Smith S, *et al.* Diagnostic and therapeutic laparoscopy for penetrating abdominal trauma: a multicentre experience. *Journal of Trauma* 1997; **42**: 825–31.
9. Sosa JL, Sims D, Martin L, Zeppa R. Laparoscopic evaluation of tangential gunshot wounds. *Archives of Surgery* 1992; **127**: 109–10.
10. Oreskovich SR, Carrico CJ. Stab wounds to the anterior abdomen. Analysis of a management plan using local wound exploration and quantitative peritoneal lavage. *Annals of Surgery* 1983; **198**: 411–19.
11. Jurkovich GJ. Injury to the duodenum and pancreas. In: Feliciano DV, Moore EE, Mattox KL (eds), *Trauma* (3rd edn). Stamford, Conneticut: Appleton & Lange, 1996, pp. 573–94.
12. Dalal SA, Burgess AR, Siegel JH, *et al.* Pelvic fracture in multiple trauma: Classification by mechanism is the key to pattern of organ injury, resuscitative requirements and outcome. *Journal of Trauma* 1989; **29**: 98–102.
13. Carrillo EH, Platz A, Miller FB, Richardson JD, Polk HC Jr. Non-operative management of blunt hepatic trauma. *British Journal of Surgery* 1998; **85**: 461–8.
14. Sclafani SJ, Shaftan GW, Scalea TM, *et al.* Non-operative salvage of computed tomography diagnosed splenic injuries: utilization of angiography for triage and embolization for hemostasis. *Journal of Trauma* 1995; **39**: 818–27.
15. Carrillo EH, Platz A, Miller FB, Richardson JD, Polk HC Jr. Non-operative management of blunt hepatic trauma. *British Journal of Surgery* 1998; **85**: 465–8.
16. Smith JS Jr, Wengrovitz MA, Delong BS. Prospective validation of criteria, including age, for safe, non-surgical management of the ruptured spleen. *Journal of Trauma* 1992; **33**: 363–8.
17. *Surgical Clinics of North America* 1997; **77**.

18. Rotondo MF, Schwab CW, McGonigal MD, *et al*. 'Damage control': an approach for improved survival in exsanguinating penetrating abdominal injury. *Journal of Trauma* 1993; **35**: 375–83.
19. Morris JA Jr, Eddy VA, Rutherford EJ. The trauma celiotomy: the evolving concepts of damage control. *Current Problems in Surgery* 1996; **33**: 611–700.

8

Head injuries

OBJECTIVES

- To understand the pathophysiology of head injury
- To carry out/oversee the initial assessment and management of the patient with a head injury
- To monitor the initial investigations required following a head injury
- To be able to consult effectively with a neurosurgeon
- To perform the safe transfer of a head-injured patient

INTRODUCTION

Serious head injuries are most often the result of falls (40%), violence (20%) and road traffic accidents (RTAs) (13%). They are more common in males, and are not infrequently associated with consumption of alcohol. In an average year in the UK, approximately one million people will attend an Emergency Department with a head injury, and almost half of these will be aged less than 16 years. The vast majority of these patients (90%) will have only minor head injuries and can be safely discharged, but the remaining 100 000 patients will need to be admitted. Of these, 10 000 (or 1%) of all head injuries will need to be transferred to the care of a neurosurgeon. Ultimately, each year 5000 people will die in the UK of a head injury, while in 50% of all trauma deaths, a head injury will have played a significant role. The overall mortality rate from head injuries for all ages in the UK is 9 per 100 000 of the population, while 63% of moderate and 85% of severely head-injured patients remain disabled after one year. Such devastating statistics serve to emphasize the overwhelming need for all healthcare professionals who deal with trauma to be competent at managing all head-injured patients.

> **The key to successful management of patients with serious head injuries is based upon minimizing secondary brain injury**

PATHOPHYSIOLOGY OF HEAD INJURY

Following whatever cause, the injuries sustained by the brain are classically divided into primary brain injury (immediate) and secondary brain injury (delayed). The primary injury is the damage which results from the causative event, for example shearing of brain tissue following rapid deceleration in an RTA, or a violent blow to the head fracturing the skull and driving bone fragments into the brain. As clinicians, there is little we can do once this damage has been done, and such injuries can only be attenuated by appropriate legislation, such as motor-cycle helmet and seat belt laws. Secondary injury is completely different. It is the subsequent neurological injury resulting from an inadequate supply of oxygen and substrates to the brain, whatever the cause (Table 8.1). Clearly, many of these causes are amenable to prevention and treatment. In order to understand how this is best achieved it is necessary to review some fundamental physiological principles governing blood flow and oxygenation of the brain.

Table 8.1 *Causes of inadequate cerebral oxygenation (secondary brain injury)*

Systemic	Intracranial
• Hypoxia	• Haematoma
• Hypotension	• Cerebral contusion
• Hypercapnia	• Brain oedema
• Hypocapnia	• Seizures
• Anaemia	• Hyperpyrexia
	• Infection (late)

Intracranial contents

The intracranial contents consist of approximately 1300 g of brain (including interstitial fluid), 150 ml of blood (50 ml arterial, 100 ml venous) and 75 ml of cerebrospinal fluid (CSF), all held within a rigid container of fixed volume. While the volume of the brain tissue is fixed, those of the blood and CSF are variable, and this results in the relative stability of the intracranial pressure (ICP) under normal circumstances. Shifts of CSF and/or venous blood out of the cranial cavity in response to normal physiological events such as coughing, straining or changes in posture keep the ICP between 5–10 mmHg. Following a head injury, the development of a mass within the skull – for example a haematoma – will initially be compensated for in the same manner. Ultimately, the point is reached when no more CSF or blood can be displaced. As the container cannot expand, there is an acute rise in the ICP (reducing cerebral blood flow; see below) and eventually distortion and herniation of the brain tissue, often referred to as coning. A typical example of this is seen when the medial temporal lobe herniates through the tentorial hiatus and compresses the third nerve and the corticospinal tracts, causing an ipsilateral third nerve palsy and contralateral hemiplegia respectively. If unrelieved, further compression of the brainstem causes a bradycardia, hypertension and decreased respiratory rate, usually known as Cushing's response.

Cerebral blood flow

AUTOREGULATION

In the uninjured brain, cerebral blood flow (CBF) is approximately 700 ml/min, some 15% of the total cardiac output. Under normal circumstances, this is kept constant by a process termed autoregulation, in which the cerebral arterioles vasoconstrict in response to a fall in pressure and vasodilate in response to a rise in pressure. The trigger for the autoregulatory response is the cerebral perfusion pressure (CPP), the difference between mean arterial pressure (MAP) and ICP. Autoregulation functions between a CPP of approximately 50–150 mmHg, and outside this range CBF varies directly with arterial pressure. When the ICP and systemic blood pressure are both normal, the cerebral perfusion pressure is very close to the systemic mean arterial blood pressure (MAP).

CPP = MAP – ICP

Following a head injury, autoregulation is disturbed and the relationship between CBF and CPP is variable. CBF is much more dependent upon CPP, and consequently it becomes much more important to maintain or even increase CPP in order to ensure adequate cerebral perfusion. In the presence of an elevated ICP this is usually achieved initially by ensuring an adequate MAP. Clearly, either a fall in systemic blood pressure, an increase in ICP, or both, will result in a fall in CPP and thereby significantly compromise cerebral oxygenation.

CARBON DIOXIDE AND OXYGEN

The cerebral arterioles are very sensitive to the partial pressure of carbon dioxide in arterial blood ($PaCO_2$), and there is a linear relationship between vascular diameter and $PaCO_2$ over the range 2.7 to 10.7 kPa (20–80 mmHg). Although these vessels are only small, they can change their diameter by 200–300%, with a consequent change in volume of 400–900%, which in a normal brain results in an increase in CBF. Paradoxically, in an injured brain, where compensation for an extra mass is already maximal, increases in the $PaCO_2$ (hypercapnia) and subsequent vasodilatation increase ICP, reducing CPP and CBF. Conversely, a reduction in $PaCO_2$ (hypocapnia) will cause vasoconstriction, reduce ICP and may increase CPP and CBF. However, extremes of hypocapnia can cause profound vasoconstriction, compromising CBF.

The cerebral arterioles are relatively little affected by changes in the partial pressure of oxygen in arterial blood (PaO_2) until it falls below 8 kPa (60 mmHg). At this point, vasodilatation occurs in an attempt to maintain CBF and oxygenation. In the injured brain this has a similar effect to the vasodilatation induced by hypercapnia, and paradoxically may actually reduce blood flow.

> **Following serious head injury, the avoidance of hypoxia, hypercapnia and hypotension are essential in order to reduce secondary brain injury**

The devastating effect of hypoxia and hypotension on eventual outcome is clearly shown in Table 8.2. Mortality is increased three-fold when both are present in patients with head injuries on arrival at hospital. It now becomes clear why the initial management of the head-injured patient follows the same principles as for all trauma patients namely; the maintenance of a clear secure airway, ensuring adequate oxygenation and ventilation and restoration of the circulation.

Table 8.2 *Effect of hypoxia and hypotension on outcome after head injury*[1]

Secondary insults	Number of patients	% of total patients	Outcome (%)		
			Good or moderate	Severe or vegetative	Died
Neither	456	65.2	51.1	21.9	27.0
Hypoxia	78	11.2	44.9	21.8	33.3
Hypotension	113	16.2	25.7	14.1	60.2
Both	52	7.4	5.8	19.2	75.0
Total cases	699	100.0	42.9	20.5	36.6

INITIAL ASSESSMENT AND MANAGEMENT OF PATIENTS WITH SEVERE HEAD INJURIES

This comprises two main objectives:

1. Prevention of hypoxia, hypotension and hypercapnia.
2. Identification of those patients with a surgically treatable intracranial haematoma.

These are achieved by following the ABC principles used for all trauma patients.[2] An initial assessment or 'primary survey' is performed, with the aim of identifying and treating immediately life-threatening injuries as they are found. This is followed by a secondary survey. Obvious head injuries may at first appear to be ignored as problems with the airway, breathing and circulation take priority. However, adopting these principles will also ensure that factors playing a significant role in the development of secondary brain injury (outlined above) are eliminated.

Airway with control of the cervical spine

Initially, this may be achieved by basic manoeuvres supplemented with simple adjuncts such as an oropharyngeal airway and oxygen via a facemask with a reservoir. Early tracheal intubation is indicated in the comatose patient (Glasgow Coma Score < 9) or where there is loss of the laryngeal reflexes. Once they are intubated, these patients must not be allowed to breathe spontaneously. Manual, or preferably mechanical, ventilation should be commenced (see below).

Tracheal intubation is more difficult and hazardous in a patient with a head injury for a number of reasons:

- Immobilization of the cervical spine prevents optimal positioning to facilitate intubation by preventing neck flexion and head extension (see below).
- Facial trauma may cause swelling, and bleeding making laryngoscopy more difficult.
- Tracheal intubation is very stimulating, causing hypertension and a rise in ICP.
- Coughing or gagging during or after intubation causes dramatic rises in ICP.
- There is the risk of regurgitation and aspiration.

To achieve intubation safely and effectively, help from an anaesthetist or doctor with appropriate training in anaesthesia should be requested urgently in all patients with severe head injuries. The most commonly used technique is to administer an intravenous anaesthetic agent, such as thiopentone, etomidate or propofol, followed by suxamethonium, a rapidly-acting muscle relaxant. The risk of aspiration is minimized by one assistant applying cricoid pressure and another applying in-line stabilization (see below).[3] This combination is often referred to as rapid sequence induction (RSI). A small dose of a potent analgesic (e.g. fentanyl) may also be given intravenously, to attenuate the hypertensive response to laryngoscopy and intubation.[4,5] Familiarity with intravenous anaesthetic agents is essential, as they can all cause profound hypotension, compromising cerebral perfusion. Furthermore, once a muscle relaxant has been administered the patient is totally dependent on the anaesthetist to provide ventilation. If this fails and intubation cannot be achieved, it will be necessary to create a surgical airway to allow oxygenation.

Whatever techniques are used to maintain the airway, care must be taken to protect the cervical spine as there is an increased risk of injury in a patient with a severe head injury.[2,6] During the initial assessment, and particularly when the airway is compromised, there will not be time to assess the cervical spine. It is therefore safer to assume that it is injured until proved otherwise, and it must be protected using a semi-rigid collar, sandbags and tapes.[7] However, this significantly impedes tracheal intubation and therefore during intubation the collar, sandbags and tape must be replaced with manual in-line stabilization.[8,9] Once the airway is secure, the above can be re-applied.

> **The most important factors are the maintenance of a clear and secure airway and administration of a high concentration of oxygen**

Breathing and ventilation

Because of the importance of avoiding hypoxia and hypercapnia in this group of patients, the need to monitor the adequacy of oxygenation and ventilation is a priority. This is best achieved by arterial blood gas analysis. Pulse oximetry is often unreliable during the initial assessment (due to factors such as poor peripheral circulation, extraneous light and patient movement), and provides no information about adequacy of ventilation. The identification of either hypoxia or hypercapnia is an indication for intubation and controlled ventilation. Additional indications for instituting ventilation in a patient with head injuries are well established and are listed in Table 8.3. Once again, anaesthetic help should be sought early. In addition, sedation and muscle relaxation will need to be maintained to allow effective ventilation. This is usually achieved either by intermittent boluses of a hypnotic (e.g. midazolam) or an infusion of an intravenous anaesthetic agent (e.g. propofol) along with a long-acting muscle relaxant (e.g. atracurium or vecuronium) and an analgesic. The latter is particularly important if there are associated injuries.

Although hypocapnia due to deliberate hyperventilation will cause vasoconstriction of the cerebral arterioles and reduce ICP, if used to excess, this may compromise cerebral perfusion.[10] Initially ventilation should be adjusted to achieve a $PaCO_2$ of 4.5 kPa. Any attempt to reduce ICP further by a greater reduction in $PaCO_2$ should only be made after consultation with a neurosurgeon.

Table 8.3 *Indications for urgent intubation and ventilation in head-injured patients*[11]

- Coma (GCS <9)
- Loss of protective laryngeal reflexes
- Ventilatory insufficiency
  Hypoxaemia: PaO_2 <9 kPa breathing air
   PaO_2 <13 kPa breathing oxygen
  Hypercapnia: $PaCO_2$ >6 kPa
- Spontaneous hyperventilation causing $PaCO_2$ <3.5 kPa
- Irregular breathing

Circulation and control of haemorrhage

It is essential to maintain an adequate systemic blood pressure (strictly the MAP) in head-injured patients because of the deleterious effects of hypotension (see above). Adequacy of volume is more important than the type of fluid administered. In the presence of hypotension, an initial bolus of 1–2 l of warmed Hartmann's solution or normal saline should be given. Further fluid requirements, including blood, will be dictated by the patient's response. There is no place for the use of glucose-containing solutions or restriction of fluids in head-injured patients (see below). Apart from in children, scalp lacerations rarely bleed sufficiently to cause hypovolaemia. Other sources such as chest, abdomen, pelvic and long-bone fractures should be sought. Once identified, rapid measures should be taken to control the haemorrhage. This will take preference over surgical management of the head injury (see below).

Hypertension is not uncommon in patients with an isolated head injury, and usually indicates compression of the brainstem, particularly if associated with a bradycardia. Urgent measures should be instituted to try and reduce the ICP. This may involve hyperventilation, the use of mannitol, or urgent surgical decompression. The hypertension must *not* be treated, as it is simply a reflection of the brain trying to maintain perfusion in the face of a rising ICP.

DIURETICS

In a patient with an isolated head injury and signs of raised ICP, neurosurgeons may request that mannitol (or frusemide) is administered in an attempt to reduce ICP and 'buy time' during transfer. In addition to the effects on the brain, there will also be a significant diuresis, depleting the circulating volume and causing hypotension. Such fluid losses must be replaced in order to prevent inappropriate hypotension. In the multiply injured patient, resuscitation of the circulation and MAP is more effective in maintaining cerebral perfusion than administering mannitol to reduce ICP.

Disability or neurological assessment

This is performed only when any problems with the airway, breathing and circulation have been identified and corrected and consists of:

- assessment of the conscious level;
- assessment of the pupils; and
- identification of focal or lateralizing neurological signs.

The aim is to try and identify those patients with an intracranial lesion, usually a haematoma, which is surgically treatable.

CONSCIOUS LEVEL

In the primary survey, the AVPU system is used to assess conscious level:

Alert
Responds to **V**oice
Responds to **P**ain
Unresponsive

In the secondary survey it is assessed using the Glasgow Coma Scale (GCS) (Table 8.4).[12] The patient's eye-opening, best verbal and best motor responses are graded using an unambiguous description of their response. A numerical score can also be assigned to each response, the sum of which gives the GCS score. This is generally felt to be less useful when communicating a patient's condition than the description of responses. Coma is defined as no eye-opening, no verbalization and not obeying commands (GCS <9). Although an impression of the patient's conscious level can often be made early on during resuscitation, any hypoxia, hypercapnia or hypotension will contribute to a reduction in the patient's level of consciousness. Therefore, an accurate assessment can only be made once these have been corrected. The initial GCS must always be documented, and it should be repeated every 10 min to establish the trend. Hypothermia and a variety of biochemical disturbances (particularly hypo/hyperglycaemia) may also contribute to, or be the cause of, a reduced level of consciousness and must always be considered. Although there is also a strong association between head injuries and the use of alcohol or drugs, it is essential that they are never assumed to be the cause of a patient's reduced level of consciousness.

Table 8.4 *The Glasgow Coma Scale and score in adults*

Response	Score
Eye-opening	
• Spontaneously	4
• To speech	3
• To pain	2
• None	1
Best verbal response (adult)	
• Orientated	5
• Confused	4
• Inappropriate words	3
• Incomprehensible sounds	2
• None	1
Best motor response	
• Obeys commands	6
• Localizes to a painful stimulus	5
• Withdraws from a painful stimulus	4
• Abnormal (spastic) flexion	3
• Extension	2
• None	1

Always check a BMstix® in the unconscious head-injured patient

---

A modified scale for best verbal response is used in young children less than 4 years of age to allow for their limited comprehension of speech and language development:

• Smiles and follows, interacts   5
• Cries consolably, inappropriate interactions   4
• Cries occasionally consolably, moaning sounds   3
• Irritable, inconsolable   2
• No response   1

When assessing the GCS, there are a number of pitfalls to avoid:

1. Eyes closed by swelling does not automatically mean 'no eye-opening'. Record that the assessment cannot be made.

2. Intubated does not mean 'no verbal response'. Record that the patient is intubated.
3. If the patient is unable to obey commands, a painful stimulus must be applied to establish the motor response. The best site is the supraorbital nerve. A painful stimulus to the lower limbs may evoke a false flexion response from a spinal reflex, while pain applied to the upper limb may evoke no response in the presence of an undiagnosed injury to the cervical spinal cord.
4. In determining the patient's response to such a painful stimulus, a hand must reach above the level of the clavicle to merit 'localizes to a painful stimulus'. Less than this is 'withdraws from a painful stimulus'.
5. Remember that injuries to limbs and the application of splints may hinder the response. If there is a true difference between left and right, record the best response, but be aware of the significance of the difference in response (see below).

The patient's conscious level gives an indication of cerebral function, and any deterioration suggests increasing impairment. This may be due to a global effect, for example the development of cerebral oedema, or a local effect such as an expanding intracranial lesion. The latter is strongly suggested when there are accompanying pupillary abnormalities and focal neurological signs

ASSESSMENT OF THE PUPILS

The pupils are examined for their symmetry of size and reaction to light. Asymmetry of more than 1 mm, with a sluggish reaction or no reaction to light, is highly suggestive of the presence of an expanding intracranial haematoma requiring urgent surgical intervention. If allowed to progress, there will also be deterioration in the patient's level of consciousness. Direct trauma to the eye may also cause similar abnormalities, but the pupil is usually irregular in shape and there is usually adjacent soft tissue injury.

FOCAL OR LATERALIZING NEUROLOGICAL SIGNS

A unilateral motor deficit, usually identified when determining the patient's best motor response, is also highly suggestive of an expanding intracranial lesion. The weakness is classically on the opposite side to the lesion (and abnormal pupil), and is caused by compression of the corticospinal tracts proximal to their decussation. There may be an accompanying sensory disturbance. Occasionally, isolated cranial nerve palsies may be seen, but these are usually detected during the secondary survey.

Exposure and environment

As with any trauma patient, all clothing must be removed to ensure that no other injuries have been missed. Patients must be 'log-rolled' into the lateral position to allow examination of their back. There is no proven benefit in allowing head-injured patients to become hypothermic, and the adverse effects on cardiac function, oxygen dissociation curve and coagulation may be deleterious. Occasionally, a head-injured patient may become hyperthermic; under these circumstances, efforts should be made to actively reduce body temperature to within normal limits.

External head injuries

These need careful evaluation as they may indicate more serious internal cranial injuries. However, they are not usually managed until the secondary survey.

SCALP LACERATIONS

These can cause significant haemorrhage, although it is unusual for adult patients to become hypovolaemic from scalp wounds. These wounds require careful toilet and suturing.

OPEN AND DEPRESSED SKULL FRACTURES

These injuries require careful assessment. Open fractures are, by definition, ones that are associated with a defect in the overlying skin, and they may be associated with penetration of the dura. Depressed skull fractures are associated with injury to the underlying brain; they need early neurosurgical referral.

BASE OF SKULL FRACTURES

The clinical signs associated with a base of skull fracture are:

- CSF ottorrhoea and rhinorrhoea;
- bruising around the mastoid process (Battle's sign);
- periorbital buising; and
- haemotympanum.

Battle's sign in particular may not be apparent for 24 h. A CSF leak implies that the dura is breached, and a neurosurgical opinion should be sought in such patients.

Prophylactic antibiotics should only be given to those patients with compound depressed skull fractures in order to reduce the risk of subsequent meningitis and abscess formation.[13] The routine administration of antibiotics is not of proven value in a base of skull fracture,[14] even in the presence of a post-traumatic CSF leak.[15] Similarly, prophylactic anticonvulsants are not given routinely to head-injured patients, even those who have a single post-traumatic seizure from which they make a rapid complete recovery. If a patient has a second or prolonged seizure, then anticonvulsants are usually administered.[13] However, if there is any doubt about their use, then the advice of a neurosurgeon must be sought.

Fluid resuscitation in head-injured patients

In the past it has been advocated that a degree of fluid restriction is acceptable in those patients with isolated head injuries in order to minimize the risk of cerebral oedema.[16] However, the importance of adequate resuscitation of the circulation and prevention of hypotension is now well established. The question now frequently asked is, which fluid is most appropriate to administer during resuscitation of patients with head injuries?[17] To answer this it is important to remember that in the brain, the plasma osmotic pressure (or plasma osmolality) controls movement of water between the vascular space and the interstitium. Of those substances within plasma that generate the osmotic pressure, sodium is the most important. Compare this to the tissues in the rest of the body, where colloid osmotic pressure is the main determinant of movement of water between the vascular space and the interstitial space.

> **In head-injured patients, maintenance of the plasma osmotic pressure is the most important determinant of the fluid used**

HYPOTONIC SOLUTIONS

Examples include 5% dextrose and 4% dextrose plus 0.18% saline. The administration of these solutions will result in dilution of the plasma electrolytes, particularly sodium, lowering the plasma osmolality. This will result in movement of water into the brain, causing swelling or worsening oedema. Furthermore, the use of dextrose-containing solutions may result in hyperglycaemia, which has been associated with a worse neurological outcome.[18,19] Consequently, they should not be administered to head-injured patients.

ISOTONIC SOLUTIONS

Examples include Hartmann's solution, lactated Ringer's and 0.9% (normal) saline. These are the most widely used solutions for resuscitation. They contain concentrations of electrolytes which have approximately the same osmolality as plasma, and therefore cause no net movement of water into the brain. Thus, they are the solutions of choice in head-injured patients. Strictly speaking, Hartmann's solution is very slightly hypotonic and if administered in large volumes the plasma osmolality will fall slightly compared with the use of similar volumes of 0.9% saline.

HYPERTONIC SOLUTIONS

Examples include 10–20% mannitol and 3–7.5% saline. The administration of these solutions will cause a rise in the plasma osmolality and result in the movement of water from the brain into the vascular space, effectively reducing total brain volume. It is this effect which is utilized when mannitol is administered to those patients with acutely raised ICP. However, the diuretic effect may result in a degree of hypovolaemia and hypotension, and it is essential to maintain an adequate circulating volume with the administration of an isotonic solution. Hypertonic saline will have a similar effect, reducing cerebral water and ICP. In addition, it also transiently increases plasma volume and blood pressure by the same effect, even when administered in relatively small volumes (250 ml). It is currently being evaluated for use in the resuscitation of multiply injured patients, particularly those with head injuries.[20]

COLLOIDS

Examples include Gelofusine, Haemaccel and starches. These are suspensions of large molecules, usually in 0.9% saline. They therefore maintain plasma osmolality and can be used in patients with head injuries, but do not offer any advantage over crystalloids alone in an isolated head injury.

Laparotomy or craniotomy?

One group of patients which presents a major management dilemma are those who have sustained both a head injury and blunt trauma to the abdomen, and are hypotensive despite resuscitation. It is clearly important to decide which problem takes priority, as both are associated with significant morbidity and mortality. Unfortunately, a reduced level of consciousness will make clinical evaluation of the abdomen unreliable, while neither a reduced GCS nor neurological examination will reliably identify the presence of a surgically treatable haematoma. It has been shown, however, that in these patients, the need for urgent laparotomy to control haemorrhage is approximately eight times that of craniotomy for an intracranial haematoma.[21] Although it is tempting to argue that a computed tomography (CT) scan can quickly be undertaken to exclude a surgical remediable lesion before laparotomy, in most hospitals it is the associated transfers to and from the CT scanner which take up the time. During this time, any persisting haemorrhage may render the patient hypotensive, and thereby contribute to further secondary brain injury. In such patients, laparotomy takes precedence over craniotomy, but it is essential that intraoperatively, close monitoring of vital signs and pupillary reaction are maintained in order to identify any acute deterioration in neurological condition. In these circumstances, once haemorrhage has been controlled consideration must be given to urgent CT scanning of the head.

Head-injured patients with blunt abdominal trauma who have been resuscitated and are haemodynamically stable, should have an ultrasound scan of the abdomen performed in the Emergency Department. When combined with a scoring system to estimate the severity of intra-abdominal haemorrhage, this appears to be a sensitive indicator of the urgency of laparotomy or safety to proceed to CT scanning of the head.[22] If ultrasound scanning is not available, then diagnostic peritoneal lavage is a valid alternative that has been shown to be more reliable than the use of vital signs alone.[23] Although very sensitive, the main disadvantage of this technique is that it is not very specific, leading to a relative excess of unnecessary laparotomies.

In those patients who have both head and abdominal injuries but have been haemodynamically stable throughout and have no focal neurological signs, where the facilities are available, a CT scan of the head and abdomen can be performed sequentially.

INITIAL INVESTIGATIONS REQUIRED FOLLOWING A HEAD INJURY

After the initial assessment and resuscitation of the head-injured patient it is important to decide who needs:

- an immediate neurosurgical referral;
- a CT scan;
- subsequent neurosurgical referral;
- a skull X-ray; and/or
- admission for observation.

The following guidelines are based upon the Report of the Working Party of the Royal College of Surgeons of England.[24]

Immediate neurosurgical referral

Patients in this group are those in whom there is the actual or potential need for neurosurgical intervention, or where appropriate investigation (usually a CT scan) cannot be performed in a reasonable time in the initial receiving hospital. Although termed an immediate referral, it takes place after the initial assessment and resuscitation of the patient and, as most District General Hospitals now have access to a CT scanner, after a scan of the head has been performed. However severe the head injury, a CT scan will be required to allow a management plan to be formulated. Ideally, the referral should be accompanied by transfer of the CT images to the neurosurgeon via an image link. It should be remembered that referral does not automatically imply transfer. Some patients will have sustained injuries which are unsurvivable, and transfer of such patients to a neurosciences unit is inappropriate.

Patients of any age in the following categories should be referred:

- Coma (GCS <9) persisting after resuscitation.
- Deteriorating level of consciousness or progressive focal neurological deficit.
- Skull fracture with any of the following:
  - confusion or deteriorating level of consciousness
  - fits
  - neurological symptoms or signs.
- Open head injury:
  - depressed compound fracture of skull vault
  - base of skull fracture
  - penetrating injury.
- Any patient who fulfills the criteria for a CT scan of the head (see below), but this cannot be performed in the referring hospital within 2–4 h.

Indications for a head CT scan before referral to the neurosurgeon

A head CT scan should be performed urgently (within 2–4 h) on patients of all ages with any of the following criteria:

- fully conscious but with a skull fracture;
- fits without a skull fracture;
- confusion or neurological symptoms and/or signs persisting after assessment and resuscitation;
- uncertain or difficult diagnosis, e.g. alcohol, drug intoxication;
- significant head injury in a haemodynamically stable patient requiring general anaesthesia; or
- tense fontanelle or suture diastasis in a child.

After the CT scan has been performed, if an abnormality is found to be present then a neurosurgical opinion should invariably be sought, preferably with the transfer of the CT images electronically to the neurosurgeon. Even if the CT scan is normal, when a patient does not respond as anticipated, fails to make satisfactory progress or deteriorates neurologically, they should be referred as further investigations such as angiography may be required to eliminate vascular injury such as dissection of the internal carotid artery as a cause of brain injury.

In the past, large doses of steroids have been administered to head-injured patients on the basis of results from *in-vivo* investigations. These findings have not been substantiated in clinical trials. There is, however, a renewed interest in this subject, and an international multicentre trial (CRASH) is currently being conducted to assess the effects of high-dose steroids in patients with head injuries.

Indications for skull X-radiography

Although skull fractures are relatively uncommon in patients with a head injury (approximately 5%), they are a significant finding as they increase the risk of an intracranial haematoma (see Table 8.5). A skull X-ray should be performed on head-injured patients with:

- a history of amnesia or loss of consciousness;
- an altered level of consciousness at hospital;
- focal neurological signs;
- difficulty in assessment: alcohol, drug intoxication;
- marked bruising of the scalp or a laceration down to bone or longer than 5 cm;
- a penetrating skull injury;
- CSF or blood loss from the nose or ear;
- A mechanism of injury resulting from:
  - high velocity, e.g. fall from a height, RTA
  - assault with a weapon.

In children, the above recommendations should be extended to include:

- fall from greater than twice the child's own height;
- a fall onto a hard surface; and
- suspected non-accidental injury.

Clearly, those patients who on clinical grounds merit a CT scan will not also require a skull X-ray.

Table 8.5 *Relative risk of an intracranial haematoma in head-injured patients with a skull fracture*[25]

	Risk of haematoma in the Emergency Department
No skull fracture	
• Orientated	1:5983
• Not orientated	1:121
Skull fracture	
• Orientated	1:32
• Not orientated	1:4

Care of the head-injured patient not requiring transfer to a neurosurgical unit

All patients who have sustained a head injury must undergo a full initial assessment, resuscitation as necessary and then have a secondary survey. Patients with any of the following signs or symptoms must be admitted for a period of observation:

- an impaired level of consciousness, including confusion;
- persisting neurological signs or symptoms;
- skull fracture or sutural diastasis;

- difficulty in assessment, e.g. alcohol or drug intoxication, epilepsy, altered mental state;
- lack of a responsible adult to supervise the patient if discharged;
- suspected non-accidental injury; and/or
- a history of coagulopathy or therapeutic use of anticoagulants.

Local agreements will dictate the care of patients whose signs or symptoms persist. After admission, any patient whose confusion, neurological signs or symptoms, CSF leak, headache or vomiting persist, should be considered for referral to the neurosurgeons, and will probably need to undergo a CT scan.

Patients who can be discharged

Although this is by far the greatest number of patients with head injuries, all of the following criteria must be fulfilled:

1. Normal conscious level (GCS 15).
2. Normal neurological examination.
3. No evidence of a skull fracture clinically or radiologically.
4. Presence of a responsible adult at home or at the place discharged to.

It is essential that clear verbal and written instructions are provided, both to the patient and the carer, detailing the indications for return to hospital.

HOW TO CONSULT EFFECTIVELY WITH THE NEUROSURGEON

One of the major pitfalls when referring head-injured patients to neurosurgeons is the failure by the referring team to convey an adequate amount of information. Although the patient may require the specialist services of the neurosurgeon, it is essential that the full picture is presented. This will then allow the neurosurgeon to decide on the relative importance of the head injury, and to ensure that there are adequate local facilities for dealing with any associated problems. The receiving neurosurgeon will require the following information at the time of referral:

- Patient details – name, age, sex.
- History of injury – time, mechanism.
- Initial neurological status – witnesses, paramedics' assessment of GCS.
- Significant changes in neurological status during transfer to hospital.
- Initial assessment on arrival at hospital:
  - airway and cervical spine
  - breathing/ventilation
  - circulatory status
  - neurological status
  - obvious neurological injuries
  - other injuries.
- Treatment administered and response:
  - need for intubation and ventilation, adequacy of oxygenation
  - volume of fluid/blood administered, pulse and blood pressure, CVP
  - drugs administered
  - improvement/deterioration in neurological status, GCS, pupils, lateralizing signs
  - management of associated injuries.
- Results of any other investigations:
  - haematology, biochemistry, arterial blood gases
  - X-rays
  - CT scan.
- Past medical history of note.

When using the GCS, it should be broken down into its three components rather than a single number be given. A description of the patient's best responses is perfectly acceptable if the numbered values cannot be remembered, and this will also convey to the neurosurgeon that a proper assessment has been made. Having this information immediately to hand is an essential part of a good referral, and will facilitate the neurosurgeon's assessment of the urgency of transfer.

SAFE TRANSFER OF PATIENTS WITH HEAD INJURIES

Each year, approximately 10 000 patients are transferred between Intensive Care Units in the UK.[11] Patients with head injuries account for 55% of these patients,[26] and this number is certainly higher if patients who are transferred directly from the Emergency Department are also considered.

Transferring patients with head injuries and other injuries between different departments of the same hospital, or between hospitals, is a hazardous process and is often associated with the deterioration of patients.[27-30] There are two types of transfer:

1. Patients with head injuries presenting to the Emergency Departments of district hospitals who need to be transferred for neurosurgical treatment; this is termed 'inter-hospital transfer'.
2. Patients may also be transferred within the primary receiving hospital, from the Emergency Department to the CT scanner, to operating theatres or to the Intensive Care Unit; these are called 'intra-hospital transfers'.

During either type of transfer the patient's condition may deteriorate, most commonly as a result of:

- hypoxia as a result of a poorly managed airway; and/or
- hypotension as a result of haemorrhage from overlooked or inadequately managed extracranial injuries.

Other problems include: (i) inadequate monitoring during transfer; (ii) inappropriate medical escorts during transfer; and (iii) poor communication between transferring and receiving hospitals, and between hospital departments.

Inter-hospital transfer

Recognition of the problems of transporting patients with serious head injuries to neurosurgical centres has led to the establishment of guidelines for the inter-hospital transfer of such patients,[11,31] and these are summarized in the following section:

THE NEED FOR COMMUNICATION

Details of communication incorporate three main points:

1. There should be designated consultants at both the referring hospital and the receiving hospital who are responsible for the transfer of patients with head injuries.
2. Local guidelines should be drawn up to establish which patients need urgent transfer, and for the care of patients being transferred.
3. All notes, laboratory investigations, X-rays and CT scans should accompany the patient to the receiving hospital, together with a comprehensive summary of treatment carried out before transfer.

THE NEED FOR ADEQUATE RESUSCITATION AND STABILIZATION BEFORE TRANSFER

The following requirements should be adhered to:

1. All patients should be fully resuscitated.
2. All patients with altered levels of consciousness must be intubated and ventilated.
3. Once intubated and ventilated, patients should be appropriately sedated and paralysed.

4. Adequate fluid resuscitation must be carried out.
5. Any surgical causes of haemorrhage should be corrected before transfer; in some cases this may involve surgery at the base hospital before transfer.

THE NEED FOR APPROPRIATE MONITORING DURING TRANSFER

The following monitors are recommended as essentials during transfer:

- ECG
- Invasive blood pressure
- Non-invasive blood pressure as a back-up
- Pulse oximetry
- Capnography.

Also suggested, depending on the clinical condition are:

- central venous pressure monitoring;
- temperature monitoring; and
- peripheral nerve stimulation to assess efficacy of the paralysing agents used.

THE NEED FOR APPROPRIATELY TRAINED STAFF TO TRANSFER THE PATIENT

The following points relating to staff experience/training should be adhered to:

1. When patients are intubated they should be accompanied by an anaesthetist of at least 2 years' experience who has had training in the transfer of head-injured patients.
2. Doctors from specialties other than anaesthetics may also transfer patients, but they must have undergone appropriate training.
3. An appropriately trained operating department assistant/practitioner or nurse should also accompany the patient, to assist the doctor during the transfer.
4. Personnel involved in transferring patients should have adequate medical indemnity insurance, either personal or provided by their hospital, when they are transferring patients.

Transferring patients with head injuries is therefore a highly specialized process. It can be very time-consuming, requiring stabilization of the patient, the establishment of monitoring, and assembly of the transfer team. It is however vital to remember that prompt neurosurgical treatment is life-saving in patients with head injuries, and too long a delay to get the transfer 'sorted out' may be detrimental. The report by the Royal College of Surgeons[24] suggests that patients requiring emergency decompressive surgery should have their operation within 4 h of the time of injury. Ideally, the protocols, equipment and personnel for performing transfer of head injuries should be organized and defined by the Emergency Department, so that as soon as a patient requiring transfer arrives, the process can be set in motion to facilitate rapid transfer.

Intra-hospital transfer

The requirements defined above for inter-hospital transfer of patients also apply to transferring patients between departments within the same hospital. Moving patients on trolleys along corridors and into remote areas such as X-ray departments and CT scan rooms can all be fraught with hazard. Lines and tubes can easily become disconnected, and careful monitoring is essential to ensure that patients remain stable.

SUMMARY

Head injury is common in United Kingdom practice and is associated with preventable deaths and disability. The most important features of management are prevention of hypoxia, hypercapnia and hypotension. Accurate assessment and early consultation with the neurosurgeon are also key elements in effective management.

REFERENCES

1. Chestnut RM, Marshall LF, Klauber MR, Blunt BA, Baldwin N, Eisenberg HM, Jane JA, Marmarou A, Foulkes MA. The role of secondary brain injury in determining outcome from severe head injury. *Journal of Trauma* 1993; **34**: 216–22.
2. The American College of Surgeons Committee on Trauma. *Advanced Trauma Life Support Program for Physicians: Instructor Manual*. Chicago: American College of Surgeons, 1997.
3. Criswell JC, Parr MJA, Nolan JP. Emergency airway management in patients with cervical spine injury. *Anaesthesia* 1994; **49**: 900–3.
4. Cork RC, Weiss JC, Hameroff SR, Bentley J. Fentanyl preloading for rapid sequence induction of anesthesia. *Anesthesia and Analgesia* 1984; **63**: 60–4.
5. Donegan MF, Bedford RF. Intravenous administration of lidocaine prevents intracranial hypertension during endotracheal suctioning. *Anesthesiology* 1980; **52**: 516–18.
6. Hills MW, Deane SA. Head injury and facial injury: is there an increased risk of cervical spine injury? *Journal of Trauma* 1993; **34**: 549–53.
7. Podolsky S, Baraff LJ, Simon RR, Hoffman JR, Larmon B, Ablon W. Efficacy of cervical spine immobilisation methods. *Journal of Trauma* 1983; **23**: 461–5.
8. Holley J, Jorden R. Airway management in patients with unstable cervical spine fractures. *Annals of Emergency Medicine* 1989; **18**: 1237–9.
9. Heath KJ. The effect on laryngoscopy of different cervical spine immobilization techniques. *Anaesthesia* 1994; **49**: 843–5.
10. Marion DW, Firlik A, McLaughlin MR. Hyperventilation therapy for severe traumatic brain injury. *New Horizons* 1995; **3**: 439–47.
11. Gentleman D, Deaden M, Midgley S, Maclean D. Guidelines for resuscitation and transfer of patients with serious head injury. *British Medical Journal* 1993; **307**: 547–52.
12. Teasdale G, Jennett B. Assessment of coma and impaired consciousness. *Lancet* 1974; **ii**: 81–4.
13. Dunn LT, Foy PM. Anticonvulsant and antibiotic prophylaxis in head injury. *Annals of the Royal College of Surgeons of England* 1994; **76**: 353–4.
14. Villalobos T, Arango C, Kubilis P, Rathmore M. Antibiotic prophylaxis after basilar skull fractures: a meta analysis. *Clinical and Infectious Diseases* 1998; **27**: 264–9.
15. Choi D, Spann R. Traumatic cerebrospinal fluid leakage: risk factors and the use of prophylactic antibiotics. *British Journal of Neurosurgery* 1996; **10**: 571–5.
16. Shenkin HA, Bezier HS, Bouzarth WF. Restricted fluid intake: rational management of the neurosurgical patient. *Journal of Neurosurgery* 1976; **45**: 432–6.
17. Zornow MH, Prough DS. Fluid management in patients with traumatic brain injury. *New Horizons* 1995; **3**: 488–98.
18. Lanier WL, Stangland KJ, Scheithauer BW, Milde JH, Michenfelder JD. The effects of dextrose infusion and head position on neurologic outcome after complete cerebral ischemia in primates: examination of a model. *Anesthesiology* 1987; **66**: 39–48.
19. Lam AM, Winn HR, Cullen BF. Hyperglycaemia and neurological outcome in patients with head injuries. *Journal of Neurosurgery* 1991; **75**: 545–51.
20. Wade CE, Kramer GC, Grady JJ, Fabian TC, Younes N. Efficacy of hypertonic 7.5% saline and 6% dextran-70 in treating trauma: a meta-analysis of controlled clinical studies. *Surgery* 1997; **122**: 609–16.
21. Thomason M, Mesick J, Rutledge R, *et al.* Head CT scanning versus urgent exploration in the hypotensive blunt trauma patient. *Journal of Trauma* 1993; **34**: 40–4.
22. Huang M-S, Shih H-C, Wu J-K, *et al.* Urgent laparotomy versus emergency craniotomy for multiple trauma with head injury patients. *Journal of Trauma* 1995; **38**: 154–7.
23. Prall JA, Nichols JS, Brennan R, Moore EE. Early definitive abdominal evaluation in the triage of unconscious normotensive blunt trauma patients. *Journal of Trauma* 1994; **37**: 792–7.
24. *Report of the Working Party on the Management of Patients with Head Injuries*. London: The Royal College of Surgeons of England, 1999.
25. Teasdale GM, Murray G, Anderson E, Mendelow DA, MacMillan R, Jennett B, Brookes M. Risk of traumatic intracranial haematoma in children and adults, implications for managing head injuries. *British Medical Journal* 1990; **300**: 363–7.
26. Mackenzie PA, Smith EA, Wallace PGM. Transfer of adults between intensive care units in the United Kingdom: postal survey. *British Medical Journal* 1997; **314**. 1455–6.

27. Rose J, Valtonen S, Jennett B. Avoidable factors contributing to death after head injury. *British Medical Journal*; **ii**: 615–18.
28. Gentleman D, Jennett B. Hazards of inter-hospital transfer of comatosed head-injured patients. *Lancet* 1981; **ii**: 853–5.
29. Gentleman D, Jennett B. Audit of transfer of unconscious head-injured patients to a neurosurgical unit. *Lancet* 1990; **335**: 330–4.
30. Lambert SM, Willett K. Transfer of multiply-injured patients for neurosurgical opinion: a study of the adequacy of assessment and resuscitation. *Injury* 1993; **24**: 333–6.
31. The Neuroanaesthesia Society of Great Britain and Ireland and The Association of Anaesthetists of Great Britain and Ireland. *Recommendations for the Transfer of Patients with Acute Head Injuries to Neurosurgical Units*. London: The Association of Anaesthetists of Great Britain and Ireland, 1996.

9

Musculoskeletal trauma

OBJECTIVES

- To understand who is at risk of musculoskeletal trauma
- To identify the risks to life, limb and function
- To detail the initial management of the trauma victim with musculoskeletal injuries

EPIDEMIOLOGY

Injuries to the limbs comprise by far the greatest number of trauma cases, the limbs being injured in about 85% of victims of blunt trauma. Limb injuries do not, in isolation, account for the majority of deaths, but will be present in the majority of fatalities. The majority of patients who present to Accident and Emergency Departments have a limb injury. These injuries vary across the spectrum, from the benign and seemingly trivial through to the truly life- or limb-threatening.

Limb injury, in the survivors of major trauma, is a common source of disability. These disabling injuries may often be subtle and distally situated in the limb, for instance involving the carpus, tarsus or phalanges.[1] Such injuries may present little threat to life in the early stages following trauma, but have a major impact on the casualty's eventual return to pre-injury function.

> Limb injury may be present in the majority of trauma victims, but is not the priority in terms of immediate management, as the life-threatening injuries are likely to be elsewhere
> Limb injuries will compromise return to pre-existing function if not appropriately diagnosed and treated

THREATS TO LIFE, LIMB AND FUNCTION

Trauma to the musculoskeletal system may represent a threat to life, place the limb at risk, or interfere with eventual return to full function and activity.

Life-threatening injuries

Musculoskeletal injuries to the limbs may be life-threatening by virtue of the trauma itself, for instance a major pelvic disruption or traumatic amputation of a limb. Severe, high-energy injuries may also be an indication of the severity of trauma to the body as a whole, and may hence be associated with a poor outcome, rather than being a direct cause of that poor outcome.[2–5]

A further danger lies in the fact that the severe mutilating injury to the limb may distract attention from covert, life-threatening injuries elsewhere. Care and the use of a structured system is essential in order to prevent this.

> **Do not be distracted by limb injuries, remember ABCDE.......**

Life-threatening complications arising from the limb wound itself include haemorrhage, fat embolism, venous thromboembolism and infection. Some of the complications of musculoskeletal injuries which may be life-threatening are summarized in Table 9.1.[6–8]

Table 9.1 *Life-threatening musculoskeletal trauma*

Life-threatening complication	Example of causative musculoskeletal injury
Concealed, non-compressible haemorrhage	Pelvic fracture
Obvious, compressible haemorrhage	Groin wound involving femoral artery
Concealed, compressible haemorrhage	Closed femoral shaft fracture
Venous thromboembolism	Pelvic fracture
Fat embolism syndrome	Femoral shaft fracture
Sepsis (gangrene, streptococcal sepsis, tetanus)	Contaminated wounds

Limb-threatening injuries

Some injuries may threaten the viability of a limb, or a portion of that limb. Such injuries often involve compromise of the blood supply to the limb that may arise from:

- direct vascular damage (penetrating or blunt intimal damage);
- vascular occlusion in the distorted limb (for example due to a dislocated joint or severely displaced fracture); or
- microcirculatory compromise caused by contained swelling (leading to compartment syndrome).

The limbs tolerate vascular compromise poorly, and irreversible damage to the metabolically active tissues such as muscle is likely to occur if the limb remains ischaemic for more than about 6 h. Nerves are also likely to be damaged, and the effects of muscle repair with fibrosis will lead to 'ischaemic' contracture.

Over a longer time-scale, of days to weeks, established infection may lead to tissue destruction and limb loss. Devitalized tissue, from ischaemic damage, will contribute to the risk of infection, acting as a culture medium.[9–12]

Threats to limb function

Many major injuries will, of course, threaten limb function. The limb that is skeletally unstable, has a compromised vascular supply, or has major neurological damage cannot be expected to function properly. There are, however, lesser injuries which can threaten limb function, often in quite subtle ways. Small, low-energy injuries, often situated peripherally in the limb, can bring about a major impairment to function.[1] Such injuries include:

- digital nerve injuries;
- dislocation of small (for example carpal/tarsal or phalangeal) joints;
- tendon injuries; and
- peri-articular and ligamentous injuries.

The effects of these injuries are compounded several-fold, with potentially devastating functional results, if the injuries remain unrecognized or neglected for days after the trauma.

MANAGEMENT OF THE CASUALTY WITH MUSCULOSKELETAL TRAUMA

Although limb injuries are very common, an enormous range of them exists, and the doctor to whom they are presented therefore needs a rational approach to their assessment and treatment. This includes assessment of:

- the casualty;
- the limb as a whole; and
- the traumatized structures and the extent of injury.

A thorough, rational and recorded assessment of the patient identifies, in turn, the life-, limb- and function-threatening injuries.

Identifying life-threatening injuries

The initial assessment of the casualty should proceed using the ABC system, identifying and treating life-threatening injuries as they are found. This examination identifies injuries and conditions compromising the airway, breathing and circulation. Attention should be paid to the limbs when addressing the 'C' (circulation) component. Immediately life-threatening haemorrhage may result from severe fractures to the pelvis and proximal, large long bones with either open or closed fractures.

Further major injuries to the limbs will be identified under 'E' in the structured system. The limbs are exposed and examined to identify or exclude these injuries. Life-threatening injuries in the limbs are listed in Table 9.2, together with their immediate treatment. The table also highlights features of the injuries which will be identified on examination and special investigation. More detailed examination of the limbs will be carried out in the secondary survey, looking for the injuries which might compromise the limbs' viability and function. These injuries are discussed in greater detail below.

Table 9.2 *Diagnosis and treatment of life-threatening limb injuries*

Injury	Diagnostic Features	Immediate Treatment*
Pelvic fracture	Mechanism of injury may be suggestive Lower-limb deformity Characteristic perineal/genital bruising Pain on palpation (gentle 'springing' of pelvis) X-radiogram appearances	Orthopaedic consultation (evaluation of stable versus unstable injury pattern) Temporary splintage (Mast trousers, binding feet together, pelvic wrapping) Skeletal stabilization (pelvic Ex-fix, clamp) Assessment of related injuries (visceral, rectal, urological)
Major limb haemorrhage	Open wound and frank blood loss Concealed loss with limb swelling, bruising and tension Peripheral neurovascular deficit (pulses, paraesthesia, paresis, pallor, coldness)	Direct pressure on sites of compressible haemorrhage Dressings and compression applied to wounds Splintage of limbs Alert vascular surgeons (consideration of angiography when stabilized)
Large/contaminated open wound	Obvious wound	Sterile wound dressing Splintage Antibiotics (to include penicillin or other effective cover against *Clostridium* sp.) Irrigation if appropriate Attention to tetanus immune status Alert orthopaedic surgeons
Fat embolism (usually later)	Confusion Petechiae Fat globules in urine Blood gas derangement	Oxygenation Fracture immobilization (the more rigid the better – external fixation or definitive fixation of femoral fractures) Discussion with intensivists

*Treatment is likely to include fluid resuscitation, blood replacement, monitoring (pulse, blood pressure, ECG, urinary output) in all cases.

Identifying limb- and function-threatening injuries (Table 9.3)

Identification of other injuries to the limbs takes place during the secondary survey, which requires a complete, thorough examination of the casualty to be made from top to toe.

The examination of the limbs proceeds in the same manner for all parts of the limb, following the standard pattern:[13]

- *Look*: for deformity, discoloration, wounds, swelling, shortening.
- *Feel*: for abnormal movement, crepitus, pulses, temperature, sensation.
- *Move*: assess the ranges of active and passive movement as well as joint stability.
- *X-ray* (where indicated): to include the joint above and below a suspected fracture on two views (usually orthogonal). Initial X-rays should be supplemented when indicated with other special investigations such as computed tomography (CT) scanning or magnetic resonance imaging (MRI) (in the stable patient).[14,15]

Table 9.3 *Limb injuries threatening limb viability or limb function*

Injury	Diagnosis	Management
Dislocations and fractures	Pain, deformity, abnormal movement/loss of active movement, swelling, later bruising. Confirm with X-ray	Inform orthopaedic surgeons Reduce and splint, where possible Plan stabilization, plan rehabilitation
Open fractures	Wound in association with pain, deformity, abnormal movement/loss of active movement, swelling, later bruising. Confirm with X-ray	Inform orthopaedic surgeons, cover wound with sterile dressing Reduce and splint, where possible Commence i.v. antibiotics Plan wound toilet, stabilization, and rehabilitation
Vascular injuries	Open wound and frank blood loss Concealed loss with limb swelling, bruising and tension Peripheral neurovascular deficit (pulses, paraesthesia, paresis, pallor, coldness)	Direct pressure on sites of compressible haemorrhage Dressings and compression applied to wounds Splintage of limbs Alert vascular surgeons (consideration of angiography when stabilized)
Compartment syndrome[16–19]	Pain (out of proportion to injury and/or not settling with analgesia and splintage) Loss of sensation and movement, loss/painful passive movement of distal parts, tense compartment, swelling (Loss of peripheral pulses is a late, grave sign)	Alert surgeons to need for urgent fasciotomy
Peri-articular fractures	Bruising, swelling and deformity Loss/painful movement X-rays confirm	Alert orthopaedic surgeons Reduction (where possible) and splintage
Nerve injury*	Loss of sensation or active movement	Alert orthopaedic/plastic surgeons Splintage for the injured limb
Tendon injury*	Loss of active movement Pain, swelling and bruising	Alert orthopaedic/plastic surgeons Splintage for the injured limb

*Some of these injuries are particularly difficult to diagnose in the unconscious patient.

The segments of the limb and the joints are all tested in turn. It has already been emphasized that the injuries threatening function may be very peripheral in the limb. Classic examples of this include the dislocated forefoot/midfoot (Lisfranc-type injury) in the driver who has been trapped in a vehicle, and subtle joint injuries in the hand, such as the ulnar collateral ligament injury to the metacarpophalangeal joint of the thumb in the motor-cyclist thrown over the handlebars.

The practicalities of acute trauma care are such that this secondary examination may not be completed within the first few hours of admission. Indeed, on some occasions, due for example to the need for urgent life-saving surgery, it will not be completed on the first day. It is important that the examination, however, should be carried out and fully documented as soon as possible. This must be accepted, but careful documentation will show how far examination has progressed, and it may be helpful for the team managing the patient to include records such as 'Feet swollen, but not yet formally assessed', so that the team continuing care is able to continue the survey.

> **Ensure that a complete musculoskeletal examination
> is performed and recorded**

There is considerable evidence that, particularly in high-energy polytrauma, injuries will be overlooked on the first examination; the secondary survey should therefore (at a convenient time) be repeated in its entirety, and this is particularly important in the unconscious patient, or the patient who has previously been unconscious.

SPECIFIC ASPECTS OF EARLY TREATMENT

The importance of a structured assessment of the casualty, with treatment of life-threatening injuries as they are identified, has already been stressed. This will always involve attention to the airway, breathing and circulation, with control of the spine, administration of oxygen and commencement of monitoring.

Specific musculoskeletal problems demanding early treatment include the following:

- *Pelvic fracture*: splintage is often required (external fixation may be the most appropriate provisional fixation method); orthopaedic surgeons are required as an emergency.[4,20] In open-book fractures, some initial temporary control can be achieved by compression of the pelvis by wrapping a bed sheet round it (pelvic 'wrapping').
- *Compressible haemorrhage*: direct pressure to the limb and application of splintage helps to control blood loss.
- *Limb fractures and dislocation*: early reduction and splintage reduces associated blood loss, improves the distal neurovascular condition, and reduces pain. Orthopaedic expertise will be required urgently.[21–24]
- *Open fractures and large soft tissue injuries*: splintage and the application of a sterile dressing help to reduce the ultimate infection rate.[25] Antibiotics and antitetanus prophylaxis should be commenced promptly,[26] and orthopaedic input is urgently required.[27–29]

Splintage

From the points made above it is evident that splintage plays an important part in the management of limb injuries, helping to: (i) reduce haemorrhage; (ii) prevent further tissue damage; (iii) aid analgesia;[20] and (iv) reduce the incidence of fat embolism.

Specific splints for the limbs include the Thomas splint and its variations, providing traction and splintage for fractures of the femoral shaft and more distally.[30] The Sager® splint is recommended for ease of use and because it can be used to splint both legs. Traction splints should not be used if the patient has also suffered a significant pelvic fracture.

Temporary splintage for the lower leg and the upper limb may be provided by padded wire frames (Kramer splints), pneumatic splints, box splints or plaster-of-Paris back-slabs. The key points are:

- immobilization of the limb, including the joint above and below the fractured segment;
- realignment of the limb;
- application so as not to compromise arterial supply or venous return; and
- application to allow examination and re-assessment of distal neurovascular status.

Dislocations, for example of the ankle joint or elbow, which are causing or threaten to cause distal neurovascular compromise should be reduced in the Accident and Emergency Department under analgesia and sedation as a matter of urgency. A decision regarding pre-reduction X-radiography should be taken on the grounds of clinical urgency.

Analgesia

Analgesia is important both psychologically and physiologically. Details of appropriate analgesia in trauma are discussed in Chapter 18. It is important to remember that intravenous analgesia will have a prompt effect, and can be titrated to an effective dosage in small increments. Analgesia can be considerably enhanced by the local use of anaesthetics, most markedly the use of a femoral nerve block in femoral fractures, which is effective in reducing muscle spasm and making the application of splintage very much easier and more comfortable for the patient. Splintage itself can, as mentioned above, provide effective pain relief.

Wound management

Open injuries should be covered as soon as possible with a sterile dressing. This approach has been shown to reduce the long-term morbidity of wound infection and deep sepsis/osteomyelitis. The wound should be covered with an antiseptic, such as Betadine® (povidone-iodine), and the dressing then applied. Attempts at cleaning the contaminated wound should not, in general, be made in the Accident and Emergency Department setting; thorough wound toilet is a surgical procedure and requires urgent surgical involvement.[31,32] Saline irrigation may occasionally be indicated.

It is helpful to provide a record of the wound before it is covered, and Polaroid photography can be used so that an image of the wound is available to doctors attending the patient after the wound has been dressed. It is inadvisable to remove the sterile dressing, once applied, until the patient is taken to the operating theatre for formal wound inspection and cleaning.

Antibiotics aimed at the early life-threatening infections (clostridial and streptococcal) should be commenced as soon as possible; benzyl penicillin provides such cover.[26] The addition of flucloxacillin or a similar antibiotic aimed at cover against staphylococci may also be used, as may an agent active against anaerobes such as metronidazole (Flagyl®) in faecally contaminated wounds. Local antibiotic policies may modify this approach, and should be followed; these may also provide guidance when wounds are contaminated in a particular way, such as human or animal bites. The advice of a microbiologist may be sought in cases where there is a threat from a specific contaminant, such as unusual animal bites or wounds sustained in a marine or riverine environment.

> **Photograph significant wounds, then apply a sterile dressing**

Antitetanus prophylaxis is important and can be life-saving. The patient's immune status (based on their time of last immunization) should be established; where it cannot be established, the patient should be assumed not to be covered. Immunoglobulin is administered to those requiring a boost, but in particularly contaminated wounds or non-immune individuals the use of antitetanus serum should be considered. Expert advice from the local clinical bacteriologist should be sought.

ALERTING OTHERS

It will be apparent from the treatment considerations outlined in this chapter, that specialist input from other surgeons is often required at an early stage in the management of the patient with limb trauma. It is helpful to have a structured approach to this communication. The following points may be helpful:

- Patient age, sex (name later)
- Mechanism of injury
- ABC criteria, spine clearance status
- Injured limb
  - Open or closed injury?
  - Which bone, which part of the bone (proximal, diaphyseal, distal, intra-articular)
  - Joint injury
  - Associated injuries identified (neurovascular status)
  - Compartment syndrome suspected?
- Treatment so far (reduction, splintage, antibiotics, dressings)
  - Investigations so far
- Other teams involved (vascular surgeons, general surgeons, etc.)
- Where the patient is now!

MANAGEMENT OF TRAUMATICALLY AMPUTATED PARTS

The technical feasibility of re-planting traumatically amputated parts can allow excellent functional and aesthetic recovery after devastating injury. Successful re-plantation relies on having a well-resuscitated patient, a viable part and surgical expertise.

It is important to remember that the first priority in managing amputated parts is to manage the person from whom the part was amputated. The ABCDE approach must be used. Good first aid and vascular spasm may have reduced the bleeding, while compensatory mechanisms may be maintaining the blood pressure. A careful assessment of the circulatory state must be made to avoid underestimating the degree of hypovolaemia.

Careful attention should be paid to haemorrhage control. Small arteries and venous ooze can be controlled with elevation and a pressure dressing, but larger-diameter arteries will require focused direct pressure. Tourniquets should only be used as a last resort in order to save life. The clamping of vessels causes further damage and can be more difficult than anticipated. It is better to apply direct digital pressure and summon expert surgical help.

Management of these injuries is often hampered by a fixation with the part rather than the person. The patient is likely to be in significant distress, and adequate intravenous analgesia should be administered early. Associated injuries should not be overlooked, and a full and thorough secondary survey must be performed. It is essential that X-radiography be carried out on both the residual stump and the part.

Re-plantation surgery draws heavily on operating theatre resources. The re-implantation team should be informed as early as possible, thus maximizing the time available to organize the necessary facilities.

Management of the amputated part is focused on reducing warm ischaemia time. Urgent transfer of the patient and the part must be organized unless the patient is already in a specialist centre. The temperature of the part should be lowered as much as possible, without allowing it to freeze. This is best achieved by taking the following steps:

- gross contamination is gently removed, but damage caused by rubbing is avoided;
- the part is covered in a single layer of damp (not dripping-wet) gauze;
- the covered part is placed in a plastic bag and the bag is sealed; and
- the sealed bag is placed in a container of water/ice mix.

The amputated part should never be allowed to come into direct contact with ice as this will cause frostbite.

Digits have little muscle volume and are more tolerant of warm ischaemia. Surgical techniques continue to improve, and crushed or avulsed tissue may be salvageable. Similarly, if the part cannot be implanted, effective use may be made of undamaged skin. It is inappropriate for the non-expert to deny the patient possible re-plantation based on time since injury or mechanism of injury. Expert surgical advice should always be sought.

SUMMARY

Limb injuries are common: they may be massive, life-threatening and obvious, or they may be subtle and easy to miss. Early management of the life-threatening injuries requires a team approach with the early involvement of orthopaedic advice. Splintage, including external fixation of pelvic fractures, may be life-saving. Prompt reduction, splintage, dressing and antibiotics can reduce the morbidity from limb trauma. The lesser injuries require a careful and systematic examination to identify them; this is not always possible in the early phase of trauma care, but must be carried out and documented as soon as possible. Clear communication with the orthopaedic surgeons helps to identify and prioritize injuries.

REFERENCES

1. Kenzora JE, Burgess AR. The neglected foot and ankle in polytrauma. *Advances in Orthopedic Surgery* 1983; **7**: 89–98.

2. Bone L, Bucholz R. The management of fractures in patients with multiple trauma. *Journal of Bone and Joint Surgery* 1986; **68A**: 945–9.

3. Sanders R, Swiontkowski M, Nunley J, Spiegel P. The management of fractures with soft-tissue disruptions. [Review]. *Journal of Bone and Joint Surgery, American Volume* 1993; **75**: 778–89.

4. Dalal SA, Burgess AR, Siegel JH, *et al.* Pelvic fracture in multiple trauma: classification by mechanism is key to pattern of organ injury, resuscitative requirements, and outcome. *Journal of Trauma* 1989; **29**: 981–1002.

5. Harviel JD, Champion H. Early assessment of the acutely injured patient. *Current Orthopedics* 1988; **2**: 99–103.

6. Gustilo RB, Merkow RL, Templeman D. Current Concepts review: the management of open fractures. *Journal of Bone and Joint Surgery* 1990; **72A**: 299.

7. Riska EB, Myllynen P. Fat embolism in patients with multiple injuries. *Journal of Trauma* 1982; **22**: 891–4.

8. Riska EB, von Bonsdorff H, Hakkinen S, Jaroma H, Kiviluoto O, Paavilainen T. Prevention of fat embolism by early internal fixation of fractures in patients with multiple injuries. *Injury* 1976; **8**: 110–16.

9. Coupland RM. *War Wounds of Limbs: Surgical Management.* Oxford: Butterworth-Heinemann Ltd, 1993.

10. Gray R. *War Wounds: Basic Surgical Management.* Geneva: International Committee of the Red Cross, 1994.

11. Gustilo RB, Anderson JT. Prevention of infection in the management of one thousand and twenty five open fractures of long bones. *Journal of Bone and Joint Surgery* 1976; **58A**: 453–8.

12. Burgess AR. Emergency evaluation. In: Yaremchuk MJ, Burgess AR, Brumback RJ (eds). *Lower Extremity Salvage and Reconstruction: Orthopedic and Plastic Surgical Management*, Chapter 3. New York: Elsevier Science Publishing Co., Inc., 1989, pp. 31–40.

13. Apley AG, Solomon L. Principles of fractures. In: *Apley's System of Orthopedics and Fractures* (6th ed.). London: Butterworths, 1982, pp. 333–68.

14. Sampson MA. Emerging technologies – trauma imaging. In: Greaves I, Ryan JM, Porter KM (eds). *Trauma.* London: Arnold, 1998, pp. 103–25.

15. Raby N, Berman L, de Lacey G. *Accident and Emergency Radiology: a Survival Guide.* London: W B Saunders Co., 1995.

16. Cohen MS, Garfin SR, Hargens AR, Mubarak SJ. Acute compartment syndrome. Effect of dermotomy on fascial decompression in the leg. *Journal of Bone and Joint Surgery, British Volume* 1991; **73**: 287–90.

17. Blick SS, Brumback RJ, Poka A, Burgess AR, Ebraheim NA. Compartment syndrome in open tibial fractures. *Journal of Bone and Joint Surgery* 1986; **68A**: 1348–53.

18. McQueen MM, Court-Brown CM. Compartment monitoring in tibial fractures. The pressure threshold for decompression. *Journal of Bone and Joint Surgery, British Volume* 1996; **78**: 99–104.

19. McQueen MM, Christie J, Court Brown CM. Acute compartment syndrome in tibial diaphyseal fractures. *Journal of Bone and Joint Surgery, British Volume* 1996; **78**: 95–8.

20. Burgess AR. External fixation in the multiply injured patient. *AAOS Instructors Course Lectures* 1990; **39**: 229–32.

21. Schatzker J, Tile M. *The Rationale of Operative Fracture Care.* (2nd ed.). Berlin: Springer, 1996.

22. Goris RJA, Gimbrere JSF, van Niekerk JLM, Schoots FJ, Booy LHD. Early osteosynthesis and prophylactic mechanical ventilation in the multitrauma patient. *Journal of Trauma* 1982; **22**: 895–903.

23. Bone LB, Johnson KD, Weigelt J, Scheinberg R. Early versus delayed stabilization of femoral fractures. A prospective randomized study. *Journal of Bone and Joint Surgery* 1989; **71A**: 336–40.

24. Pape H-C, Auf'm'Kolk M, Paffrath T, Regel G, Sturm JA, Tscherne H. Primary intramedullary femur fixation in multiple trauma patients with associated lung contusion – a cause of posttraumatic ARDS? *Journal of Trauma* 1993; **34**: 540–8.

25. Esterhai JL, Jr, Queenan J. Management of soft tissue wounds associated with type III open fractures. [Review]. *Orthopedic Clinics of North America* 1991; **22**: 427–32.

26. Mellor SG, Easmon CSF, Sanford JP. Wound contamination and antibiotics. In: Ryan JM, Rich NM, Dale RF, Morgans BT, Cooper GJ (eds). *Ballistic Trauma*. London: Edward Arnold, 1997, pp. 61–71.

27. Caudle RJ, Stern PJ. Severe open fractures of the tibia. *Journal of Bone and Joint Surgery, American Volume* 1987; **69A**: 801–7.

28. Court-Brown CM, McQueen MM, Quaba AAR. *Management of Open Fractures*. London: Martin Dunitz, 1996.

29. Bowyer GW, Rossiter ND. Management of gunshot wounds to limbs. *Journal of Bone and Joint Surgery, British Volume* 1997; **79B**: 1031–6.

30. Coombs R, Green S, Sarmiento A (eds). *External Fixation and Functional Bracing*. London: Orthotext, 1989.

31. Bowyer GW, Ryan JM, Kaufmann CR, Ochsner MG. General principles of wound management. In: Ryan JM, Rich N, Dale R, Morgans B, Cooper GJ (eds). *Ballistic Trauma*. London: Edward Arnold, 1997, pp. 105–19.

32. Rowley DI. *War Wounds with Fractures: a Guide to Surgical Management*, Geneva: International Committee of the Red Cross, 1996.

10

Spinal injuries

OBJECTIVES

- To understand the anatomical basis of patterns of spinal injury
- To detail the initial management of the patient with a definite or suspected spinal injury
- To identify the role of investigations in spinal injury
- To understand the principles of definitive management in spinal injury

INTRODUCTION

Acute spinal cord injury primarily affects young, otherwise healthy males (with a typical age range of 18 to 35 years, and a male to female ratio of 3 to 1). The annual incidence of acute spinal cord injury in the UK is approximately 10–15 per million population.[1,2] The permanent paralysis experienced by these 800 or so patients a year leads to major disability, a shorter life expectancy and significant economic costs. Lifetime costs for a representative person with complete paraplegia injured at age 27 were estimated to be US$1 million in 1992.[3] Road traffic accidents (RTAs) and falls from heights account for the majority of patients (approximately 40% and 20%, respectively), but sports and leisure activities such as gymnastics, rugby, horse-riding, skiing and diving into shallow water are also associated with spinal cord injury.[4] Perhaps surprisingly, spinal injury resulting from penetrating trauma is as common as that resulting from sports activities.[2,5]

Advances in the management of spinal cord-injured patients have resulted in an improvement in overall survival and quality of life. Nonetheless, there is still scope to reduce the consequences of secondary injury and further neurological deterioration in the acute phase.[4,6]

CLINICAL ANATOMY

Vertebral column

The vertebral column usually consists of 33 vertebrae, but only the upper 24 (seven cervical, 12 thoracic and five lumbar) articulate. The five sacral and four coccygeal vertebrae are fused to form the sacrum and coccyx, respectively. The vertebral column is most vulnerable to injury at the cervicothoracic, thoracolumbar and, less commonly, lumbosacral junctions. These are transition zones in terms of mobility and curvature. The thoracic vertebrae are relatively immobile compared with the cervical and lumbar vertebrae because of the alignment of the facet joints and attachment to the thoracic cage.[7] The sacral vertebrae are relatively fixed within the bony pelvis.

The stability of the spinal column depends primarily on the integrity of the ligaments and intervertebral discs connecting the vertebrae.[4] When assessing the injured spine, the concept of stability is important, as it refers to the ability of the vertebral column to withstand further stress without further deformity or neurological damage. Stability can be determined by considering all the bony and ligamentous elements of the spinal column in three vertical regions or columns. The anterior column comprises the anterior longitudinal ligaments, the anterior part of the annular ligament and the anterior half of the vertebral body. The posterior column comprises the ligamentum flavum, supraspinous, interspinous, intertransverse and capsular ligaments (together referred to as the posterior ligament complex) along with the neural arch, pedicles and spinous processes of the vertebrae. The middle column consists of the posterior longitudinal ligament, the posterior part of the annular ligament and the posterior wall of the vertebral bodies. Instability occurs when the middle column along with either the anterior or posterior columns is injured to the extent that ligamentous or bony integrity is lost. When this occurs, the entire vertebral column should be considered unstable. It is important to appreciate that instability may be purely ligamentous.[4]

The stability of the spine is dependent on the integrity of the anterior, middle and posterior columns. If two of these are injured, then the spine is unstable and any movement may damage the cord

---

Spinal canal

The spinal cord extends from the foramen magnum, through the spinal canal to terminate anywhere between T12 and L3 (usually the lower margin of the L1 vertebral body). Thereafter, the canal contains the lumbar, sacral and coccygeal spinal nerves (the cauda equina). Between the bony canal and the spinal cord is a potential space which contains extradural fat and blood vessels. The space varies along the length of the spine, and is narrowest in the thoracic area. Fractures of the thoracic spine are thus frequently complicated by spinal cord injury.[8] In contrast, there is a large potential space at the level of C1 behind the odontoid peg, and bony injuries in this area may not involve the cord.

Spinal cord

The spinal cord is divided into 31 segments each with a pair of anterior (motor) and dorsal (sensory) spinal nerve roots. On each side, the anterior and dorsal nerve roots combine to form the spinal nerves as they exit from the vertebral column. Each segmental nerve root supplies motor innervation to specific muscle groups (myotomes) and sensory innervation to a specific area of skin (dermatome). By testing sensory modalities and motor functions it is possible to localize any neurological abnormality to specific spinal levels. The neurological level of injury is the lowest (most caudal) segmental level with normal sensory and motor function. A patient with a C5 level exhibits, by definition, abnormal motor and sensory function from C6 down. It is important to remember that the spinal cord segments do not correspond with the vertebral levels.

The neurological level of injury is the lowest (most caudal) segmental level with normal sensory and motor function

---

The spinal cord is organized into paired bundles of nerve fibres or 'tracts' that carry motor (descending) and sensory (ascending) information. These tracts are specifically organized anatomically within the cord. The most important are the corticospinal and spinothalamic tracts and the dorsal or posterior columns. Within the tracts, the more centrally situated fibres innervate more proximal areas of the body (e.g. the arms) and the more lateral fibres innervate the distal areas (e.g. sacrum). The corticospinal tracts carry descending motor fibres and are located anteriorly within the cord. These tracts decussate (cross the midline) in the medulla before descending into the spinal cord. Injuries to the corticospinal tracts therefore produce signs on the same side (ipsilateral) as the injury. The dorsal columns carry ascending sensory fibres and are located posteriorly in the cord. They transmit light touch, proprioception and vibration sense. As they ascend through the medulla, the dorsal columns also decussate. Signs following injury are therefore also ipsilateral. The spinothalamic tracts lie in two areas: the lateral spinothalamic tracts transmit pain and temperature, while the anterior spinothalamic tracts transmit light touch. In contrast to the corticospinal tracts and dorsal columns, the anterior and lateral spinothalamic tracts usually decussate within three spinal segments (or two vertebral bodies' height). Injuries therefore tend to affect sensation on the opposite (contralateral) side. These anatomical and functional differences are important in determining both the level and the nature of cord injury.[4]

Sympathetic autonomic nervous system fibres exit from the spinal cord between C7 and L1, while parasympathetic pathways exit between S2 and S4. Progressively higher spinal cord lesions cause increasing degrees of autonomic dysfunction. Severe autonomic dysfunction, resulting in hypotension, relative bradycardia, peripheral vasodilation and hypothermia causes neurogenic shock (see below).

The spinal cord is supplied with blood by three longitudinal vessels: one anterior spinal artery and two posterior spinal arteries. The anterior spinal artery runs down the midline in the anterior median fissure of the cord. It supplies the anterior two-thirds of the cord along its whole length. The calibre varies according to its proximity to a major radicular artery, and the narrowest part is in the mid-thoracic area. The two posterior spinal arteries primarily supply the posterior third of the cord, and frequently anastomose with each other and the anterior spinal artery. These three arteries are augmented by numerous radicular arteries along the length of the cord. Ischaemic injury to the cord may be caused by arterial occlusion secondary to trauma or a period of profound hypotension. Although the principal watershed area of the spinal cord is the mid-thoracic region, at any given level of the spinal cord, the central cord is also a watershed area. Thus ischaemic injury can produce a variety of clinical syndromes depending on the vessels involved, the segmental level and the degree of damage in watershed areas. A vascular injury may also cause ischaemia which extends to several segments higher than the initial injury.

PATHOPHYSIOLOGY OF SPINAL INJURY

Mechanism of injury

Combinations of abnormal flexion, extension, rotation and compression will injure the spine in predictable ways. Extension or flexion with rotation is the main cause of injury in the cervical spine, whereas compression with flexion or rotation is the main mechanism of injury in the thoracic and lumbar spine. Although minor degrees of injury may cause significant damage in patients who have pre-existing spondylosis, an abnormally narrow spinal canal or instability from diseases such as rheumatoid arthritis, the mechanisms are broadly the same. Whatever the mechanism, approximately 14% of all spinal injuries will result in cord damage.[9] Of these, 40% occur in the cervical region, 10% in the thoracic area, 35% at the thoracolumbar junction, and 3% in the lumbar region.

FLEXION

Hyperflexion injuries are typically caused by flexion about an axis anterior to the vertebral bodies. In countries where lap-type seat belts are used (rather than combined lap and diagonal belts as in the UK), hyperflexion injuries in RTAs are common. Rapid deceleration in the flexed position, falls on the back of the head with flexion of the neck, diving and contact sports such as rugby may also produce flexion injuries. Anterior column compression and, more importantly, posterior ligament complex distraction and failure of the middle column occur. The typical bony lesion associated with this mechanism is a horizontal fracture extending through the body, pedicle and posterior elements of the vertebra (Chance fracture). Pure hyperflexion injuries in the cervical vertebrae are less common because flexion is limited by the chin abutting the chest. Extreme cervical hyperflexion can fracture the anterior superior corner of the inferior vertebrae (Tear-drop fracture) and tear all the posterior ligaments. This unstable injury is usually found in the C5/6 region. The odontoid peg of C2 may also be fractured by sudden severe flexion.

FLEXION WITH ROTATION

The combination of hyperflexion with rotation is much more likely to produce significant injury to the cervical and thoracic spine than other mechanisms. Between 50% and 80% of all cervical spine injuries and most thoracolumbar injuries are caused by this mechanism. Such injuries often follow RTAs or direct trauma. There is significant disruption of the posterior ligament complex and the posterior column. The facet joints, lamina, transverse processes and vertebral bodies may fracture. In the cervical region the relatively flat facet joints may dislocate, without causing a fracture. The spinous processes of C6/7 can also be avulsed by the interspinous ligaments (the clay-shoveller's fracture). With greater shearing forces, all the intervertebral ligaments may tear and the upper vertebral body can be displaced relative to the one below.

EXTENSION

Hyperextension injuries tend only to be found in the cervical and lumbar region. Hyperextension damages the anterior column, and an avulsion fracture of the anterior inferior aspect of the vertebral body may be seen. The posterior aspect of the vertebral body may also be crushed, with a risk of retropulsion of bony fragments or intervertebral disc into the vertebral canal. A special type of hyperextension fracture occurs through the pedicles of C2 following hyperextension with distraction or compression (the 'hangman's fracture'). This may occur with judicial hanging (rather than conventional suicide attempts which usually result in asphyxiation), or striking the chin on a steering wheel in a collision.

ROTATION

Rotation rarely occurs in isolation. Whether associated with flexion or extension, these forces primarily injure the posterior ligament complex and are frequently associated with instability. There may be an associated facet joint dislocation.

COMPRESSION

Wedge fractures are the commonest type of fracture of the lumbar and thoracic vertebral bodies and are usually stable because the posterior ligaments remain intact. They result from forward or lateral flexion around an axis which passes through the intervertebral disc. If the force was sufficient to compress the anterior vertebral body to half the height of the posterior vertebral body, the posterior ligaments must also be considered to be damaged and the injury regarded as unstable. If the direction of force is such that lateral flexion occurs, there will be a compression fracture of the lateral part of the vertebral column. An axial stress which causes both the anterior and middle columns to fail is referred to as a burst fracture. In these injuries, retropulsion of the posterior vertebral wall or intervertebral disc into the canal places the cord at risk.

A specific compression fracture is the Jefferson's fracture of C1 (the atlas). A weight falling on the head, landing on the head after a fall or striking the top of the head will compress the atlas between the occipital condyles and C2 (the axis). The lamina and pedicles are fractured and, in addition, the transverse ligament holding the odontoid peg in position can be torn. The transverse ligament prevents posterior excursion of the odontoid peg. The skull and C1 may then slide forward on C2. Despite this, significant displacement must occur before the odontoid impinges on the cord (the anterior third of the spinal canal of the atlas is occupied by the odontoid peg, the posterior third is occupied by the spinal cord and the middle third is occupied by areolar tissue).

Primary neurological damage

Primary cord injury results from mechanical disruption of neural elements. There is a transient or permanent reduction in spinal canal volume by bone fragments, haematoma or soft tissue, with direct impingement on the spinal cord. Penetrating injuries may also cause direct injury. Primary spinal cord injury without radiological abnormality (SCIWORA) occurs in children who are less than 8 years old. The unique hypermobility and ligamentous laxity of the paediatric bony cervical and thoracic spine predisposes to SCIWORA.[10] Regardless of mechanism, the primary cord injury causes pericapillary haemorrhages that coalesce and enlarge, particularly in the grey matter. Infarction of grey matter and early white matter oedema are evident within 4 h of experimental blunt injury. At 8 h after injury, there is global infarction at the injured level, and only at this point does necrosis of white matter and paralysis below the level of the lesion become irreversible. The necrosis and central haemorrhages subsequently enlarge to occupy one or two levels above and below the point of primary impact.[11] The extent of this primary neurological damage depends on the spinal level of the injury.

Secondary neurological damage

Major contributing factors to neurological injury are secondary phenomena occurring in the minutes and hours following injury.[6] Secondary damage leads to interstitial and intracellular oedema, which may further complicate any reduction in spinal perfusion. As this oedema spreads, neurons are compressed and further clinical deterioration can result. With high spinal injuries, this process can lead to respiratory failure. Even when a complete transverse myelopathy is evident immediately after injury, some secondary damage will occur which is avoidable. The common causes of secondary injury to the spinal cord are:

- hypoxia;
- hypoperfusion; and
- further mechanical disturbance of the spine.

Although there is little evidence that mishandling of patients is a common cause of secondary mechanical injury, neurological damage can result from malpositioning of the spine in uninjured patients,[12] so extreme caution should be exercised in moving and positioning patients with proven or potential spinal injury.

HYPOXIA

Hypoxia can result from head, chest and upper airway injuries, although spinal injury itself can directly impair ventilation or lead to respiratory failure (Table 10.1). There is a direct relationship between the level of cord injury and the degree of respiratory dysfunction. With lesions above C5, there is weakness or paralysis of the diaphragm, vital capacity is reduced (10–20% of normal) and cough is weak and ineffective. Thus, patients with lesions above C5 will usually require mechanical ventilation. Patients with high thoracic cord injuries (T2 to T4) have vital capacities at 30–50% of normal, and a weak cough. With descent to lower-cord injuries, respiratory function improves and at T11 respiratory dysfunction is minimal, vital capacity is essentially normal and cough is strong.[13] To reduce secondary hypoxic damage, impairment in ventilation must be recognized and normal oxygenation and ventilation must be maintained.

Table 10.1 *Respiratory failure in spinal cord injury*

- Intercostal muscle and phrenic nerve paralysis
- Atelectasis secondary to decreased vital capacity (VC)
- Ventilation/perfusion (V/Q) mismatch from sympathectomy/adrenergic blockade
- Increased work of breathing (because compliance is decreased)
- Decreased coughing with inability to expectorate (with risk of atelectasis and pneumonia)
- Muscle fatigue

HYPOPERFUSION

The early phases of primary injury are associated with reduced regional blood flow from direct capillary damage. Further secondary hypoperfusion may result from either systemic hypotension due to bleeding elsewhere, or a failure of autoregulation. Without autoregulation, a fall in mean arterial pressure will result in a reduction in spinal perfusion.

Conversely, if the pressure is increased too much, then a spinal haemorrhagic infarct or haematoma could develop. Secondary damage from hypoperfusion is reduced by early recognition and treatment of hypoxia, hypovolaemia and neurogenic shock.

NEUROGENIC SHOCK

In acute spinal cord injury, shock may be neurogenic, haemorrhagic, or both. Following injuries at or above T6 there is significant loss of the sympathetic autonomic (adrenergic) outflow. Consequently vasomotor tone is reduced and, if the lesion is high enough, sympathetic innervation of the heart ceases. This loss of sympathetic tone results in hypotension and also enhances vagal reflexes, causing profound bradycardia. The triad of hypotension, bradycardia and peripheral vasodilatation resulting from the interruption of sympathetic nervous system control is termed *neurogenic shock*. It is important to consider this cause of shock in the patient with spinal injuries. However, spinal injuries are frequently associated with other major injuries and hypovolaemia must be excluded before attributing persistent hypotension to neurogenic shock. Hypotension associated with injury below T6 is invariably caused by haemorrhage. Similarly, hypotension in the presence of a spinal fracture alone, with no neurological deficit, is also likely to be due to haemorrhage. To complicate matters, patients with injury above T6 may not show the classical physical findings associated with haemorrhage (tachycardia and peripheral vasoconstriction). Thus, neurogenic shock may mask the normal response to hypovolaemia caused by other injuries. The onset of neurogenic shock can take minutes to hours to develop, because spinal injury can initially result in a pressor response due to the release of catecholamines. It may be 24 h before levels of catecholamines fall and neurogenic shock is unmasked.

Spinal shock

For each mechanism of injury described above, there may be complete or incomplete (partial) cord injury. The distinction between complete and incomplete cord injury cannot, however, be made until the patient has recovered from *spinal shock*. Spinal shock is defined as the complete loss of all neurological function, including reflexes, rectal tone and autonomic control below the level of spinal cord injury. Spinal shock is unrelated to hypovolaemia or neurogenic shock. It usually involves a 24- to 72-h period of complete loss of sensory, motor and segmental reflex activity with flaccid paralysis and areflexia below the level of the injury. Despite this profound paralysis, areas of the cord are still capable of a full recovery.

> **Spinal shock is a neurological, not a cardiovascular condition**

Within the spinal cord, sacral fibres are positioned more laterally than corresponding fibres from other regions of the body. Spinal injuries (particularly anterior and central) which primarily affect the midline of the spinal cord may not affect the sacral fibres. This results in 'sacral sparing' in which sensation is retained over the sacral and perineal area. Preservation of sacral function may indicate an incomplete cord lesion. However, definitive characterization of the nature of the injury cannot occur until spinal shock has resolved. This is usually indicated by return of reflex activity below the level of injury.

> **Complete and incomplete cord injury cannot be distinguished in the presence of spinal shock**

ASSESSMENT AND MANAGEMENT OF PATIENTS WITH SPINAL INJURY

The possibility of spinal injury should be considered in all trauma patients.[14] Common reasons for missing significant spinal injuries include failing to consider injuries in patients who are either unconscious, intoxicated or have pre-existing risk factors (such as arthritis), failing to examine patients adequately, and errors in the interpretation of radiographs.[15–18]

Primary survey

AIRWAY WITH CERVICAL SPINE CONTROL AND BREATHING

During assessment of Airway, Breathing and Circulation, efforts must be made to protect the spinal cord from potential secondary injury. This is assisted by early immobilization of the whole spine. Thereafter, evaluation of the spine can be safely deferred until immediately life-threatening conditions have been assessed and resuscitation is under way. The majority of trauma patients will have been immobilized during the pre-hospital phase.[19] The adequacy of immobilization and the position of any cervical collars, head blocks and other extrication devices should be checked. If none is in place, immobilization can be achieved by holding the head in the neutral position, or by the use of improvised or commercially available head blocks and tape. Patients who are agitated and moving around should not have their cervical spine immobilized in isolation. Long spine boards should be removed as soon as possible in a controlled way, usually as part of the log-roll. This will decrease the risk of pressure sore development in the spinally injured.

> **Do not leave patients on long spine boards: remove them during the log-roll**

The airway is the first priority. A jaw thrust, clearing of oral secretions and insertion of an oral or nasal airway may be all that is required initially to maintain the airway. Supplemental oxygen should be administered to prevent secondary damage from hypoxia. Throughout this, the whole spine must be maintained in neutral alignment after gentle controlled movement to a neutral position if this is necessary. Attempts to bring the head into neutral alignment against palpable resistance or if the patient complains of pain should be abandoned and the head immobilized as it is found.

Unconscious trauma patients should then have their airway secured by early orotracheal intubation. In conscious patients with signs of a high spinal cord injury (for example, weakness in arms and legs, neurogenic shock or diaphragmatic breathing) early intubation and ventilation should be considered. Indications for ventilation include CO_2 retention and poor respiratory effort with a low vital capacity.

Intubation is not contraindicated in the presence of spinal injury. The ideal technique is fiberoptic intubation with cervical spine control. However, there is little evidence that a properly performed orotracheal intubation with manual in-line immobilization will cause further cervical spine injury.[20,21] Oral suction, laryngoscopy and intubation may precipitate severe bradycardia from unopposed vagal stimulation in patients with autonomic disruption from cervical or high thoracic spinal cord injury. Atropine should be immediately available.

CIRCULATION

Persistent signs of shock must not be attributed to spinal cord injury until haemorrhage has been excluded. Almost 80% of patients with spinal cord injury have multiple injuries.[5] The most common sources of occult haemorrhage are:

- chest injuries (often associated with thoracic spine fractures);
- mediastinal injuries;
- intra-abdominal haemorrhage;
- retroperitoneal haemorrhage; and
- pelvic fractures and long-bone fractures.

Signs of peritonism (guarding, rigidity and rebound tenderness) may be absent in a patient with spinal injuries. Referred shoulder tip pain may be the only indication of intra-abdominal injury, and ultrasound or diagnostic peritoneal lavage are essential to exclude intra-abdominal bleeding. Urgent correction of any continuing bleeding is required to reduce the risks of hypoperfusion and secondary nerve damage.

Once occult sources of haemorrhage have been excluded, initial treatment of neurogenic shock involves cautious fluid resuscitation. Excessive fluid administration may precipitate pulmonary oedema. The therapeutic goals for neurogenic shock are adequate perfusion with a systolic blood pressure of 90–100 mmHg (acceptable for patients with complete cord lesions), a heart rate of 60–100 beats per minute, urine output above 30 ml/h, and normothermia. Patients with persisting bradycardia should be given atropine 0.5–1 mg intravenously, this being repeated if necessary until the heart rate is acceptable. If these measures fail, inotropic support with full haemodynamic monitoring may be required. This should be reserved for patients who have decreased urinary output despite adequate fluid resuscitation.

THE LOG-ROLL

A log-roll should be performed at the end of the primary survey. This allows assessment of the back and spinal column and, as stated above, the removal of the long spine board if one is present. Before the log-roll is commenced, mechanical stabilization of the cervical spine should be removed and replaced by manual in-line immobilization by the log-roll team leader. At the same time, the neck can be checked for any deformity, tenderness, bogginess or spasm. To examine the remainder of the vertebral column the patient must be 'log-rolled'. This technique requires at least five people. One person is responsible for maintaining the in-line stabilization of the head and neck and coordination of the log-roll (the team leader). A second person holds the patient's shoulder with one hand and places the other hand on the pelvis. The third person holds the pelvis with one hand and places the other hand under the patient's opposite thigh. The fourth person places both arms under the opposite lower leg and supports it during the roll. The fifth person is responsible for examining the back, conducting a rectal and perineal examination, observing pressure areas, and clearing debris. Further staff will be needed to assist with the removal of a long spine board. The team leader must give clear audible instructions and indicate in advance what these will be:

'The instruction will be ready, steady, move'.

The examination of the back includes looking for evidence of bruising or swelling, palpation over the spinous processes for deformity, swelling, wounds or increased tenderness down the whole length of the spine. Local tenderness at any point should be used to guide radiographic examination. Percussion of the spine using the thenar eminence may reveal injuries which are not initially tender to palpation (e.g. anterior column injuries). Examination of the perineum should identify sacral sparing, assess anal tone and check for the presence of priapism (a sustained penile erection secondary to spinal injury). Sacral sparing has such great prognostic value that preservation of perianal sensation, rectal motor function, and activity of the long flexors of the great toe should be actively sought. If there is some distal motor or sensory function or sacral sparing then the injury is likely to be an incomplete (or partial) cord lesion and there is considerable scope for neurological improvement.

Patients with altered level of consciousness or other distracting injuries may not have any features on examination of the back to suggest spinal injury, and may be unable to cooperate with neurological examination. Other signs which suggest spinal injury in these patients are listed in Table 10.2. Despite these, spinal injury cannot be absolutely excluded until a full neurological and radiological examination has been completed. In the interim, these patients will require spinal immobilization until they regain consciousness.

Table 10.2 *Signs of spinal injury in the unconscious patient*

- Diaphragmatic breathing
- Neurogenic shock (hypotension and bradycardia)
- Flaccid areflexia (spinal shock)
- Flexed posture of the upper limbs (loss of extensor innervation distal to C5)
- Response to pain above the clavicles only
- Priapism (the erection may be incomplete)

Once the 'log-roll' is completed, the patient can be rolled back to the supine position.

Secondary survey

The secondary survey in conscious patients involves a focused history to establish pre-existing medical conditions, the mechanism of injury, and the presence of back or neck pain, limb weakness and sensory disturbance. Most conscious patients with spinal injury will complain of pain in the region of the injury.[22–24] If there is no pain in the back or neck, the patient should be asked to cough, and then have their heels tapped.[25] This can occasionally reveal a painful area, particularly if there are distracting injuries. The patient should then be asked to move each limb in turn, provided that there is no pain or discomfort in the limb or spinal column. In addition, direct questions should be asked regarding absent or abnormal sensation in the limbs or trunk. The spectrum of symptoms and signs associated with incomplete cord lesions is so varied that any sensory or motor symptoms should be taken seriously. At this stage, a more thorough neurological examination should be carried out. Each dermatome should be tested for sensitivity to a sterile pin or similar stimulus (pain) and cotton wool (light touch). Coordination, tone, power and deep tendon reflexes must then be tested and any asymmetry noted. The root values of dermatomes and myotomes must be known in order to interpret the findings (Table 10.3). Assessment of power should be standardized to allow comparison over time and between limbs (Table 10.4).

Table 10.3 *Segmental values for dermatomes and myotomes*

Segment	Representative Dermatomes	Representative Myotomes
C5	Sensation over deltoid	Deltoid muscle
C6	Sensation over thumb	Wrist extensors
C7	Sensation over middle finger	Elbow extensors
C8	Sensation over little finger	Middle finger flexors
T1	Sensation over inner aspect of elbow	Little finger abduction
T4	Sensation around nipple	–
T8	Sensation over xiphisternum	–
T10	Sensation around umbilicus	–
T12	Sensation around symphysis	–
L1	Sensation in inguinal region	–
L2	Sensation anterior upper thigh	Hip flexors
L3	Sensation anterior mid thigh	Knee extensors
L4	Sensation on medial aspect leg	Ankle dorsiflexors
L5	Sensation between 1st and 2nd toes	Long toe extensors
S1	Sensation on lateral border of foot	Ankle plantar flexors
S3	Sensation over ischial tuberosity	–
S4/5	Sensation around perineum	–

Table 10.4 *Muscle power*

- 0 = no flicker of movement
- 1 = a flicker of contraction, but no movement
- 2 = movement, but not against gravity
- 3 = movement against gravity
- 4 = movement against resistance
- 5 = normal power

The aim of the neurological examination is to determine the level and nature of the lesion, document the deficit, and identify the need for emergency treatment. Injuries above C5 cause quadriplegia and respiratory failure. At C5 and C6 the biceps are also weak, and at C4 and C5 the deltoid, supraspinatous and infraspinatus are weak. C7 injuries cause weakness of the triceps, wrist extensors, and forearm pronators. Injuries at T1 and below cause paraplegia; the precise level can be determined from the level of sensory loss. Injuries from T10 down can cause a cauda equina syndrome. The cauda equina includes the terminal spinal cord and the spinal roots from T12 to S5. Acute compression may cause bilateral leg pain, flaccid paralysis and retention of urine. Pain in the sacral dermatomes may also be present. A burst fracture of L1 is a typical cause of acute cauda equina syndrome.

A complex situation can arise where there is an incomplete cord injury. In general, it is not possible to determine the precise nature of the injury in the acute phase, and inappropriate attempts to do so may distract from more immediate clinical priorities. However, any motor or sensory sparing revealed by meticulous examination in the acute phase may have enormous prognostic value.[26] There are three principal patterns of incomplete cord injury which can sometimes be recognized – anterior, central, and lateral cord syndromes:

1. An *anterior cord syndrome* is due to direct mechanical compression of the anterior cord or obstruction of the anterior spinal artery. It affects the spinothalamic and corticospinal tracts, resulting in variable loss of motor function (corticospinal tracts) and impaired pain/temperature sensation (spinothalamic tracts). There is preservation of light touch, proprioception and vibration sense (dorsal columns).
2. *Central cord syndromes* are produced by brief compression of the cervical cord and disruption of the central grey matter. They usually occur in patients with an already narrow spinal canal, either congenitally or from cervical spondylosis. There is weakness of the arms, often with pin-prick loss over the arms and shoulders, and relative sparing of leg power and sensation on the trunk and legs. Abnormality of bladder function and dysaesthesias in the upper extremities (burning hands or arms) are common. There is usually sacral sparing. This pattern is, as with sacral sparing, due to the anatomical arrangement of fibres within the cord. The more centrally situated fibres supply the arms and these are therefore the most affected by central lesions in the cervical cord.
3. Penetrating trauma may cause a *lateral cord syndrome* (Brown–Séquard syndrome). All sensory and motor modalities are disrupted on the side of the wound at the level of the lesion. Below this level however, there is ipsilateral loss of muscle power and tone, proprioception, vibration sense and motor function with contralateral loss of pain and temperature sensation.

Differentiation of an isolated nerve root injury from an incomplete spinal cord injury can also be difficult. The presence of neurological deficits that indicate multilevel involvement is suggestive of spinal cord injury rather than a nerve root injury. In the absence of spinal shock, motor weakness with intact reflexes indicates spinal cord injury, while motor weakness with absent reflexes indicates a nerve root lesion.

By the end of the secondary survey, there should be a clear indication of the presence and immediate consequences of any spinal injury. The patient should also have a nasogastric tube and urinary catheter *in situ*. These help to prevent bladder and gastrointestinal distention developing after spinal injury. Urinary catheterization must be performed under strictly aseptic conditions in order to reduce the incidence of infection.

RADIOGRAPHY

Patients who are not under the influence of alcohol or drugs and are fully conscious with no neck pain or tenderness, no abnormal neurological symptoms or signs and no major distracting injuries (such as major limb, chest or abdominal injury) do not require cervical spine radiographs.[27–32] Under these circumstances the spine can be cleared clinically. There are currently trials underway to develop clearer decision rules for these patients.[33] Patients with symptoms or signs, altered consciousness, intoxication or major distracting injuries require three cervical spine radiographs: a lateral to include the top of T1 vertebral body; a long anteroposterior (AP) view; and an open-mouth AP view to show the C1/C2 articulation.[22,23,29,34–36] The combination of these three views has a very high sensitivity for spinal injury,[37] although injuries may still be missed.[38] All radiographs should be interpreted using the ABCDS system (Table 10.5).

Table 10.5 *The ABCDS system of radiographic interpretation*

- Adequacy and alignment
- Bones
- Cartilage and joints
- Disc space
- Soft tissue

Lateral cervical spine radiograph

The lateral view will reveal approximately 90% of cervical spine injuries, with a sensitivity of over 90%.[35,37] To interpret a lateral cervical spine radiograph, the adequacy of the film should be checked first. An adequate lateral cervical spine includes the top of T1 (cervicothoracic junction).[39] Missed injuries mainly occur at this point, so alternative techniques such as pulling the shoulders down during the exposure or taking 'swimmers' or trauma oblique views may be necessary.[40] The 'swimmers' view is taken with the patient lying supine, with one arm directly above the head and the other by the side. Oblique views (at 30°) show the intervertebral formina, the pedicles and the facet joints.[41] They can also be used to image the odontoid peg in an unconscious patient if an open-mouth view is unobtainable.[42] If these views fail to show the cervicothoracic junction, then a computed tomography (CT) scan must be considered, depending on the clinical picture.[34,43]

The next step is to check alignment by tracing three imaginary lines (or arcs) on the film: the anterior longitudinal line is a smooth unbroken arc along the anterior margins of the vertebral bodies; and the posterior longitudinal line lies along the posterior margins of the vertebral bodies. The spinolaminar line lies along the bases of the spinous processes. All three lines should be traced as smooth arcs on the lateral film. The loss of the normal cervical lordosis is non-specific, and may be due to muscle spasm, old injuries, age-related changes, a semi-rigid cervical collar or radiographic positioning. Apparent forwards movement of a vertebra on the vertebra below is suggestive of facet joint dislocation. If the displacement is more than one-half of the width of a vertebral body then a bilateral facet joint dislocation should be suspected. If the displacement is less, then unifacet dislocation is likely. Pseudospondylolisthesis may be seen in children at C2/C3 and, more rarely, C3/C4.[40]

The third step is to evaluate the individual vertebrae. Fractures of C1 and C2 can be difficult to see. The odontoid peg should be visible immediately posterior to the arch of C1. The normal distance between the bones at this point is 3 mm in adults and 5 mm in children. Widening of this distance and displacement of the posterior arch of C1 from its expected alignment along the smooth arc of the spinolaminar line should be sought. Fractures in the pedicles of C2 (hangman's fracture) can be subtle and should be looked for specifically. The vertebral bodies of C3 to T1 have a uniform rectangular shape, and the heights of the anterior and posterior aspects of each vertebral body should be the same. A difference of greater than 2 mm indicates a compression fracture.[40] A difference greater than 25% of the height of the vertebrae can only occur if the middle and posterior columns have been damaged. A 'tear-drop' fracture tends to occur on the anterior superior corner of the vertebral body of C5 or C6. There is interspinous widening and marked soft tissue swelling, which can be used to distinguish it from a simple avulsion fracture. In contrast, hyperextension of the neck can lead to avulsion of the anterior inferior corner of the vertebral body along with opening of the intervertebral space anteriorly and narrowing posteriorly. The spinal canal should be over 13 mm wide, and is measured from the posterior longitudinal line to the spinolaminar line. Narrowing of the canal occurs following dislocations and compression fractures which displace segments of bone posteriorly. Pre-existing disease and degeneration may also lead to a narrowing of the canal.

Narrowing of the anterior intervertebral disc space, with widening posteriorly, indicates that there has been a hyperflexion injury. Conversely, hyperextension produces widening of the anterior disc space with narrowing posteriorly. The facet joints normally have parallel articular surfaces with a gap of less than 2 mm between them. A unifacet dislocation will be accompanied by soft-tissue swelling and rotation of the vertebrae above the dislocation. Both facet surfaces can then be seen on the lateral view (the 'bow-tie' sign). A bilateral facet dislocation is associated with extensive forward displacement of the vertebral body, widening of the interspinous processes, disc space narrowing and soft-tissue swelling.[40,44] However, there is no rotation of the vertebrae.

Finally, the soft-tissue shadow anterior to the vertebral bodies has characteristic appearances and dimensions.[45] Anterior to C1 to C4, the soft-tissue shadow should be less than 7 mm (or a maximum of 30% of the width of the vertebral body). From C5 to C7, the oesophagus increases the gap between the trachea and the bones to 22 mm in the adult (or one vertebral body width), and to 14 mm in the child. In children this gap can be wider due to crying, neck flexion and pre-sphenoidal adenoidal enlargement. Although the absence of soft-tissue swelling does not rule out significant injury,[46] pre-vertebral swelling is present in over 50% of patients with fractures.

A significant neck injury may still be present despite no evidence of fracture or dislocation on the lateral film. Given that the stability of the vertebral column is dependent on radiolucent ligaments,[47] the film should also be checked for radiological indicators of potential ligamentous injury (Table 10.6).

Table 10.6 *Signs of possible ligamentous injury on lateral cervical spine radiographs*

- Facet joint over-riding
- Facet joint widening
- Interspinous fanning
- Greater than 25% compression of the vertebral body
- Over 10° angulation between vertebral bodies
- Over 3.5 mm vertebral body over-riding with fracture

Anteroposterior and open-mouth cervical spine radiographs

There is rarely any difficulty with the adequacy of the long AP view. However, the open-mouth view may have to be repeated in order to clearly show the C1/C2 articulation. In the long AP view, the spinous processes and pedicles should be aligned in a straight (vertical) line, and the distances between spinous processes should be approximately equal. Lateral deviation may indicate a unifacet dislocation. Abnormal widening of an interspinous distance compared with the spaces above and below may indicate instability. The vertebral bodies should be rectangular with a regular internal trabecular pattern and equal soft-tissue spacing between articulating surfaces.

In the open-mouth view, the distances between the lateral masses of the atlas and the odontoid peg should be symmetrical, with less than 2 mm of lateral overhang of C1 on C2 in adults. The articulating surfaces should also be parallel. Fractures of the odontoid peg can occur in the peg itself, at its base, or through the body of C2. Most fractures are at the base of the peg and are unstable. Common errors include misreading the shadows of the arch of C1, the overlying teeth, or the epiphyseal plate as a fracture. The epiphysis is V-shaped, and has usually fused by age 12. The interpretation of all three standard cervical spine radiographs is summarized in Table 10.7.[44,48]

Additional radiography

Given that up to one-quarter of patients with spinal injury have damage at more than one level, it is usually necessary to obtain further radiographs once resuscitation is complete. Combinations of cervical and thoracic fractures or thoracic and lumbar fractures are most common.[49] In conscious patients, these should be guided by symptoms and signs, but additional films typically include AP and lateral thoracic or lumbar spine radiographs. All five lumbar vertebrae should be clearly visible along with the lumbosacral junction and the thoracic vertebrae under investigation. The alignment can be assessed on lateral films using the three lines described for the cervical spine. These change from kyphotic to lordotic at the T1/L1 junction. In the lumbar region, a line running through the facet joints should also trace out a smooth curve, although this is difficult to see in the thoracic region because of the overlying ribs.

Table 10.7 *Interpretation of cervical spine radiographs*

Lateral view
- top of T1 must be visible
- the three longitudinal arcs should be maintained
- the vertebral bodies should be of uniform height
- the odontoid peg should be intact and closely applied to C2

Anteroposterior view
- spinous processes should be in a straight line and equally spaced

Open-mouth view
- base of the odontoid peg is intact
- lateral margins of C1 and C2 align
- spaces on either side of the odontoid peg are equal

An anterior displacement greater than 25% on the lateral film is associated with fractures of the facets and damage to ligaments in all three columns. Hyperflexion with rotation can produce anterior displacement due to subluxation or dislocation of the facet joints. Unilateral or bilateral facet dislocation is associated with widening of the interspinous gaps, fractures of the articular surface (best seen on the AP view) and soft-tissue swelling. Subluxation occurs when the upper articular surface is riding high on the one below but they are still in contact with one another. This is also associated with widening of the interspinous gaps.

On the AP views, vertical alignment of the spinous processes should also be checked. In addition, the distance between the two lateral borders of the vertebra, the pedicles and the facet joints increases progressively down the vertebral column. Malalignment may indicate a unifacet dislocation or a fracture of the lateral articular surface. In these cases, the spinous process tends to rotate towards the side of the injury.

Each vertebra must be assessed individually for steps, breaks or loss of the normal posterior concavity. In the upper thoracic region the facet joints, spinous processes and transverse processes normally cannot be seen because of overlying ribs, soft tissues and the alignment of the facet joints. Chance fractures of the vertebral bodies and tear-drop fractures (mainly at T12/L1/L2 in adults or T4/5 in children) should be visible on lateral views. A discrepancy of 2 mm or more in the height of the anterior and posterior vertebral bodies indicates a fracture, except in T11 to L1 where this difference is normal. On AP views, the superior and inferior surface of the vertebral bodies should be parallel. A crush fracture may be detected by noting loss of trabecular pattern, overlapping of bone fragments and widening of the interpedicular distance. An anterior/superior wedge fracture indicates that the spine has been subjected to either a hyperflexion or hyperextension injury. With hyperflexion, there is associated soft-tissue swelling, anterior disc space narrowing, widening of the posterior disc space, loss of the anterior vertebral height, and in extreme situations, subluxation of the facet joints. Rarely there is lateral wedging of the vertebral bodies due to lateral flexion and rotation.

Hyperextension injuries can lead to widening of the anterior disc space with fracture and posterior displacement of the posterior aspects of the vertebrae. Isolated fractures of the transverse and spinous processes can occur following direct trauma, as well as being part of the pattern of injuries resulting from hyperflexion and hyperextension mechanisms.

The intervertebral discs should be similar and even throughout, and their height usually increases progressively down the spine to L4/L5. Commonly the disc at L5/S1 is narrower than that at L4/L5, and is associated with dense sclerosis of the underlying cortical surfaces and marginal osteophytes. The soft-tissue shadows around the vertebral column may be the only clue to an underlying bony or ligamental injury. Soft-tissue changes on AP films following fractures of the upper thoracic vertebrae can mimic a ruptured thoracic aorta. The interpretation of thoracic and lumbar spine radiographs are summarized in Table 10.9.

Table 10.9 *Interpretation of thoracic and lumbar spine radiographs*

Lateral views
- the three longitudinal arcs should be maintained
- the vertebral bodies should be of uniform height
- loss of height or wedging should be sought
- normal posterior concavity of vertebral bodies maintained

Anteroposterior views
- spinous processes should be a straight line and equally spaced
- soft-tissue paraspinal line does not bulge
- the vertebral bodies should be of uniform height
- distance between pedicles shows normal slight widening

FLEXION/EXTENSION VIEWS

Conscious patients who have well-localized severe neck pain but no neurological or radiographic abnormalities may have an unstable ligamentous injury.[47,50] Such injuries are much more common in the cervical spine. Flexion views of the cervical spine may be useful in demonstrating any instability; these are achieved by asking the patient to flex their neck voluntarily during exposure, after which the film should be examined for evidence of subluxation. CT should be undertaken before flexion/extension views if there is any suggestion of abnormality on the plain films.[33]

COMPUTED TOMOGRAPHY (CT)

CT scanning has become the mainstay for definitive imaging of vertebral column injuries. Middle and posterior column fractures can be clearly visualized,[51] although fractures, subluxations and dislocations which parallel the plane of the scan (typically involving the odontoid peg, facets or pedicles), may be better visualized on plain films as they can be missed by CT.[52] There is evidence that routine imaging of the upper cervical spine in patients undergoing CT for head injury will reveal abnormalities not detected on the plain film.[43]

MAGNETIC RESONANCE IMAGING (MRI)

MRI is ideal for imaging the contents of the spinal canal and detecting ligamentous and intervertebral disc damage,[53] as well as vascular injury. MRI will also identify extradural spinal haematomas and spinal cord haemorrhage, contusion and oedema.[54,55] Sagittal T2-weighted images are regarded as most useful in defining ligamentous injury. MRI scanning is currently only suitable for haemodynamically stable patients.

EMERGENCY TREATMENT

The aim of emergency treatment in spinal injury is to reduce secondary injury, improve motor function and sensation and reduce the extent of permanent paralysis. Emergency treatment options include high-dose steroids and surgical decompression.

STEROIDS

Methylprednisolone sodium succinate is the only pharmacological treatment for acute spinal cord injury that has been extensively studied. The three US National Acute Spinal Cord Injury studies (NASCIS) have shown that the administration of methylprednisolone within 8 h of blunt spinal injury significantly improves neurological outcome.[56,57] Additional benefit can be obtained in patients whose treatment was delayed to between 3 and 8 h after injury by extending the maintenance dose to 48 h.[58,59] The critical factors for recoverable function appear to be the extent of initial deficit and the time from injury to initiation of therapy. Complete axonal disruption following the primary or secondary injury is not associated with an improvement in neurological recovery after steroids.

With the exception of penetrating injuries, the high-dose steroids do not appear to be related to any increased risk of medical complications in the short term (such as hypoglycaemia, pancreatitis or gastric ulcers). With penetrating injuries (especially gunshot wounds), there is an increased risk of infection and higher mortality when patients are given high-dose steroids. Although the need for further trials is recognized, high-dose methylprednisolone has been accepted as the standard emergency therapy in many countries;[60] the dose regimen is given in Table 10.10.

Table 10.10 *Dose regimen for methylprednisolone in acute spinal cord injury*

- 30 mg/kg i.v. bolus over 15 min immediately
- 5.4 mg/kg/h over 23 h (commenced 45 min after the bolus) in patients receiving treatment during the first 3 h after injury
- 5.4 mg/kg/h over 47 h (commenced 45 min after the bolus) in patients receiving treatment between 3 and 8 h after injury

---

SURGERY

Although open wounds require surgical exploration, the timing of surgery in patients who have sustained a closed acute spinal cord injury remains controversial.[61] Surgically remediable and potentially reversible cord compression due to dislocation of a vertebral body or displaced bone fragments must be treated urgently. Decompression within 2 h may allow some recovery of spinal cord function. However, even stable injuries can be associated with significant cord compression and may benefit from decompression. Early decompression is also advocated for incomplete lesions, especially if the limbs are becoming progressively weaker. Detailed clinical, radiographic, MRI and CT evaluation will usually be required in order to make informed treatment decisions.

DEFINITIVE CARE

Although some fractures heal with immobilization and time (usually 2–3 months), many patients with complex vertebral fractures will require closed or open reduction and internal fixation to ensure stability. This is usually undertaken by neurological or orthopaedic surgeons with a specialist interest in spinal surgery. Skull traction may be required in the interim, or may be used as definitive treatment. Manipulative reduction in experienced hands can have dramatic effects.[62] When spinal cord injury is present, the patient should be discussed with and, preferably managed by, a specialist spinal injuries unit. If this requires transfer, the patient should be fully resuscitated and accompanied by appropriately trained staff to maintain immobilization and manage any complications (such as respiratory failure).

> **Obtain early specialist advice**

SUMMARY

The management of suspected spinal cord injury involves early immobilization of the whole spine, and the institution of measures to prevent secondary injury from hypoxia, hypoperfusion or further mechanical disturbance. Early ventilation and management of neurogenic shock are the key elements of resuscitation specific to spinal injuries. All spinal injuries should be considered unstable and incomplete until proven otherwise. Careful and informed neurological assessment, together with appropriate plain radiography, will identify the majority of spinal injuries. Emergency treatment involves high-dose steroids for blunt injuries and early consideration for surgical decompression. CT and MRI imaging may be required to define the extent and nature of the injury. Definitive care is best undertaken in specialist multidisciplinary units, and may involve further operative stabilization of the spine.

REFERENCES

1. Swain A. Trauma to the spine and spinal cord. In: Skinner D, Swain A, Peyton R, Robertson C (eds). *Cambridge Textbook of Accident and Emergency Medicine*. Cambridge: Cambridge University Press 1997; pp. 510–32.

2. Leggate JRS, Driscoll PA, Gwinnutt CL, Sweeby CA. Trauma of the spine and spinal cord. In: Driscoll P, Skinner D (eds). *Trauma Care: Beyond the Resuscitation Room*. London: BMJ Books, 1998, pp. 135–55.

3. Berkowitz M, Harvey C, Greene CG, Wilson SE. *The Economic Consequences of Traumatic Spinal Cord Injury*. New York: Demos Publications, 1992.

4. Grundy D, Swain A. ABC of Spinal Cord Injury (3rd ed.). London: BMJ Books, 1996.

5. Burney RE, Maio RF, Maynard F, Karunas R. Incidence, characteristics and outcome of spinal cord injury at trauma centers in North America. *Archives of Surgery* 1993; **128**: 596–9.

6. Toscano J. Prevention of neurological deterioration before admission to a spinal cord injury unit. *Paraplegia* 1988; **26**: 143–50.

7. Savitsky E, Votey S. Emergency approach to acute thoracolumbar spine injury. *Journal of Emergency Medicine* 1997; **15**: 49–60.

8. Burt AA. Thoracolumbar spinal injuries: clinical assessment of the spinal cord injured patient. *Current Orthopedics* 1988; **2**: 210–13.

9. Riggins RS, Kraus JF. The risks of neurologic damage with fractures of the vertebrae. *Journal of Trauma* 1977; **17**: 126–33.

10. Kriss VM, Kriss TC: SCIWORA Spinal Cord Injury Without Radiographic Abnormality in infants and children. *Clinical Pediatrics (Philadelphia)* 1996; **35**: 119–24.

11. Janssen L, Hansebout RR. Pathogenesis of spinal cord injury and newer treatments: a review. *Spine* 1989; **14**: 23–32.

12. Merli GJ, Staas WE Jr. Acute transverse myelopathy: association with body position. *Archives of Physical Medicine and Rehabilitation* 1985; **66**: 325–8.

13. Ali J, Qi W. Pulmonary function and posture in traumatic quadriplegia. *Journal of Trauma* 1995; **39**: 334–7.

14. Cohn SM, Lyle WG, Linden CH, *et al*. Exclusion of cervical spine injury: a prospective study. *Journal of Trauma* 1991; **31**: 570–4.

15. Ravichandran G, Silver JR. Missed injuries of the spinal cord. *British Medical Journal* 1982; **284**: 953–6.

16. Reid DC, Henderson R, Saboe L. Etiology and clinical course of missed spine fractures. *Journal of Trauma* 1987; **27**: 980–6.

17. Gerritis BD, Petersen EU, Mabry J, *et al*. Delayed diagnosis of cervical spine injuries. *Journal of Trauma* 1991; **31**: 1622–6.

18. Davis JW, Phraener DL, Hoyt DB, *et al*. The etiology of missed cervical spine injuries. *Journal of Trauma* 1993; **34**: 342–6.

19. Faculty of Pre-hospital Care of the Royal College of Surgeons of Edinburgh and Joint Royal Colleges Ambulance Service Liaison Committee. Joint position statement on spinal immobilization and extrication. *Pre-hospital Immediate Care* 1998; **2**: 168–72.

20. Majernick TG, Bieniek R, Houston JB, Hughes HG. Cervical spine movement during oro-tracheal intubation. *Annals of Emergency Medicine* 1986; **15**: 417–20.

21. Mcleod ADM, Calder I. Spinal cord injury and direct laryngoscopy – the legend lives on. *British Journal of Anaesthesia* 2000; **84**: 705–9.

22. Ringenberg BJ, Fischer AK, Urdaneta LF, *et al*. Rational ordering of cervical spine radiographs following trauma. *Annals of Emergency Medicine* 1988; **17**: 792–6.

23. Ross SE, O'Malley KF, de long WG, *et al*. Clinical predictors of unstable cervical spine injury in the multiply injured patient. *Injury* 1992; **23**: 317–19.

24. Roberge RJ, Wears RC. Evaluation of neck discomfort, neck tenderness and neurological deficits as indicators for radiography in blunt trauma. *Journal of Emergency Medicine* 1992; **10**: 539–44.

25. Cooper C, Dunham M, Rodriquez A. Falls and major injuries are risk factors for thoracolumbar fractures: cognitive impairment and multiple injuries impede the detection of back pain and tenderness. *Journal of Trauma* 1995; **38**: 692–6.

26. Folman Y, Masri W. Spinal cord injury: prognostic indicators. *Injury* 1989; **20**: 92–3.

27. Kriepke DL, Gillespie KR, McCarthy MC, *et al*. Reliability of indications for cervical spine films in trauma patients. *Journal of Trauma* 1989; **29**: 1438–9.

28. Saddison D, Vanek VW, Racanelli JL. Clinical indications for cervical spine radiographs in alert trauma patients. *American Surgeon* 1991; **57**: 366–9.

29. Hoffman JR, Schriger DL, Mower W, *et al.* Low risk criteria for cervical radiography in blunt trauma: a prospective study. *Annals of Emergency Medicine* 1992; **21**: 1454–60.

30. Roth BJ, Martin RR, Foley K, *et al.* Roentgenographic evaluation of the cervical spine. A selective approach. *Archives of Surgery* 1994; **129**: 643–9.

31. Royal College of Radiologists. *Guidelines for Use of the Radiology Department.* London: Royal College of Radiologists, 1995.

32. Velmahos GC, Theodorou D, Tatevossian R, *et al.* Radiographic cervical spine evaluation in the alert asymptomatic blunt trauma victim: much ado about nothing? *Journal of Trauma* 1996; **40**: 768–74.

33. Clancy MJ. Clearing the cervical spine of adult victims of trauma. *Journal of Accident and Emergency Medicine* 1999; **16**: 208–14.

34. Ross SE, Schwab CW, Eriberto TD, *et al.* Clearing the cervical spine: initial radiologic evaluation. *Journal of Trauma* 1987; **27**: 1055–9.

35. MacDonald RL, Schwartz ML, Mirich D, *et al.* Diagnosis of cervical spine injury in motor vehicle crash victims: how many X-rays are enough? *Journal of Trauma* 1990; **30**: 392–7.

36. West OC, Anbari MM, Pilgram TK, Wilson AJ. Acute cervical spine trauma: diagnostic performance of single-view versus three-view radiographic screening. *Radiology* 1997; **204**: 819–23.

37. Streitweser DR, Knopp R, Wales LR, *et al.* Accuracy of standard radiographic views in detecting cervical spine fractures. *Annals of Emergency Medicine* 1993; **12**: 538–42.

38. Woodring JH, Lee C. Limitations of cervical radiography in the evaluation of acute cervical trauma. *Journal of Trauma* 1993; **34**: 32–9.

39. Annis JA, Finlay DB, Allen MJ, *et al.* A review of cervical spine radiographs in casualty patients. *British Journal of Radiology* 1987; **60**: 1059–61.

40. Pope TL, Riddervold HO. Spine. In: Keats TE (ed.). *Emergency Radiology* (2nd ed.). St Louis, MO: Mosby, 1989.

41. Ireland AJ, Britton I, Forrester AW. Do supine oblique radiographs provide better imaging of the cervicothoracic junction than swimmer's views? *Journal of Accident and Emergency Medicine* 1998; **15**: 151–4.

42. Turestsky DB, Vines FS, Clayman DL, Northup HM. Technique of use of supine oblique views in acute cervical spine trauma. *Annals of Emergency Medicine* 1993; **22**: 685–9.

43. Kirshenbaum KJ, Nadimpalli SR, Fantus R, *et al.* Unsuspected upper cervical spine fractures associated with significant head trauma: role of CT. *Journal of Emergency Medicine* 1990; **8**: 183–98.

44. Kathol MH. Cervical spine trauma. What is new? *Radiologic Clinics of North America* 1997; **35**: 507–32.

45. Sistrom CL, Southall EP, Peddada SD, Schaffer HA. Factors affecting the thickness of the cervical prevertebral soft tissues. *Skeletal Radiology* 1993; **22**: 167–71.

46. Miles KA, Finlay D. Is prevertebral soft tissue swelling a useful sign in injury of the cervical spine? *Injury* 1998; **19**: 177–9.

47. Wilberger JE, Maroon JC. Occult post-traumatic cervical ligamentous instability. *Journal of Spinal Disorders* 1990; **3**: 156–61.

48. Raby N, Berman L, de Lacey G. *Accident and Emergency Radiology: A Survival Guide.* London: WB Saunders, 1995.

49. Keenan TL, Antony J, Benson DR. Non-contiguous spinal fractures. *Journal of Trauma* 1990; **30**: 489–91.

50. Lewis LM, Docherty M, Ruoff BE, *et al.* Flexion/extension views in the evaluation of cervical spine injuries. *Annals of Emergency Medicine* 1991; **20**: 117–21.

51. Borock EC, Grabram SG, Jacobs LM, *et al.* A prospective analysis of a two year experience using computer tomography as an adjunct for cervical spine clearance. *Journal of Trauma* 1991; **31**: 1001–6.

52. Woodring JH, Lee CL. The role and limitations of computerised tomography scanning in the evaluation of cervical trauma. *Journal of Trauma* 1992; **33**: 698–708.

53. Benzel EC, Hart BL, Ball PA, *et al.* Magnetic resonance imaging for the evaluation of patients with occult cervical spine injuries. *Journal of Neurosurgery* 1996; **85**: 824–9.

54. Flanders A, Schaefer D, Doan H, Mishkin M, Gonzales C, Northrup B. Acute cervical spine trauma: correlation of MR findings with degree of neurological deficit. *Radiology* 1990; **177**: 25–33.

55. Johnson G. Early imaging of spinal trauma. *Trauma* 1999; **1**: 227–34.
56. Bracken MB, Shepard MJ, Collins WF, *et al*. Methylprednisolone or naloxone in the treatment of acute spinal cord injury. Results of the second National Acute Spinal Cord Injury Study. *New England Journal of Medicine* 1990; **322**: 1405–11.
57. Bracken MB, Shepard MJ, Collins WF, *et al*. Methylprednisolone or naloxone treatment after acute spinal cord injury: 1 year follow up data. Results of the second National Acute Spinal Cord Injury Study. *Journal of Neurosurgery* 1992; **76**: 23–31.
58. Bracken MB, Shepard MJ, Holford TR, *et al*. Administration of methylprednisolone for 24 or 48 hours or tirilazad mesylate for 48 hours in the treatment of acute spinal cord injury. Results of the third National Acute Spinal Cord Injury randomized controlled trial. *Journal of the American Medical Association* 1997; **277**: 1597–604.
59. Bracken MB, Shepard MJ, Holford TR, *et al*. Methylprednisolone or tirilazad mesylate administration after acute spinal cord injury: 1-year follow up. Results of the third National Acute Spinal Cord Injury randomized controlled trial. *Journal of Neurosurgery* 1998; **89**: 699–706.
60. Bracken MB. *Pharmacological Interventions for Acute Spinal Cord Injury*. The Cochrane Library, Issue 1, Oxford, 2000.
61. Tator CH, Fehlings MG, Thorpe K, Taylor W. Current use and timing of spinal surgery for management of acute spinal injury in North America: results of a retrospective multicentre study. *Journal of Neurosurgery* 1999; **91**: 12–18.
62. Duke RFN, Spreadbury TH. Closed manipulation leading to immediate recovery from cervical spine dislocation with paraplegia. *Lancet* 1981; **i**: 577–8.

11

Ophthalmic injury

OBJECTIVES

- To understand the importance of ophthalmic injury
- To learn to take an ophthalmic history
- To interpret ophthalmic signs
- To identify ophthalmic injuries which indicate neurological damage
- To understand management decisions
- To learn to triage ophthalmic injuries

INTRODUCTION

Ophthalmic injury is common in the workplace, during interpersonal violence, and following road traffic accidents. If the patient has multiple injuries or is unconscious, ophthalmic injuries are easily overlooked. The signs may be subtle and the consequences of a missed diagnosis can lead to blindness.

THE MULTIPLY INJURED PATIENT

The first priority is a thorough correctly performed primary survey with appropriate attention to the airway, breathing, circulation and disability. Obvious eye injuries will be noted under E of the primary survey, or during the performance of airway and other interventions.

> The first priority is always ABC with cervical spine stabilization

An essential part of trauma management is the secondary survey, which must be thorough and include an assessment of the eyes. If this is difficult, then ophthalmic assistance should be sought, since the signs can be subtle and even missed.

If the face is injured, the eye may also be injured, and if the eye is injured the brain may also be injured, particularly with penetrating injury.

> - ABC with neck stabilization comes first
> - A thorough secondary survey should be performed, including the eyes
> - The possibility of occult eye or brain injury must be considered

History

A detailed history of the injury is essential, although such information may not be immediately available in the early stages of the management of a patient with multisystem trauma. The following questions should be considered:

- Is there a possibility of penetrating injury?
- Was there direct blunt trauma or gouge injury?
- Was there a missile injury?
- Was there a chemical injury or burn?
- Is there a past history of ophthalmic disease?
- Is there a history of spectacle or contact lens wear?
- Is the patient taking any eye medication?

Common weapons that cause penetrating injuries include broken glass, knives, snooker cues and pencils. It is especially important to be aware of the possibility of cranial penetration. The presence of direct blunt trauma or gouge injury suggests the possibility of severe ocular injury, with or without fracture of the facial skeleton.

Fragment formation from a hammer hitting a metal chisel, or from snapping metal may result in intraocular foreign bodies which may be very difficult to see. These patients should always undergo X-radiography. Protruding foreign bodies which have penetrated the globe should never be removed in the resuscitation room.

If there is any possibility of a radio-opaque foreign body, always perform an orbital X-radiograph

---

Chemical burns to the eyes are an ophthalmic emergency whether caused by an acid or an alkali, and in either case the eye should be immediately and copiously washed out using at least 1 l of normal saline through a giving set. Alkalis are particularly associated with severe ocular damage, and will rapidly cause severe tissue damage. The possibility of airway injury should also be considered, since chemical vapour can burn the airway and cause laryngeal oedema.

Previous ophthalmic surgery, such as for cataracts, will predispose the patient to rupture of the globe. A history of spectacle wearing raises the possibility of injury from glass fragments, and will affect the future assessment of acuity. Contact lenses should be identified and removed for safe-keeping (for example, in saline in a labelled mid-stream urine pot).

It is important to determine whether the patient is receiving any eye medication, particularly drops which influence pupil size or produce systemic effects (Table 11.1). The taking of any systemic medication for ophthalmic conditions should also be noted.

Table 11.1 *Ophthalmic medications which affect the pupil*

Miosis (constricted pupil)
  Pilocarpine
  Phospholine iodide (also inhibits pseudocholinesterase – beware general anaesthetic)

Mydriasis (dilated pupil)
  Atropine
  Phenylephrine
  Cyclopentolate
  Tropicamide

It should also be noted that a number of eye medications such as beta-blocker eye drops may have systemic effects, while drugs such as opiates or atropine, though given for other reasons, will affect pupillary size.

Symptoms

Wherever possible, an appropriate history should be obtained regarding the onset and development of symptoms. The following facts should be established:

- Has there been any loss of vision and if so, how quickly has it occurred?
- Is the eye painful?
- Is the patient photophobic?

The examination

A formal and detailed examination of the eyes and surrounding structures forms part of the secondary survey; however, signs of significant ophthalmic and facial trauma should be noted as part of the primary survey and investigations should be directed accordingly.

The examination should follow a pre-defined format:

- Record the visual acuity
- Check for a relative afferent pupillary defect (RAPD) (swinging torch test)
- Check facial, lid and ocular symmetry and appearance
- Examine the anterior and posterior segments (the globe).

VISUAL ACUITY

The most basic assessment of visual function is the visual acuity,[1] and this is measured by asking the patient to read a standard reading chart (a Snellen chart). Visual acuity is recorded as a fraction with the distance from the chart recorded as the numerator, and the best line achieved on the chart as the denominator. The patient should wear his/her spectacles, but if they are not available then a pin-hole should be used to overcome any spectacle error. The eyes are tested one at a time, with one eye carefully occluded. Very poor vision is recorded as the ability to count fingers, see hand movements or perceive light.

In the patient with polytrauma, early formal assessment of visual acuity using a Snellen chart is rarely possible, and a less formal estimation will be required pending later re-assessment.

> **Record the visual acuity**

THE SWINGING TORCH TEST

This tests for a relative afferent pupillary defect (RAPD),[2] which assesses optic nerve function and gross retinal function.

1. In reasonable general illumination the direct and consensual reflexes of each pupil are checked with a bright light. The pupils should be of equal size, and should both react to light. It is important not to forget the effects on pupillary activity of any drugs which might have been given previously.
2. The light is shone onto the first pupil for 2 s, and then swung to the other pupil, taking 1 s to swing across. The light is then swung back to the first pupil after 2 s. This movement is repeated for several cycles and the reaction of the pupils is observed.

The pupils should react equally, but if either pupil dilates when the torch is shone on it, that eye has poor retinal or optic nerve function (an afferent pupillary defect).

ASSESSMENT OF FACIAL APPEARANCE

The majority of patients will have a generally symmetrical face. Trauma can cause a fracture of the facial skeleton around the orbit or significant soft-tissue swelling. This may distort the bony and soft-tissue structure, resulting in facial asymmetry.

The horizontal alignment of the pupils and lateral canthi are checked by careful inspection. A more formal method, which is not usually appropriate in the resuscitation room, can be performed by holding a transparent ruler in front of the face. The eyes and lateral canthi should be level. An inferiorly displaced eye indicates a fracture of the floor of the orbit.

The presence of double vision on upwards or downwards gaze and loss of sensation in

the area of the infraorbital nerve should also be sought. These signs are suggestive of an orbital floor fracture with involvement of the inferior rectus muscle and infraorbital nerve.[3] An inferiorly displaced lateral canthus may indicate a fracture of the zygoma. Depression of the zygomatic fracture resulting in an abnormal facial contour on the affected side may also be found, although zygomatic fractures are more commonly associated with swelling. Sensation over the cheek should also be assessed.

The anteroposterior position of the globe should be assessed.[4] Both eyes should appear to be equally prominent, but possible abnormalities include: (i) a sunken eye (*enophthalmos*); and (ii) a protruding eye (*exophthalmos* or *proptosis*). The degree of proptosis or enophthalmos should initially be assessed by careful observation, although subsequent formal assessment with an exophthalmometer will be required following specialist referral.

Fractures of the facial skeleton will require semi-urgent specialist referral unless they involve the airway, or are associated with neurological problems or an orbital haematoma – all of which require urgent intervention. Orbital haematoma is associated with blunt trauma and often with a fracture of the facial skeleton. The haematoma can cause a pressure rise in the posterior part of the orbit, compressing the optic nerve; this is an urgent sight-threatening problem and requires urgent ophthalmic referral.[5] The signs of orbital haematoma are listed in Table 11.2.

Table 11.2 *Signs of orbital haematoma*

- Proptosis
- Reduced or absent ocular movements
- RAPD if the optic nerve is compressed
- Reduced visual acuity
- Tense orbit

RAPD, relative afferent pupillary defect.

Orbital tension is assessed by gently palpating over the swelling through the upper lid. It is important never to press on a penetrated eye as the pressure rise may cause the intraocular contents to extrude.

Never press on a perforated eye

Investigations of facial fractures, which include plain X-radiography and computed tomography (CT) scanning, are unlikely to be a high priority in the patient with multisystem trauma. Nevertheless, appropriate plans should be made for the correct initial and definitive investigations. Definitive investigations will be arranged following referral to the appropriate specialist surgical team.

Facial X-radiographs can be difficult to read, and if there is any doubt then expert advice should be taken. As well as showing soft-tissue swelling and fractures, the presence of fluid (blood) in the sinuses and the so-called tear-drop sign (due to prolapse of the orbital fat pad through an orbital floor fracture) are useful indicators of orbital trauma. CT scanning is particularly good at demonstrating fractures of the floor of the orbit, and the optic canal which can compress the optic nerve (the patient will have reduced vision and a RAPD).

LID INJURIES

Blunt injury can cause a ptosis from avulsion of the levator palpebrae superioris tendon. These patients are treated conservatively. However, it is important to be aware that a third-nerve palsy can also cause a ptosis, and therefore the ocular movements and pupils should be examined in order to exclude this.

Always consider that the eye or brain may be penetrated if the eyelids have a penetrating injury, especially with glass or knife injuries.

Lid lacerations

The wound must be searched for foreign bodies and X-radiographs taken if necessary (it should be remembered that small wounds can hide large foreign bodies). The threshold for performing X-radiographs should be low.

The contour of the lid margins, which should be smooth and continuous should be inspected, and the lids gently retracted in order to examine the eye. This should be done very carefully and may require ophthalmic referral and surgical lid retractors. It is vital not to press on the eye as it may also be penetrated. Penetration of the sinuses should be considered, and such cases will require systemic antibiotics in order to prevent infection.

> • **Always consider damage to underlying structures**
> • **Examine the eye very gently**
> • **If suturing is required, request the ophthalmologist to do this**

ANTERIOR AND POSTERIOR SEGMENTS (THE GLOBE)

Examination of the globe of the eye requires practice and, ideally, the use of a slit lamp. If the use of a slit lamp is not possible, as in the case of major multisystem trauma, a bright penlight and close inspection of the eye, or a magnifier such as the plus 10 lens in the ophthalmoscope, should be used. The fundus should always be examined using an ophthalmoscope. An informal assessment of whether the intraocular pressure is raised can be made by the application of gentle pressure to the closed eye. However, this should never be attempted in the penetrated eye.

> **Never apply an eyepad to a ruptured globe, since this may inadvertently apply pressure and cause extrusion of the contents of the eye**

The anterior segment

The conjunctiva should be smooth and transparent, but blood may have collected underneath it. Following blunt trauma, if the posterior aspect of the haemorrhage cannot be seen, this indicates that blood may have tracked forward from a base of skull fracture. A CT scan should be considered to exclude this, as base of skull fractures are associated with long-term morbidity, and there may be intracranial injury.[6] Subconjunctival blood may also hide a penetration or a rupture of the globe.[7] If there is any suspicion that this may be the case, expert assistance should be sought.

The cornea should be transparent and perfectly smooth, and should give off a bright, even reflection of light. The cornea should be examined carefully for abrasions, lacerations or foreign bodies. Iris pigment may be seen where it has prolapsed forward to plug a hole in the cornea.[8]

The upper lid should be inverted in order to check for foreign bodies. This should not be attempted if the eye is perforated.

Eversion of the upper lid should be carried out in step-wise fashion:

1. The patient is asked to look down.
2. The lashes are grasped between the thumb and forefinger.
3. A cotton bud is placed at the top of the tarsal plate (10 mm from the lid margin).
4. The cotton bud is pushed down and the lashes pulled up; the upper lid should then evert.

> **Do not evert the eyelids if the globe is perforated**

The iris should be flat and have a round pupil at its centre. A distorted iris indicates significant damage to the anterior segment of the eye. Blunt trauma can result in a dilated pupil due to rupture of the sphincter pupillae muscle. Occasionally blunt trauma will cause miosis (pupil constriction).[9]

The presence of blood in the anterior segment indicates damage to the iris, lens, ciliary body or drainage angle. This is called an *hyphaema*, and requires urgent ophthalmic assessment as an uncontrolled rise in intraocular pressure can develop.[10]

Assessment of hyphaema   The lens should be clear; this is best assessed by looking at the red reflex with an ophthalmoscope. Any opacity will appear as a dark area in the reflex. More formal assessment can be carried out with a magnifier or a slit lamp. All ocular trauma patients should have the intra-ocular pressure measured, although this may have to be delayed based on other treatment priorities.

The posterior segment

The fundus should be examined with an ophthalmoscope. Blunt trauma can cause:

- vitreous haemorrhage and a cloudy view;[11]
- comotio retinae, seen as greyish oedema and haemorrhages;[12] and
- retinal tears and detachment (this usually occurs 2 weeks post-trauma).[13]

If it is impossible to examine the eye as a result of severe peri-orbital swelling, specialist advice should be sought from an ophthalmologist.

- **Always suspect a ruptured globe**
- **Always consider cranial penetration**[14]
- **Always record the Glasgow Coma Score**
- **Always perform an appropriate neurological examination**

CHEMICAL INJURY

Chemical injuries are an absolute emergency,[15] and require immediate and copious irrigation with sterile normal saline. Both eyelids should be everted and the conjunctival fornices irrigated. Particles such as lime or cement should be sought and removed. Topical anaesthesia should be applied.

ASSOCIATED INTRACRANIAL INJURY

If there is intracranial injury, then the intracranial pressure can rise. This may be seen as swollen optic discs which should always be sought.[16] The pupils can enlarge due to uncal herniation through the tentorium cerebelli pressing on the third nerve,[17] and so the pupil reactions must always be recorded. The pupils should not be dilated, but if this is done the neurosurgeons should be told as it may mislead them!

The cranial nerves can be damaged, and the ocular movements should be assessed to identify intracranial injury. The patient may not be conscious or cooperative, so these tests may have to be performed later. The cranial nerves and general nervous system should always be examined for associated signs.

NON-ACCIDENTAL INJURY[18]

Although fortunately relatively rare, non-accidental injury to children does occur and there are a number of specific ophthalmological manifestations which should not be missed. Infants generally do not get black eyes accidentally, and corneal cigarette burns may be deliberately inflicted despite apparently plausible explanations. Retinal haemorrhages occur in shaken babies. It is important to be aware that children do not 'malinger', and reduced vision with a normal examination may indicate psychological problems. If there is any doubt, the child should be admitted and the ophthalmologist and the paediatrician involved.

INVESTIGATIONS

Fractures

Suspected facial or orbital fractures require plain X-rays to be taken of the orbits and face; these may demonstrate the fracture directly or show associated signs such as a fluid level in the maxillary sinus. The best investigation for these fractures is a CT scan, but this should be organized as a routine investigation.[19] A tense orbital haematoma does not need urgent CT scanning as this will delay the appropriate management – which is urgent decompression of the orbit.

Lid lacerations

Lid lacerations should be assessed critically for any chance of cranial penetration with a low threshold for X-ray and CT scanning.[20] A base of skull fracture will only normally be demonstrated by CT scanning, but this examination does not need to be ordered urgently.

Foreign bodies

All ocular foreign bodies should be treated as being potentially intraocular, and there should be a low threshold for performing X-ray of the eye in such cases. If a view of the fundus is not possible, an ultrasound can provide details of retinal detachment, intraocular foreign body or posterior scleral rupture.

TREATMENT

Corneal or subtarsal foreign body

These should be removed carefully with a needle, using the slit lamp biomicroscope. Corneal foreign bodies may be buried in the corneal stroma and require quite vigorous débridement, which is a specialist procedure. If there is any doubt about the situation, ophthalmic assistance should be sought.

Corneal abrasions

These are very painful but heal quickly. The pupil should be dilated in order to ease ciliary muscle spasm, antibiotic ointment instilled, and a firm double eye-pad applied. The eye must be shut before the pad is applied. The patient can remove the pad the next day and instil antibiotic drops four times a day. Topical anaesthetic drops should not be given for use at home since they inhibit corneal epithelial cell division and hence healing.[21]

Penetrating injury[22]

This is a surgical emergency. The patient should not have topical medication applied to the eye. The eye should be covered with an eye-shield (not a pad, as this will press on the eye and cause the contents to extrude).

The patient should be nursed sitting up, and adequate pain relief must be given. A tetanus booster must be given if appropriate, and the patient should also be given systemic antibiotics (ciprofloxacin penetrates the eye well and has a broad spectrum of activity). The patient must remain nil-by-mouth, and arrangements should be

made for the ophthalmologist to take the patient to the operating theatre as soon as possible.

Orbital haematoma[5]

This is usually a mild problem which requires only conservative management.

If the orbit is very tense, urgent ophthalmic advice should be obtained. The patient may require orbital decompression through the upper lid and/or high-dose systemic steroids. These patients can be difficult to assess, and ophthalmological assistance is essential.

Orbital fractures[3]

Patients with orbital fractures should be told not to blow their nose, and treatment with systemic antibiotics with a broad spectrum (including anti-anaerobic cover) should be started. Further management can be delayed if there is no airway compromise.

Hyphaema[10]

The presence of a hyphaema indicates significant intraocular trauma, and as such should be assessed by an ophthalmologist. The management includes bed-rest sitting up, pupil dilatation with atropine drops and, if the intraocular pressure is raised, appropriate medical management. If necessary, anterior chamber washout can be considered, although this is potentially hazardous.

Lid lacerations[23]

These all require appropriate plastic surgical techniques for effective closure; therefore they should be referred after the administration of a tetanus booster[24] and systemic antibiotics as indicated.

The polytrauma patient

Although the immediately life-threatening problems should be addressed first, ophthalmic injury can lead to severe lifetime disability, and the presence of an ophthalmic injury should be sought in all polytrauma patients.

It is important to note that the eyes may be damaged by remote injury. For example, crush injuries to a limb or the chest can result in retinal damage from emboli or Purtscher's retinopathy.[12] Episodes of hypotension can result in infarction of the occipital cortex or the optic nerves.[25]

Useful ophthalmic preparations

For the prescription of ophthalmic preparations, prefixes are used to denote whether the formulation is an ointment, or should be used as drops.

- Oc indicates an ointment formulation.
- Gutt or G indicates a drop formulation.

Topical preparations contain preservatives which are toxic to the inside of the eye and thus should not be applied to eyes that may have been penetrated.

The most common ophthalmic drugs used in the casualty department (and their uses) are listed in Table 11.3.

Table 11.3 *Ophthalmic preparations*

Drug	Use
Amethocaine, benoxinate	Topical anaesthetic. For examination of the patient with corneal foreign body or corneal abrasion. Stings on application.
Fluorescein	Orange dye which adheres to areas of cornea with no epithelium. This fluoresces as yellow green under a blue light when dilute, and is adherent to de-epithelialized cornea. Will stain soft contact lenses yellow.
Cyclopentolate, tropicamide	Dilate the pupil. Pale irises dilate quickly and dark irises dilate slowly. Always record in the notes which drug was used to dilate pupils and when it was given.
Chloramphenicol, fucithalmic	Broad-spectrum topical antibiotics. Used as prophylaxis in cases of corneal abrasion and foreign bodies.
Ofloxacin	Broad-spectrum, strongly bactericidal antibiotic used in cases of severe corneal infection.
Betagan, acetazolamide, pilocarpine	Used to reduce intraocular pressure. Betagan can cause asthma; acetazolamide is a systemic preparation and should not be used in patients with renal failure. Pilocarpine will cause the pupil to constrict.
Dexamethasone	Steroid used to reduce anterior segment inflammation. Beware side effect of raised intraocular pressure.
Ciprofloxacin	Broad-spectrum bactericidal systemic antibiotic which penetrates the eye through the blood–retinal barrier. Used in penetrating ocular injury.
Cefuroxime, metronidazole	Systemic antibiotics used in orbital fractures and lid lacerations. Note metronidazole is useful in sinus injury. Cefuroxime may not cover streptococci.

Note: atropine and homatropine last for a long time (up to several days) and should not be used in the Accident and Emergency Department.

SUMMARY

The eye should always be assessed in a careful and systematic fashion. This can be difficult and may require specialist skills. A low threshold for seeking ophthalmological assistance is appropriate. The priorities in the management of the multiply injured patient remain those of the primary survey, but it is important to remember that ophthalmic injury can lead to lifetime visual disability that may be prevented by appropriate timely intervention. Thus, it is vital to judge the management priorities appropriately.

REFERENCES

1. Westheimer G. Visual acuity. In: Moses RA, Hart WM (eds). *Adler's Physiology of the Eye: Clinical Application*. St Louis: Mosby, 1987, pp. 415–28.
2. Thompson HS, Corbett JJ, Cox TA. How to measure the relative afferent pupillary defect. *Survey of Ophthalmology* 1981; **26**: 39–42.
3. Dutton JJ. Management of blow-out fractures of the orbit. *Survey of Ophthalmology* 1991; **35**: 279–80.
4. Orbit, eyelids, and lacrimal system. Section 7. *American Academy of Ophthalmology Basic and Clinical Science Course*. P. 113.
5. Liu D. A simplified technique of orbital decompression for severe retrobulbar haemorrhage. *American Journal of Ophthalmology* 1993; **116**: 34–7.
6. Kylstra J. Preparation of the eye trauma patient for surgery. In: Shingleton BJ, Hersh PS, Kenyon KR (eds). *Eye Trauma*. St Louis: Mosby, 1991, p. 53.

7. Kylstra J, Lamkin JC, Runyan DK. Clinical predictors of scleral rupture after blunt ocular trauma. *American Journal of Ophthalmology* 1993; **115**: 530–5.

8. Barr CC. Prognostic factors in corneoscleral lacerations. *Archives of Ophthalmology* 1983; **101**: 919–24.

9. Kennedy RH, Brubaker RF. Taumatic hyphaema in a defined population. *American Journal of Ophthalmology* 1988; **106**: 123–30.

10. Little BC, Aylward GW. The medical management of traumatic hyphaema. *Journal of the Royal Society for Medicine* 1993; **86**: 458–9.

11. Cinotti AA, Maltzman BA. Prognosis and treatment of perforating ocular injuries. *Ophthalmic Surgery* 1975; **6**: 54–61.

12. Bressler SB, Bressler NM. Traumatic maculopathies. In: Shingleton BJ, Hersh PS, Kenyon KR (eds). *Eye Trauma*. St Louis: Mosby, 1991, pp. 187–94.

13. Cox MS, Schepens CL, Freeman HM. Retinal detachment due to ocular contusion. *Archives of Ophthalmology* 1966; **76**: 678–85.

14. De Villiers JC, Sevel D. Intracranial complications of transorbital stab wounds. *British Journal of Ophthalmology* 1975; **59**: 52–6.

15. Pfister R. Chemical injuries of the eye. *Ophthalmology* 1983; **90**: 1246-53.

16. Frisen L. Swelling of the optic nerve head: a staging scheme. *Journal of Neurology, Neurosurgery and Psychiatry* 1982; **45**: 13–18.

17. Leigh RJ, Zee DS. Diagnosis of peripheral oculomotor palsies and strabismus. In: *The Neurology of Eye Movements*. Philadelphia: FA Davis Co., 1991, p. 331.

18. Harley RD. Ocular manifestations of child abuse. *Journal of Pediatric Ophthalmology and Strabismus* 1980; **17**: 5013–28.

19. Grove AS. Computed tomography in the management of orbital trauma. *Ophthalmology* 1982; **89**: 433–40.

20. Thompson JT, Paarver LM, Enger C, and National Eye Trauma Study (NETS). Endophthalmitis after penetrating ocular injuries with retained intra-ocular foreign bodies. *Ophthalmology* 1993; **100**: 1468–74.

21. Abelson MB. The final points of corneal abrasion management. *Reviews in Ophthalmology* 1995; **February**: 111–12.

22. Esmaeli B, Elner S, Schork MA, Elner VM. Visual outcome and ocular survival after penetrating trauma. *Ophthalmology* 1995; **102**: 393–400.

23. Eyelid and lacrimal trauma. In: Spoor TC (ed.). *An Atlas of Ophthalmic Trauma*. London: Martin Dunitz 1997, pp. 67–94.

24. Committee on trauma of the American College of Surgeons, Prophylaxis against tetanus in wound management. *Bulletin of the American College of Surgery* 1984; **69**: 22–3.

25. Lessell S. Indirect optic nerve trauma. *Archives of Ophthalmology* 1989; **107**: 382–6.

12

Maxillofacial injuries

OBJECTIVES

- To understand the importance of facial injuries in airway obstruction and haemorrhage
- To provide a systematic approach to the assessment of facial injuries
- To describe simple and effective methods of treating maxillofacial emergencies in the resuscitation room

INTRODUCTION

Since the Second World War, interpersonal violence has overtaken road traffic accidents (RTAs) to become the most common cause of maxillofacial injuries. In a typical study of facial injuries in the UK, 52% resulted from assaults, whereas RTAs were responsible for 16% and sport 19%. Some 11% were caused by falls, and only 2% by industrial accidents.[1] Home Office statistics show that recorded violent crime against the person more than doubled between 1974 and 1990, and continues to rise.

The most common facial injury in an assault victim is a laceration, this being the situation in almost 40% of all assaults.[2] Those most commonly assaulted are young men between the ages of 18 and 25 years, and about 50% of victims have positive blood-alcohol levels. Alcohol is the most important contributory factor in assault cases, and may also complicate the initial management of the injuries.

One study has shown that 30% of all assault victims had fractures, and 83% of these were of the facial skeleton.[2] Midface fractures are more common in RTAs, whereas nasal bone fractures and fractures of the mandible and zygoma are more common in assaults.

- **Interpersonal violence is now the most common cause of a facial injury in the United Kingdom**
- **50% of assault victims with facial injuries will have raised blood-alcohol levels**

ANATOMICAL CONSIDERATIONS (Figures 12.1 and 12.2)

The airway

The most common cause of death in facial injuries is airway obstruction. This is often due to the tongue simply falling backwards in the unconscious patient and obstructing the airway. This is more likely with bilateral fractures of the mandible where the tongue may lose its anterior support. Facial injuries also commonly cause fractures of the teeth or dentures, with bleeding in the mouth. This also compromises the airway when the patient is lying on his/her back. Conscious patients with mouth and face injuries are usually more

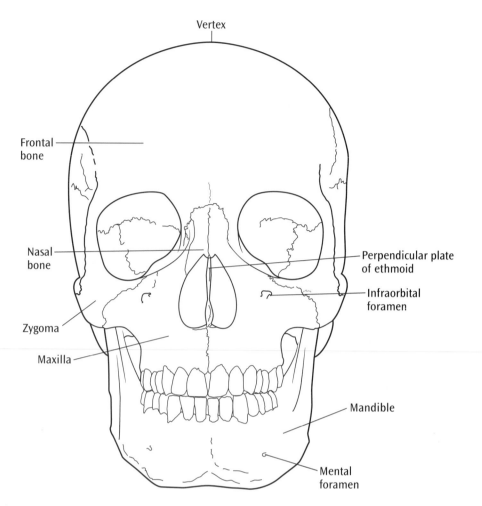

Figure 12.1 *Anterior view of the skull and facial bones.*

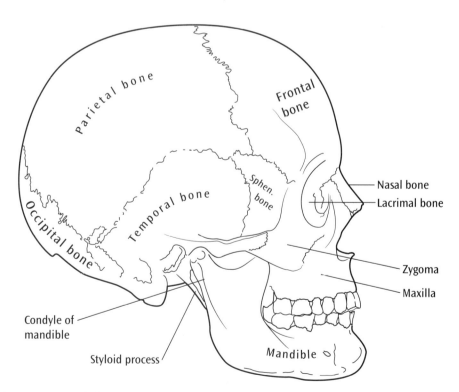

Figure 12.2 *Lateral view of the skull and facial bones.*

comfortable sitting up, with their heads forward, in order to allow blood and saliva to drain out of the mouth.

The middle third of the facial skeleton

The middle third of the facial skeleton is a complex three-dimensional structure consisting mainly of the two maxillae and nasal bones centrally, and the zygomatic bones laterally. It is attached to the base of the skull and may usefully be regarded as a 'crumple zone' like that incorporated into the design of a car. In a frontal impact, the middle third of the face will crumple and absorb some of the force which would otherwise be transmitted to the skull and brain. As it is pushed backwards, the middle third slides down the sloping base of the skull, obstructing the airway and causing an anterior open bite. Pulling the upper jaw forwards in this situation may therefore relieve the airway. The maxilla tends to separate from the skull base at one of three levels originally described by Le Fort (Figure 12.3).[3]

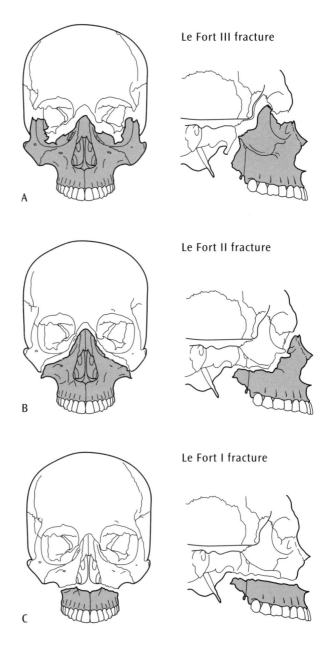

Figure 12.3 *Le Fort fracture dislocations of the maxilla.*

The mandible

The mandible, together with its attached structures, forms the lower third of the facial skeleton, and is slung beneath the skull base, articulating with the temporal bones at the temporomandibular joints. The necks of the condyles just inferior to the temporomandibular joints are a point of weakness, and fractures commonly occur here from force transmitted through the mandible from a blow on the chin. The combination of a laceration on the chin, and bilateral condylar fractures is sometimes called the 'guardsman fracture', as it might occur when fainting on parade and falling forwards on to the chin.

Soft tissues

The soft tissues which cover the facial skeleton have an excellent blood supply. This, when associated with the dramatic appearance that some facial injuries may have, can lead the inexperienced to attribute hypovolaemic shock to the facial injury, and overlook internal bleeding in the abdomen or thorax. Large lacerations of the face tend to gape because of muscle pull, and may give the impression of tissue loss, when this is not the case. It should be remembered that soft-tissue wounds of the lower neck, such as stab wounds, may involve the apex of the lung (Figure 12.4a and b).

Facial injuries, particularly those to the middle third of the face, may cause rapid soft-tissue swelling. This ballooning of the tissues can mask underlying fractures. Gross swelling of the eyelids can hide significant damage to the globe of the eye. The high incidence of missed eye injury in midface trauma has been documented.[4] The zygoma forms part of the orbit and affords protection to the globe. The greatest proportion of missed eye injuries are associated with fractures of the orbitozygomatic complex.

The cervical spine

The head is supported on the cervical spine, which is easily damaged in deceleration injuries or falls. There is therefore a relationship between facial injuries, head injuries and injuries to the cervical spine.

> **Where an unconscious patient has a significant facial injury, there is a 10–15% chance that there is an injury to the cervical spine**

The teeth

Teeth are frequently knocked out or fractured in facial injuries. They may be inhaled, especially in the unconscious patient, and cause pulmonary complications if not removed with the bronchoscope at an early stage. The anatomy of the airways is such that a tooth is more likely to be impacted in the right main bronchus, and demonstrated on chest radiographs near the right border of the heart shadow. Smaller fragments of teeth may slip down into the more peripheral airways, making their recovery more difficult. Ingested teeth will generally pass through the alimentary tract uneventfully.

Avulsed teeth may also be displaced into the soft tissues, particularly of the lip. Lip lacerations should be carefully explored before closure in the presence of missing or broken front teeth. A fracture of the crown of a tooth may expose the pulp of the tooth; this is extremely painful and frequently the main complaint of a patient with a facial injury.

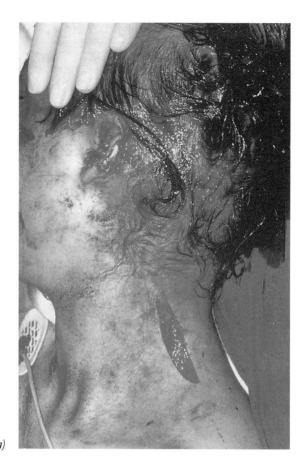

(a)

(b)

Figure 12.4 *Stab wound to the left neck (a) causing a haemopneumothorax seen on X-ray (b).*

MANAGEMENT

This section deals with the management of a facial injury from the time the casualty arrives in the Accident Unit until the maxillofacial team takes over the case for definitive management. A greater understanding of basic trauma management principles, and improved paramedic training has greatly improved the pre-hospital care of trauma victims, and the number reaching the Accident Unit alive.

The initial management of the facial injury follows the principles described earlier in this manual. Particular care should be taken to stabilize the cervical spine, in view of the association of neck injury with maxillofacial trauma. The primary survey is intended to detect and remedy immediately life-threatening injuries. The exact diagnosis of the type of facial injury is unnecessary during the primary survey, and is delayed until the secondary survey or later.

The detailed nature of each intervention during the primary survey will not be repeated here, as this has been covered in other sections of the manual (see Chapter 3). Those aspects of the primary and secondary survey particularly relevant to maxillofacial injuries will, however, be emphasized.

THE PRIMARY SURVEY

The primary survey comprises five aspects:

- Airway with cervical spine control
- Breathing
- Circulation
- Disability
- Exposure and environmental control.

For each parameter of the primary survey, the principles are to:

1. Assess
2. Control
3. Treat.

Airway with cervical spine control

The patency of the airway should be immediately assessed, as airway obstruction is the most common cause of death in facial injury. While the airway is being assessed and re-established, the cervical spine should be immobilized. It is important to speak to the casualty and to ask his/her name. The response affords immediate information on the level of consciousness, patency of the airway, and ability to breathe.

> **Many patients with facial injuries will be under the influence of alcohol or drugs. But – never assume that confusion, abusiveness or lack of cooperation is due to alcohol – it may be due to hypoxia**

At this stage it is important to:

- **look** for:
  - agitation due to hypoxia
  - cyanosis; this is best seen around the lips or lining of the mouth
  - the use of the accessory muscles of respiration.
- **listen** for:
  - the characteristic noises of airway obstruction – stridor, snoring or gurgling
  - hoarseness suggesting damage to the larynx.

ESTABLISH THE AIRWAY

Although severe facial injuries look intimidating, it is usually possible to establish an airway with simple procedures. It is unusual to have to resort to an immediate surgical airway unless there is a foreign body impacted in the vocal cords, or there is direct damage to the larynx.

- **The main cause of death in facial injury is airway obstruction**
- **The conscious patient may be more comfortable sitting up with his/her head forward. This allows blood and secretions to drain out of the mouth rather than fall to the back of the throat**

The vital stages in airway establishment are to:

- clear debris (broken teeth/dentures) from the mouth with a careful finger sweep and suction;
- chin lift and jaw thrust – the chin lift may be difficult when the face is covered with blood and slippery to the touch;
- consider pulling the tongue forwards;
- consider disimpaction of displaced maxilla; and
- consider pulling a displaced mandible forwards.

In the unconscious patient, pulling the tongue forwards is easier with a towel clip or with a suture passed through the dorsum of the tongue as far posteriorly as possible. Other instruments tend to crush the tongue and make it swell. In a fracture of the middle third of the facial skeleton, the upper jaw may have been pushed back to slide down the skull base and obstruct the airway. The inability of the front teeth to meet together vertically (anterior open bite) may suggest this. In this case the upper jaw should be held and pulled forward to disimpact it, and clear the airway. Where there is a bilateral fracture of the mandible, the central portion of the mandible to which the tongue is attached may have fallen backwards, allowing the tongue to fall back against the posterior wall of the pharynx. Again, pulling the anterior part of the mandible forward may clear the airway.

If the airway cannot be established by these simple methods, a laryngoscope should be used to check that there is not a foreign body such as a denture impacted in the vocal cords, and if there is, to remove it. If it cannot be removed quickly and easily, it should be left and a surgical airway performed. If no foreign body is seen and it is possible to pass an endotracheal tube, this should be undertaken. If there is oedema around the glottis, or the degree of bleeding is too great to enable the operator to see the vocal cords, again, a surgical airway should be performed.

Cricothyroidotomy

A cricothyroidotomy is the preferred way to establish a surgical airway in an emergency.[5] Tracheostomy should not be regarded as an emergency operation to be carried out in the Accident Unit, unless there is an experienced surgeon present.

Cricothyroidotomy should not be performed in children under the age of 12 years, because of the risk of damaging the cricoid cartilage. The cricoid is the only circumferential support for the upper trachea in this age group, keeping the trachea open. In a child, the alternative is needle cricothyroidotomy.

Tracheostomy

In laryngeal fractures, tracheostomy is preferred to needle cricothyroidotomy because of anatomical disruption. This should always be performed by an experienced surgeon. *Needle tracheostomy* may buy valuable time in the interim.

- **In an acute emergency, cricothyroidotomy is faster and safer than tracheostomy**
- **Avoid cricothyroidotomy under the age of 12 years**
- **Tracheostomy rather than cricothyroidotomy should be carried out in the presence of a fractured larynx**

Maintain the airway

Once an airway has been established, it must be maintained and frequently re-assessed. The method used will depend on the extent of the facial injury and the level of consciousness, as well as the need to protect the lower airway from blood or vomit, or both. The airway may be maintained by:

- posture;
- oropharyngeal airway;
- nasopharyngeal airway;
- intubation;
- surgical airway; or
- tongue suture.

An oropharyngeal airway is easily dislodged, and poorly tolerated in a responsive patient, while a nasopharyngeal airway is better tolerated and less likely to be dislodged. Neither will prevent the aspiration of blood or debris and either may become blocked with a blood clot. Care is required when passing a nasopharyngeal airway in a patient with fractures of the middle third of the facial skeleton, as these may be associated with skull base fractures. The tube should be passed horizontally through the nostril, and not upwards towards the skull base. Once in position, a nasogastric tube can be passed through it to aspirate the stomach contents.

In severe facial injuries, the main threat to the airway is bleeding into the mouth and oropharynx. Endotracheal intubation with a cuffed tube is preferable, as this protects the lower airways and facilitates ventilation. Depending on the level of consciousness, this may require the use of sedation and muscle relaxants. However, intubation can be difficult when there is uncontrolled bleeding into the mouth. A surgical airway should not be delayed by repeated attempts to intubate.

- **Oropharyngeal tubes may be poorly tolerated and easily displaced in the restless patient**
- **Great care is required when passing a nasopharyngeal airway in the presence of a skull base fracture**
- **Intubation may be difficult in the presence of uncontrolled bleeding in to the mouth and pharynx. Never persist with attempts at intubation if a surgical airway would be more appropriate**

IMMOBILIZE THE CERVICAL SPINE

The cervical spine should have been manually stabilized during the establishment of an airway. This is particularly important during attempts to intubate. Casualties will often arrive with the cervical spine already immobilized with a semi-rigid collar, and in general this should not be removed until a cervical spine fracture has been excluded radiographically. However, if intubation or a surgical airway is required, it will be necessary temporarily to remove the collar to allow surgical access. Careful manual immobilization is then required during the procedure.

If the casualty has arrived without a cervical collar, the cervical spine should now be immobilized with a collar, tapes and sandbags. In head and neck injuries time is saved if, just before the collar is fitted, the neck is observed for venous congestion, and the position of the trachea is palpated. If a laryngeal fracture is suspected, the larynx may be felt to detect crepitus.

However, before the collar is fitted, look at the neck for:

- swelling;
- wounds;
- surgical emphysema;
- tracheal deviation;
- laryngeal crepitus; and
- raised jugular venous pressure.

Breathing

The assessment, control and treatment of breathing difficulty is described elsewhere in this manual (see Chapter 4), and is not modified in the presence of facial and neck injuries. It is important to remember that :

- facial injuries sustained in RTAs are frequently associated with chest and abdominal injuries, including diaphragmatic rupture; and
- penetrating injuries to the lower part of the neck may involve the apex of the lung, to cause a haemopneumothorax. Damage to the phrenic nerve in the neck will also paralyse the diaphragm.

Circulation

The tissues of the head and neck have a good blood supply. However, in the absence of damage to the major vessels in the neck, or severe middle third facial fractures, the degree of bleeding is usually insufficient to cause clinical hypovolaemic shock with a reduction in blood pressure.

It is vital not to assume that hypovolaemic shock is due to maxillofacial injuries. It is easy for attention to be diverted by a severe facial injury, and to miss covert bleeding into the lungs, abdomen or pelvis. Scalp injuries may also bleed profusely; this alone is unlikely to cause hypovolaemia in an adult, but significant scalp injuries in children may be life-threatening.

> **Never assume that shock is due solely to facial or scalp bleeding**

Post-nasal bleeding into the oropharynx in severe middle third facial fractures may be torrential, and difficult to control. It often signifies a base of skull fracture.

The assessment and control of bleeding follows the principles outlined elsewhere in the manual (see Chapter 6). The following applies specifically to maxillofacial injuries.

Major bleeding from the soft tissues of the head and neck can usually be controlled by direct pressure to the bleeding site. Once the bleeding has stopped, the wound should not be probed, particularly if it is in the neck, until the casualty is in an operating environment where bleeding can be controlled surgically.

> **Probing wounds in the neck may precipitate severe recurrent bleeds**

In the Accident Unit it is important to avoid the temptation to clamp bleeding vessels in the neck, unless they can be seen clearly and cannot be controlled with pressure. Inappropriate attempts at clamping may tear blood vessels, and important nerves like the vagus or accessory nerves may be inadvertently clamped.

> **Avoid the temptation to clamp bleeding vessels**

Bleeding inside the mouth may be inaccessible to direct pressure, other than biting on a swab. If the general condition of the casualty permits, sitting them up will not only reduce venous bleeding but will also allow blood to escape through the mouth rather than fall to the back of the throat and block the airway.

Bleeding from the inferior alveolar artery within the mandible will usually be controlled once the mandibular fracture is reduced and held immobile for a few minutes. It may be helpful to pass a wire around the teeth on either side of a bleeding mandibular fracture, tightening it to pull the ends of the fracture together; in this case, maxillofacial assistance will be required.

One of the most difficult situations to manage in maxillofacial trauma is torrential bleeding from the region of the nasopharynx following trauma to the middle third of the facial skeleton. This often signifies a fracture of the skull base in this area, and can require massive resuscitation.

> **In catastrophic bleeding, intubation or a surgical airway may be necessary to secure the airway**

The following interventions may help to control severe bleeding into the nasopharynx.

- Even with good suction, blood accumulates in the back of the throat and obstructs the airway. Endotracheal intubation with a cuffed tube is required to protect the airway. If intubation cannot be achieved, a surgical airway should be inserted, again using a cuffed tube. A 6- or 7-mm cuffed tracheostomy tube can usually be inserted through a cricothyroidotomy. If the condition of the casualty permits, the head of the bed should be raised to reduce the venous pressure at the skull base.
- Consideration should be given to inserting anterior and posterior nasal packs. Alternatively, it often helps to pass a Foley catheter through each nostril, until they can be seen behind the soft palate. The catheter balloon can then be inflated and pulled forward to impact in the nasopharynx. A variation on this is the Epistat™ device with anterior and posterior balloons which can be inflated to apply pressure also to the anterior nasal cavity.
- If the maxilla is very mobile, the nasopharyngeal balloons or packs may simply press the posterior maxilla downwards, rather than apply pressure to the skull base. If this happens, it will be necessary to push firmly upwards with a finger at the back of the palate.

Disability: brief neurological examination

The assessment of the level of consciousness in the primary survey by the AVPU method is unchanged in the presence of maxillofacial injuries. However, it is important to remember that:

- pupil signs may be misleading in the presence of cranio-orbital trauma; there may, for example, be a traumatic mydriasis, causing one pupil to be larger than the other.
- the presence of blindness in one or both eyes should be established at an early stage as prompt surgical decompression of the orbit or optic nerve may be effective in some circumstances. Even if the eyes are closed by swelling, it is possible, in the conscious patient, to put a pen torch against the swollen eyelid, and ask whether the casualty can see the light.
- Approximately 50% of maxillofacial injuries are caused by assault, and 50% of those assaults are alcohol-related. The level of consciousness may be altered by alcohol or drugs. Confusion and agitation may result from hypoxia as well as from alcohol or drugs. Facial fractures with swelling of the tongue and dental malocclusion also contribute to poor speech.

In accepting the additional difficulties of AVPU assessment in the presence of maxillofacial injuries, the important principle is to establish – and record – a baseline level of deficit which can be regularly re-assessed to detect deterioration at an early stage.

Exposure and environmental control

The casualty must be completely undressed, but kept warm, in order to allow a full examination and detection of other injuries. The cervical spine must be kept immobile as the patient's clothes are cut off.

SECONDARY SURVEY

The secondary survey will only be described here as it relates to the maxillofacial region. In the absence of airway obstruction, or uncontrolled bleeding, the definitive treatment of maxillofacial injuries may usually be delayed until the patient is completely resuscitated, and the life-threatening injuries have been dealt with.

Examination of the head and face

The head and face should be inspected for swelling and bruising. Swelling may mask the deformity associated with underlying fractures of the facial bones. The bruising and swelling of a 'black eye' may mask fractures of the orbitozygomatic complex, or damage to the globe of the eye.

Examination of the skull base

Evidence of a skull base fracture should be sought. 'Panda eyes', bruising over the mastoid (Battle's sign) or subconjunctival haemorrhage associated with skull base fractures, may take some hours to develop.

Le Fort II and III fractures of the maxilla, and nasoethmoid fractures, are often associated with fractures of the cribriform plate of the ethmoid, leading to a leak of cerebrospinal fluid (CSF) down the nose. This may be difficult to detect in the early stages as the CSF is mixed with blood. A clue may be given by the 'tramlines' left by mixed blood and CSF running down the cheek (the blood tends to separate from the CSF to leave two lines of blood, separated by CSF). Subsequently, further investigations may be required to confirm the presence of CSF leak.

Examination of the ears

Evidence of haematoma, lacerations of the external canal, and evidence of skull base injury should be sought in the ears. In addition, the ears should be examined for haematoma, lacerations of the external canal, and evidence of skull base injury. Blood in the external auditory canal is often due to a tear in the anterior wall following a blow to the mandible that has forced the head of the condyle back into the canal.

If the tympanic membrane is intact in the presence of a skull base fracture, CSF will not be seen, but the tympanic membrane will bulge outwards and have a blue appearance due to blood in the middle ear.

Examination of the face and scalp

The face and scalp should be examined for lacerations. Scalp lacerations should be gently probed with a gloved finger to detect depressed fractures of the underlying skull.

It is important to make sure that branches of the facial nerve have not been damaged (Figure 12.5). The branches of the nerve should be tested by asking the casualty to raise his/her eyebrows, screw up their eyes and show their teeth. Microneural repair of the damaged branches is much easier if carried out at initial wound exploration and closure in the operating theatre.

> **When examining facial lacerations, always test the branches of the facial (7th cranial) nerve**

If the parotid salivary duct has been severed by a cheek laceration, it will require repair. If lacerations are to be sutured in the Accident Unit, the wounds should be explored to exclude the presence of foreign bodies, such as teeth fragments in lip lacerations, and

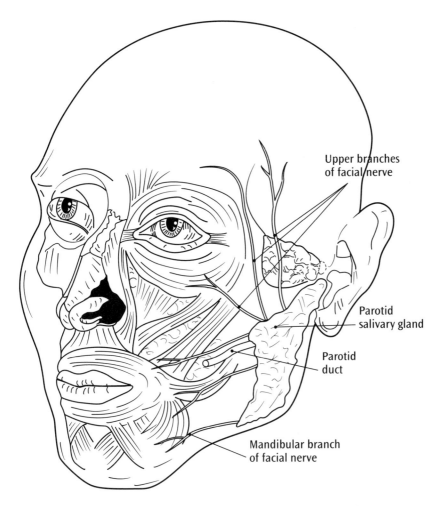

Upper branches
of facial nerve

Parotid
salivary gland

Parotid
duct

Mandibular branch
of facial nerve

Figure 12.5 *The main branches of the facial nerve and the position of the parotid duct.*

appropriate radiographs should be performed. Wounds should also be thoroughly cleaned
to prevent tattooing with debris.[5]

> **If there is any possibility of foreign body (for example, teeth and glass),
> always perform an X-radiograph**

Examination of the eyes

The eyes should always be examined to detect globe damage or fractures of the orbital walls.
The reactivity of the pupils which will have originally been noted as part of AVPU in the
primary survey should be re-checked, looking for any signs suggestive of deterioration.
When the eyelids are swollen, it is painful to force them open to allow examination of the
fundus. By shining a pen torch held against the lids, the casualty will be say whether he/she
sees light, indicating if the visual pathway is intact, or not. It may be necessary to delay a full
ophthalmological assessment until the swelling has reduced.

> **Always remove the patient's contact lenses**

There is a high incidence of missed injuries to the globe associated with fractures of the orbitozygomatic complex. Under these circumstances the casualty should have a full eye assessment performed by an ophthalmologist.

Any subconjunctival haemorrhage should be noted. If the posterior limit of the bleeding cannot be seen, this indicates that it is blood tracking forwards from a fracture. This sign may take some hours to develop. Subconjunctival bleeding with a visible posterior limit is due to direct trauma to the conjunctiva. Double vision should be recorded, as this may indicate oedema in the orbit, or a blow-out fracture of the orbital walls (usually the orbital floor) (Table 12.1). Blow-out fractures are commonly missed as they do not show readily on standard radiographs. In general, a blow-out fracture of the orbit should be suspected when double vision is associated with numbness of the skin, in the distribution of the infraorbital nerve, even if no fracture is seen on the occipitomental radiograph. There may be tethering of the globe on that side when the casualty is asked to look up.

Table 12.1 *The signs and symptoms of an orbital blow-out fracture*

- Swelling and bruising around the eye
- Diplopia, usually looking upwards; often associated with pain
- Tethering of the globe when looking up; the globe may retract backwards when looking up
- A sunken eye (enophthalmos), although this may take time to develop and may not be initially apparent
- Numbness over the cheek and upper lip on that side in the distribution of the infraorbital nerve

Isolated orbital floor fractures may not be apparent on the standard 15° occipitomental radiograph, but there will usually be blood in the associated maxillary sinus, causing opacity on the radiograph. If the sinus is not too opaque, the 'hanging-drop sign' may be present. This is a small bulging opacity below the shadow of the infraorbital margin on the occipitomental radiograph, representing herniation of the periorbital fat down through the fractured orbital floor. In practice, this injury is usually confirmed on a coronal computed tomography (CT) scan.

Palpation of the facial bones

The facial bones should be palpated in order to detect fractures. Painful bruising and swelling may mask underlying fractures. Fractures of the zygoma and orbit are particularly easy to miss when there is a swollen black eye.

> **Beware of the black eye! It is easy to overlook a fracture of the orbitozygomatic complex, or damage to the globe of the eye**

MANDIBULAR FRACTURES

Clinical features of mandibular fractures include:

- pain on movement;
- swelling and bruising;
- the teeth do not meet properly (change in dental occlusion);
- a step in the occlusal plane of the teeth;
- numbness of the chin and lower lip on that side; and/or
- bleeding from the mouth.

Radiography in mandibular fractures
These should include an orthopantomogram and PA mandible.

MAXILLARY FRACTURES

Clinical features of maxillary fractures include:

- gross swelling of the face (ballooning);
- disruption of the dental occlusion;
- nosebleed; and
- the upper jaw can be moved.

In a Le Fort I fracture, only the tooth-bearing portion of the maxilla is mobile, while in a Le Fort II fracture the bridge of the nose moves with the maxilla. In a Le Fort III fracture, both cheekbones move with the maxilla.

In maxillary fractures, the middle of the face may look flat, and CSF may leak from the nose if the cribriform plate is fractured.

Radiography in maxillary fractures

These should include a 15° occipitomental investigation (CT is desirable in Le Fort II and III fractures following consultation with maxillofacial surgeons).

ZYGOMATIC FRACTURES

Clinical features of zygomatic fractures include:

- black eye;
- bloodshot eye (subconjunctival haemorrhage);
- flat cheek unless masked by swelling;
- possible double vision;
- numbness of the skin of the cheek in the distribution of the infraorbital nerve; and
- unilateral nosebleed.

Radiography in fractures of the zygoma

This should comprise a 15° occipitomental investigation.

NASAL FRACTURES

Clinical features of fractures of the nasal bones (or nasoethmoid complex) include:

- the bridge of the nose being swollen and tender;
- the nose being deformed;
- bleeding from the nose; and
- the nasal septum being deviated, blocking the nostril.

If the nasoethmoid complex is fractured, the angle between the forehead and nose is deepened, and fractures may be felt on the infraorbital margin on each side. There may also be a CSF leak.

Radiography in nasal fractures

Standard radiographs are often of little help in the diagnosis of a broken nose. A CT scan is indicated for nasoethmoid fractures in order to determine the extent of frontal sinus involvement.

INJURIES TO THE LARYNX AND TRACHEA

Clinical features of laryngeal and tracheal injuries include:

- evidence of direct trauma to the neck;
- noisy breathing (snoring, gurgling, croaking);
- hoarseness of the voice; and
- crepitus.

Radiography in laryngeal injuries

CT scanning should be used to investigate laryngeal injury.

Examination of the teeth and mouth

If the upper and lower teeth do not seem to meet properly, this may indicate a fracture of the maxilla or mandible. Some dental malocclusions are pre-existing and are developmental in origin. A haematoma in the floor of the mouth strongly suggests a mandibular fracture. Fractured teeth exposing the pulp may be very painful and require early dental management. Broken or avulsed teeth should be accounted for. They may be:

- lost at the scene of the accident;
- intruded into the gum;
- inhaled;
- ingested; or
- lying in the soft tissues, particularly the lip, as a foreign body.

Chest radiographs should be taken to exclude the presence of a tooth in the bronchus (often the right main bronchus). Small fragments of teeth may work their way further down into the airways. It is important to identify tooth fragments in the lung and to refer for a specialist opinion.

- **Always try to account for missing teeth or pieces of broken denture, even if the casualty did not lose consciousness. If they cannot be accounted for, a chest X-radiograph should be taken**
- **Inhaled teeth must be identified and removed by bronchoscopy**

SUMMARY

Facial injuries, whether in isolation or in combination with other injuries, should be managed in accordance with the principles emphasized throughout this manual. Significant facial injuries often appear more serious than they are, but if the primary and secondary surveys are carried out carefully, more serious life-threatening conditions will not be overlooked. When death occurs from a facial injury, it is nearly always from airway obstruction.

REFERENCES

1. Crosher RF, Llewelyn J, MacFarlane A. Should patients with facial fractures be regarded as high risks for HIV? *British Journal of Oral and Maxillofacial Surgery* 1997; **35**: 59–63.
2. Shepherd JP, Shapland M, Scully C, Leslie IJ. Pattern, severity and aetiology of injury in assault. *Journal of the Royal Society of Medicine* 1990; **83**: 75–8.
3. LeFort R. Étude experimentale sur les fractures de la machoire supérieure. *Revue de Chirurgie de Paris* 1901; **23**: 208–27, 360–79, 479–507.
4. Al-Qurainy A, Stassen LFA, Dutton GN, Moos KF, El-Attar A. The characteristics of midface fractures and the association with ocular injury: a prospective study. *British Journal of Oral and Maxillofacial Surgery* 1991; **29**: 291–301.
4. Brantigan CO, Grow JB. Cricothyroidotomy: elective use in respiratory problems requiring tracheostomy. *The Journal of Thoracic and Cardiovascular Surgery* 1976; **71:** 72–81.
6. Schmelzeisen R, Gellrich NC. The primary management of soft tissue trauma. In: Ward Booth P, Schendel SA, Hausamen JE (eds). *Maxillofacial Surgery*. London: Churchill Livingstone, 1999, pp. 229–44.

13

Injuries in children

OBJECTIVES

- To understand the epidemiological, anatomical, physiological and societal differences between paediatric and adult trauma
- To offer an approach to the severely injured child
- To explain the principles of assessment and resuscitation of the injured child
- To outline the age-specific problems within body systems of the injured child
- To highlight psychological effects of trauma on children

INTRODUCTION

It is well established that trauma is the commonest cause of death in children over the age of 1 year. Injury is also a significant cause of permanent disability. It is, however, uncommon for hospital or pre-hospital staff to have to deal with a severely traumatized child. In the four years from 1994 to 1997 the UK trauma network recorded a total of 741 children with an Injury Severity Score of 16 or more presenting to Accident and Emergency (A&E) departments in England and Wales.[1] Of these 741 children, 549 (74%) were over 5 years of age. The average A&E department can, therefore, only expect to deal with two or three severely injured children per year. Severe trauma in the pre-school child is particularly uncommon.

An epidemiological study of childhood trauma deaths showed that 74% of children who died from injury had no signs of life on the arrival of the first responder.[2] Resuscitation was only of potential benefit to the 26% of children who had vital signs on the arrival of the emergency services. If this pattern of death after trauma is indeed typical, then improvements in resuscitation are likely to have a marginal effect on childhood mortality rates. This is in marked contrast to the proven benefit of preventive measures that involve a change in environment.

INITIAL ASSESSMENT AND MANAGEMENT

There are important anatomical, physiological and psychological reasons why children are not small adults. These differences are more than a matter of scale.

The arrival of a severely injured child should be preceded by a warning from the pre-hospital services. Specialist staff should be notified and age-specific equipment prepared. If the age of the child is known, an approximate weight can be calculated using the formula:

$$\text{Weight (in kg)} = (\text{age in years} + 4) \times 2$$

Drug doses and fluid volumes are calculated on a weight basis. A designated marker board can be used to display age, weight, equipment sizes, fluid bolus volumes and drug doses for the expected child. Once the child has arrived in the resuscitation room a structured and methodical approach should be followed. Life-threatening injuries are identified and treated during the primary survey. This is followed by the more detailed secondary survey. A structured approach will allow a calm environment to prevail. There is a good case for allowing the parents to remain with the child during the resuscitation to offer reassurance and to gain the child's cooperation. A designated individual should be allocated to look after the parents and explain events as they develop. The parents should be positioned where the child can see them, and physical contact between the parent and the child encouraged.

The primary survey follows the format of the mnemonic ABCDE.

Airway

An initial 15 second assessment of airway and breathing is made, and the cervical spine is simultaneously immobilized. The cervical spine should remain immobilized until a spinal injury has been excluded clinically and radiographically. Ideally the child should be immobilized with a semi-rigid collar, sand bags and tape, though this degree of immobilization may not be possible in the chubby infant or combative child.

If a child can talk, then the airway may be assumed to be patent. If there is any suspicion of airway obstruction or of altered conscious level, then further attention to the airway is required.

The jaw thrust is an important airway manoeuvre in the unconscious injured child, as it should not cause movement of the cervical spine. Airway manoeuvres such as head tilt and chin lift are best avoided because they may compromise in-line immobilization of the cervical spine.

Blood, vomitus or foreign material in the oropharnyx should be cleared by gentle suction under direct vision. All children with significant trauma should be given 100% oxygen. This is optimally achieved using a non-rebreathing facemask. If airway obstruction does not respond to a jaw thrust, a nasopharyngeal or oropharyngeal airway may be inserted. Nasopharyngeal airways are not widely available in paediatric sizes, but a shortened uncuffed lubricated endotracheal tube may serve the same purpose.

> Size of oropharyngeal tube: centre of lower incisors to the angle of the mandible (concave side upward)
> Size of nasopharyngeal tube: tip of nose to tragus of ear

If the airway cannot be secured with basic manoeuvres, then an advanced airway technique is indicated. Tracheal intubation in the injured child should be performed by an experienced practitioner, using a rapid sequence induction to avoid further rises in intracranial pressure.

> Size of oral endotracheal tube:
>   Length in cm = (age/2) + 12
>   Internal diameter = (age/4) + 4
>   In children aged less than 12 years, uncuffed endotracheal tubes should be used

Needle cricothyroidotomy may be performed as a temporizing measure, but a formal cricothyroidotomy should not be performed in a child aged less than 12 years.

Breathing

The work and effectiveness of breathing is assessed by 'looking, listening and feeling'. If respiratory efforts are inadequate, ventilation should be assisted using a bag-valve apparatus.

The chest must be examined for obvious injury, checking tracheal position, palpating for crepitus and chest expansion and auscultating for normal and abnormal breath sounds. There is a higher incidence of tension pneumothorax in children because of the more mobile mediastinum. This condition should be diagnosed clinically and requires immediate decompression with a needle thoracocentesis using a 16-gauge cannula inserted in the second intercostal space in the mid-clavicular line, followed by insertion of a chest drain (Table 13.1).

Table 13.1 *Chest drain sizes in children*

Age	Chest drain size (French gauge)
0–12 months	12–16
1–5 years	16–20
5–10 years	20–24
10–15 years	24–28

Massive haemothorax may require chest drain insertion if it is causing respiratory distress, but intravenous access and fluid resuscitation should take priority.

Circulation

It may be difficult to recognize circulatory compromise in the child. The initial signs of shock are non-specific, as the child has an enormous capacity to compensate for hypovolaemia. Deterioration and decompensation, when it occurs, may be precipitous. Peripheral perfusion can be gauged by assessing the capillary refill. The nail bed is pressed for 5 s, and the refill time should be less than 2 s. Normal values for heart rate and blood pressure in children are given in Table 13.2. Tachycardia is a non-specific response to pain and fear.

> **Any child who has cool pale skin and a tachycardia should be presumed to have hypovolaemia, irrespective of blood pressure measurements**

Table 13.2 *Heart rate in children*

Age (years)	Normal heart rate range (beats/min)
<1	110–160
2–5	95–140
5–12	80–120
>12	60–100

> **Systolic blood pressure (mmHg) = 80 + (age in years $\times$ 2)**

Any child with severe injury should have intravenous access secured, the simplest method being cannulation of a peripheral vein. Veins on the hands, cubital fossae and feet are all suitable. Intravenous access may be technically difficult, particularly in the chubby toddler.

If peripheral venous access is not possible, then intraosseous access should be considered. This technique can be easily used up to the age of 6 years, but is rarely necessary after the age of 3 as venous access is unlikely to be a major difficulty.

Intra-osseous needle sites:
    Tibia: anterior tibia 2–3 cm below tibial tuberosity
    Femur: anterolateral 3 cm above lateral condyle

Alternative forms of vascular access include:

- cannulation of the femoral vein using a Seldinger technique;
- peripheral cut-down at the long saphenous or cephalic veins; or
- cannulation of the external jugular vein.

Cannulation of the subclavian and internal jugular veins should only be attempted as a last resort, as this procedure is often technically difficult and complications are not uncommon.

Blood should be sent for routine biochemistry, haematology and cross-matching. Children have decreased glycogen stores and are more prone to hypoglycaemia than adults. Thus, the blood glucose should always be measured and hypoglycaemia treated with 5 ml/kg of 10% dextrose (0.5 g/kg of dextrose). An intravenous fluid bolus should be given to all children with evidence of shock.

> **Initial fluid bolus = 20 ml/kg**

The initial fluid bolus should be warmed crystalloid or colloid. This may be repeated once, but if there is an inadequate response then blood should be administered. Ideally this should be cross-matched, but if not available type-specific or O-negative blood should be used.

Disability

A rapid assessment of the neurological status is made using either the AVPU method (see below) or the Glasgow Coma Score (GCS), depending on the age of the child. The standard GCS is not applicable to children under the age of 5 years, in which case the modified verbal response should be utilized (see below).

- The pupillary response is tested.
- The AVPU assessment is carried out:
  A: Alert
  V: responds to Vocal stimulus
  P: responds to Painful stimulus
  U: Unresponsive

Exposure

Because of their greater body surface area children are at much greater risk of hypothermia, and therefore although they must be exposed for examination, appropriate precautions must be taken to avoid loss of heat.

Adjuncts to the primary survey

RADIOGRAPHY

The primary survey should be accompanied by X-rays of the chest, pelvis anteroposterior (AP) view, and the lateral cervical spine.

ANALGESIA

Analgesia should be administered to any injured child. Pain assessment in children is difficult, and visual analogue charts can be helpful. There is no role for intramuscular or oral opiates in the severely injured child, as absorption is unpredictable and any benefit may be delayed. Analgesia is optimally achieved by intravenous morphine at a dose of 0.1–0.2 mg/kg.

Local nerve blocks can be useful; femoral nerve blocks are particularly effective for fractures of the femoral shaft, using bupivicaine (2 mg/kg) or lignocaine (3 mg/kg).

NASOGASTRIC TUBE PLACEMENT

Children have a tendency to swallow air when frightened or in pain. This leads to acute gastric dilatation, causing abdominal pain and diaphragmatic splinting, and putting the child at risk of regurgitation and aspiration. Abdominal examination may be difficult and misleading under such circumstances. A nasogastric tube will decompress gastric dilatation. A gastric tube should be placed in any seriously injured child, while an orogastric tube should be used if a basal skull fracture is suspected.

URINARY CATHETER

If an injured child can pass urine spontaneously and urine production does not need to be measured accurately, then urinary catheterization may be avoided. However, if accurate measurement of urine output is required (for example, in a burned child), then a urinary catheter should be inserted. If urinary catheterization is indicated, the smallest silastic catheter should be used.

In children weighing less than 15 kg catheters with an inflatable balloon should not be used; rather a small-bore feeding tube should be inserted as a catheter.

If there are concerns about uretheral injury in boys, a suprapubic catheter is indicated, but this procedure should only be performed by those with appropriate experience.

Secondary survey

On completion of the primary survey any immediately life-threatening injuries should have been identified and the child stabilized. The secondary survey may then be undertaken, which entails a detailed head-to-toe examination of the child. In addition, detailed information about both the child and the circumstances of the accident should be obtained.

HEAD INJURIES

Each year in the UK, about 4000 children (male:female ratio, 2:1) per 100 000 of the population attend an A&E department with a head injury.[3] About 40% of these children have scalp lacerations, while only 9% have evidence of any brain injury (amnesia or impairment of consciousness). Head injury is the commonest cause of death in children aged between 1 and 15 years, with an annual incidence of approximately 5 per 100 000 population.[4] It is important to record the mechanism of injury; infants suffering non-accidental injury (NAI) and older children who are involved in road traffic accidents (RTAs) tend to have more extensive injuries than from other causes. Similarly, falls from more than twice the child's height are associated with severe injury. Avoidable factors have been shown to contribute to unnecessary mortality and morbidity.[5]

Pathophysiology

The initial injury gives rise to 'primary damage' (cortical contusions, lacerations, diffuse axonal injury, diffuse vascular injury) which depends largely on the force involved. Both intracranial (haematoma, brain swelling, oedema, infection) and extracranial (hypoxia, hypotension, hypercarbia, fever, metabolic disturbance) factors contribute to 'secondary damage'.

Primary damage may best be modified by prevention through public health and legal measures (use of rear seat belts, cycle helmets, playground design, 'at risk' registers), whereas secondary damage can be minimized by optimal medical and nursing management.

ASSESSMENT IN THE A&E DEPARTMENT

The airway, breathing, circulation and cervical spine (ABC) need immediate attention, and should be managed using existing guidelines.[5,6] Cervical spine injury in association with head injury (although uncommon) *must* be considered particularly where the injury was forceful (for example, following a significant fall or RTA), or where the child's level of consciousness does not allow any assessment of neck pain. While assessing the airway, examination of the posterior pharyngeal wall may reveal bruising, indicating a possible high cervical injury. A lateral and AP radiograph of the complete cervical spine to C7/T1 must be seen. Particular interest should be paid to the upper cervical spine, which is a more common site of injury in children compared with adults. A quick assessment of level of consciousness should be made using AVPU. There is a modified version for children under the age of 4 years,[6] as the verbal responses differ in the very young! Resuscitation should be instituted where necessary, followed by a second, more detailed assessment of the history, particularly from the paramedics, and a complete examination as the secondary survey.

HISTORY

The important features in the history include:

- The mechanism, time and place of injury.
- Loss of consciousness at the time or subsequently, and whether the level of consciousness has been improving, is unchanged, or is deteriorating.
- A period of amnesia after the head injury.
- Was there anything to suggest a seizure?
- Any previous medical condition likely to affect the assessment (e.g. cerebral palsy, diabetes, epilepsy), or the outcome (e.g. anticoagulants).

In infants, particularly in the first four months of life, it is important to consider if the story is credible as NAI must be considered.

EXAMINATION

The level of consciousness should be assessed (using the GCS; Table 13.3), and pupil size and reactivity, symmetry of limb movements and vital signs (respiratory rate, pulse rate, blood pressure and temperature), recorded on a standard chart. These observations should be repeated every 15 min if consciousness is impaired, and every hour for the first 4 h if it is not.

If a painful stimulus needs to be applied, pressure over the supraorbital notch is least likely to leave lasting painful bruises, and gives information through trigeminal sensory pathways relayed through the brainstem. Fingernail bed or sternal pressure may elicit motor responses through spinal pathways and so can confuse the assessment of brain function.

For eye-opening, if the eyes are closed by swelling, then c is recorded. For best verbal response if the patient has an endotracheal tube or tracheostomy *in situ*, e is charted, whereas d is given for dysphasia. In the best motor response, the limb with the best response is noted. The components of the verbal response are altered to be more age-appropriate for children under the age of 5 years (Table 13.4).

Table 13.3 *Glasgow Coma Scale*

Eye-opening:	4	Spontaneously
	3	To speech
	2	To pain
	1	No response to stimulation
Best verbal response:	5	Orientated
	4	Confused
	3	Inappropriate
	2	Incomprehensible sounds
	1	No sounds
Best motor response:	6	Obeys commands
	5	Localizes
	4	Normal flexion to pain
	3	Abnormal flexion to pain
	2	Extension to pain
	1	No response to pain

Table 13.4 *Modified verbal component of the Glasgow Coma Scale for children under 5 years*

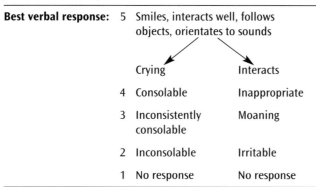

Best verbal response:	5	Smiles, interacts well, follows objects, orientates to sounds	
		Crying	Interacts
	4	Consolable	Inappropriate
	3	Inconsistently consolable	Moaning
	2	Inconsolable	Irritable
	1	No response	No response

Young children must have their height and weight measured. The scalp and face should be examined for bruising (often felt as a 'boggy' swelling), and lacerations. Penetrating injury occurs around the orbit and temporal bone and may be obvious. If the foreign body has been removed there may only be a small wound. The anterior fontanelle, if patent, should be palpated for signs of raised intracranial pressure. The fontanelle is usually closed by 9 months of age, but may remain patent until 18 months or later.

The fundi should be examined for retinal haemorrhages, particularly in infants where NAI is suspected. Restriction of external ocular movements may occur from orbital fractures or cranial nerve injury.

Fractures of the anterior cranial fossa may produce:

- CSF rhinorrhoea;
- epistaxis;
- periorbital haematoma(s);
- subconjunctival haemorrhage; or
- anosmia (this is uncommon and can be difficult to elicit in the very young).

The tympanic membrane should be examined for haemotympanum, a tear or CSF otorrhoea. There may be evidence of bruising over the mastoid region, indicative of a mastoid fracture ('Battle's sign'); this sign may become apparent some hours or days after the injury.

A full examination for other injuries should then be undertaken. In infants it is important to look for signs of neglect, shaking or previous injury.

DISCHARGE, ADMISSION OR INVESTIGATION?

Emergency computed tomography (CT) should be performed in a child with clinical or radiological evidence of a fracture, altered or deteriorating level of consciousness (GCS 14 or less), a seizure, or focal neurological signs. Children who have had a trivial injury, have not lost consciousness, are alert and orientated with no abnormal signs on examination and have good family support, may be discharged.

Further observation or imaging is required in the child who is alert, orientated and obeying commands (GCS 15) if:

- the mechanism of injury was not trivial;
- consciousness was lost;
- there is post-traumatic amnesia;
- there is persistent headache or vomiting; or
- there is a scalp haematoma or full-thickness laceration.

The initial investigation of choice is a plain skull radiograph; however, the yield from skull radiographs in children between 2 and 15 years of age is very small, as brain injury occurs without a skull fracture in children more frequently than in adults.[7,8]

The increasing availability of CT scanning offers an effective alternative to plain radiographs, and provides more information but with much higher X-ray exposure. In addition, in small children, CT scanning is often only possible after sedation or anaesthesia. Alternatively, where facilities exist, the child can be admitted for observation for at least 6 h (avoiding a skull radiograph), and CT scanning performed only if consciousness deteriorates or symptoms – particularly headache and vomiting – persist.

Imaging should be reported at the time by a radiologist, as radiologically apparent skull fractures are frequently missed. Teleradiology links to the regional neurosurgical unit are valuable in the management of the child with an abnormal scan.[9,10]

Hospital admission

The child who is alert and orientated (GCS 15) should be admitted if there are any features of the following:

- abnormal behaviour;
- persisting nausea and vomiting;
- seizures;
- focal neurological signs;
- abnormal radiology (skull fracture or abnormal CT); or
- suspicion of NAI.

Any child with a GCS of less than 15 must be admitted.

Referral to a neurosurgeon

A child should be discussed with a neurosurgeon if:

- neurosurgical assessment, monitoring and management are required;
- the CT scan shows an intracranial lesion; or
- CT cannot be performed locally within a reasonable time.

Neurosurgical assessment, monitoring and management are required in a child with a CSF leak, a suspected or definite penetrating injury, a compound depressed skull fracture, a 'growing' fracture, a seizure or focal neurological signs, persisting lowered level of consciousness after resuscitation, or deterioration in the level of consciousness. The latter is most usefully defined as a sustained drop of one point on motor or verbal scores, or two points on the eye-opening score.

Discharge from hospital

A reliable parent or guardian must be at home, the child must be alert and orientated (for 12 h), and symptoms such as nausea, headache and dizziness must be resolving.

CHEST TRAUMA

Epidemiology

Data on the incidence of paediatric thoracic trauma is particularly sparse in the UK, with figures from the UK trauma audit and research network showing that during 1996–98, of 59 443 injured children, only 0.7% sustained thoracic injuries. Of those children with an injury severity score >16, 25% had thoracic trauma,[1] this being because thoracic injuries are often associated with head or abdominal injuries.[11] Most thoracic injuries are blunt, the incidence of penetrating trauma being 3.7%. The commonest cause of chest injury is a road traffic accident (RTA), with the child being involved as a pedestrian. Thoracic trauma is a marker of serious injury and is associated with extrathoracic injuries in 70% of cases. The mortality is most closely related to these other injuries (Table 13.5).

Table 13.5 *Mortality from thoracic injuries*

Type of injury	Mortality rate (%)[12]
Overall	26
Isolated thoracic injury	5
Thoracic and abdominal injuries	20
Thoracic and head injuries	35
Thoracic, abdominal and head injuries	39

Special considerations in paediatric chest trauma

Although children may suffer the same range of injuries as seen in adults, the pattern of injury in children is different owing to anatomical and physiological differences.

THE HEART

The heart occupies a greater proportion of the anterior chest in comparison with that in adults. This is important to remember when treating penetrating trauma or inserting left chest drains.

THE RESPIRATORY SYSTEM

At birth, the lungs are relatively small and immature, with alveolar development continuing until the age of 8 years. Young children have less pulmonary reserve, and this may contribute to the high mortality from pulmonary contusions seen in children.

THE MEDIASTINUM

This is relatively more mobile; tension pneumothorax can cause the inferior vena cava to kink at the diaphragm. This leads to profound impairment of venous return to the heart; hence tension pneumothorax can cause electromechanical dissociation.

THE RIBS

The ribs are much more pliable in pre-adolescence, so fractures are seen less frequently. Significant intrathoracic injury has been shown to occur without rib fractures in up to 52% of cases.[13]

Injuries to the heart, great vessels, haemothorax and lung laceration carry the greatest mortality rates. A series studying children with blunt chest injury following RTAs reported a pulmonary contusion rate of 73%. There was an 8% death rate, principally associated with fatal brain injury.[14]

Management

Injured children should be approached in a similar manner to adults, using a system of simultaneous primary survey and treatment of immediately life-threatening conditions.

Consideration of the mechanism of injury will aid in the diagnosis of chest injuries, which although not apparent on primary survey, may well prove life-threatening later. Very few patients require surgery; most injuries can be managed with observation or a chest drain.

> **All children with chest injuries require 100% oxygen**

TENSION PNEUMOTHORAX

This is a clinical diagnosis and may present with reduced air entry, tracheal deviation, hyper-resonance, respiratory distress and hypotension. The immediate treatment is insertion of a large-bore cannula in the second intercostal space, mid-clavicular line, followed by an appropriately sized intercostal drain in the fifth intercostal space between the mid-axillary and anterior axillary lines. This drain should be directed towards the ipsilateral lung apex.

MASSIVE HAEMOTHORAX

This may be diagnosed clinically, the signs on the affected side being decreased air entry with dullness to percussion, and reduced breath sounds.

On the chest X-ray there will be the appearance of massive fluid accumulation in the relevant hemithorax, which may amount to a complete 'white out'.

Haemorrhage into the pleural cavity and compression of the lung may cause hypoxia. Management of the hypoxic child when no other cause is evident is to insert an intercostal chest drain immediately after obtaining venous access and correcting the hypovolaemia. Children with massive haemothorax will require urgent blood transfusion (O-negative or type-specific) and an appropriate surgical referral.

Precipitous drainage, in otherwise stable patients, of large haemothoraces without replacement blood and surgical support at hand can remove a tamponade effect and lead to disastrous further haemorrhage.

OPEN PNEUMOTHORAX

An open or sucking wound in the chest wall compromises respiratory mechanics, leading to hypoxia. Air may be felt flowing through the wound and signs of pneumothorax may be present. Classically, occlusion of the wound with a dressing fixed on three sides (acting as a valve) is recommended, but more recently the Ashermann chest seal has been developed. This has an integral valve which is placed over the top of the open wound and serves the same function more efficiently. An intercostal drain will subsequently be required.

CARDIAC TAMPONADE

Blood in the pericardium reduces venous return and therefore compromises cardiac output. The child will have a clinical picture suggestive of shock. The classical sign of distended neck veins may be difficult to detect or be absent, especially if hypovolaemia is present. Cardiac tamponade following trauma will usually require surgery, and the child should always be reviewed by an experienced surgeon. Intravenous fluid resuscitation may not improve the cardiac output.

> **Pericardiocentesis may be of benefit before definitive treatment, but should not delay surgery**

Pericardiocentesis is performed with a long needle of 14–16 G inserted below the xiphisternum, inclined at 45% and aimed towards the tip of the left scapula with ECG monitoring throughout. If the patient is stable and the facility is available, echocardiography can confirm the diagnosis and provide ultrasonically-directed pericardiocentesis.

Chest radiography in thoracic trauma

The portable supine chest X-ray is the mainstay initial investigation of thoracic trauma. It has been estimated that serious chest injuries are missed or underestimated in 38% of chest X-rays,[15,16] with anterior pneumothoraces and small haemothoraces being commonly missed. Thus, if an intrathoracic injury is suspected clinically and is not evident on the plain chest X-ray, a contrast-enhanced CT scan should be performed.

An injured child with blunt trauma who requires a CT scan of the abdomen, should also have the thorax scanned. This takes little extra time and may detect the thoracic injuries not seen on the plain chest X-ray. Any child sent for CT scanning must be accompanied by a team who can deal with any sudden deterioration in the child's condition

Emergency thoracotomy

There is little experience of paediatric emergency thoracotomy in the UK, but a review of 17 such cases from America suggests that it should not be performed in patients who present without signs of life.[17] Emergency thoracotomy should *only* be considered in patients with either: (i) penetrating trauma; or (ii) blunt trauma with detectable vital signs and deterioration despite maximal conventional therapy.

Injuries which are not immediately life-threatening

RIB FRACTURES

The incidence of rib fractures in pre-adolescent children with thoracic trauma is 50%.[13] This is much lower than in adults as there is less calcification in the young rib, and so increased pliability. Considerable force can therefore be transmitted to the thoracic contents without the ribs fracturing. Rib fractures require only analgesia, but their presence should alert the clinician to the possibility of other injuries, particularly pulmonary contusion.

Particular types of rib fracture should be noted:

- *Posterior rib fractures*: in infants, these are highly suggestive of NAI.
- *Flail chest*: this involves multiple rib fractures, producing an unstable section of chest wall that moves paradoxically, and usually requires mechanical ventilation.
- *First rib*: as in adults, fracture of the first rib is a particularly serious injury, and is nearly always associated with other injuries.

PULMONARY CONTUSION

This is the commonest lesion in children with blunt thoracic trauma, with an incidence of 50–70%. The alveoli fill with blood from ruptured capillaries so the affected area does not allow gaseous exchange, and instead acts as a shunt. The treatment is analgesia, oxygen therapy and judicious fluid replacement. Further management is guided by oxygen saturation and arterial blood gases. Careful fluid management is important in pulmonary contusion as over-infusion of intravenous crystalloids may cause pulmonary oedema and further impair respiratory function. Under-hydration will, however, cause inspissation of sputum and increased difficulty in clearance of bronchial secretions.

A proportion of pulmonary contusions will be associated with pneumothoraces, haemothoraces and pleural effusions. Flail chest can rarely occur with pulmonary contusion, often heralding the need for pain relief and ventilation. These should be treated appropriately.

CARDIAC CONTUSION

Severe cardiac contusion is usually fatal at the scene. Cardiac contusion presenting clinically with ECG abnormalities in thoracic trauma is rare. Prospective studies where the lesion has been sought by specific investigation have shown an incidence of 14%. Management is by ECG monitoring and the treatment of any cardiac dysrhythmias.

INJURY TO THE GREAT VESSELS

This is suggested by a widened mediastinum, though this sign is not often seen. These injuries are rarely seen, most children dying before arrival at hospital. Post-mortem studies of all trauma victims have shown that 2% of children who died from trauma had ruptured aortas. This study also showed that of those who sustained this injury as vehicle passengers, none was wearing a seat belt.[18]

Patients who reach hospital do so because the tear is contained by the adventitia of the vessel. The diagnosis is suggested by a widened mediastinum on the chest X-ray. If aortic damage is suspected, a contrast enhanced CT or aortogram is required immediately.

RUPTURED DIAPHRAGM

This usually occurs on the left. Gross herniation of abdominal viscera into the chest can cause respiratory compromise. The injury is usually (but not always) visible on the initial chest X-ray, though may not be suspected until a nasogastric tube is passed and noted to be in the chest on X-radiography.

TRACHEOBRONCHIAL INJURY

These injuries are rare, but may present with: (i) a massive and persistent air leak; or (ii) pneumothorax despite adequate intercostal drainage. If the diagnosis is suspected, the child should be referred to a cardiothoracic surgeon for investigation and repair.

> **Most thoracic injuries can be dealt with by simple interventions, dealing with airway, breathing, circulation, and the judicious use of intercostal drains**

ABDOMINAL TRAUMA

The abdomen is the third commonest site of injury after head injuries and isolated limb fractures. As pre-adolescent children have short and incompletely ossified thoracic cages and widened sternocostal angles, the abdominal organs are especially vulnerable to even minor degrees of force. In the UK, the majority of paediatric abdominal injuries result from blunt trauma. In children who have clear clinical or X-radiographic evidence of injury but no significant history of trauma, the possibility of NAI must be considered.

The vast majority of paediatric abdominal injuries can be successfully treated conservatively. Surgery is rarely required in the acute phase, and the mainstay of treatment is appropriate resuscitation. Inexpert treatment of paediatric abdominal injury (including inadequate resuscitation) accounts for up to 35% of all preventable deaths. Hence, the early involvement of an experienced paediatric surgeon and senior anaesthetic support is mandatory in this setting but only *rarely* is surgical intervention required.

The primary survey

The effects of abdominal trauma on the primary survey are discussed below.

BREATHING

Diaphragmatic splinting may be due to excess air (aerophagia, particularly if the child is distressed and in pain) or fluid in the peritoneum.

CIRCULATION

The abdomen is a common site for occult blood loss and can contribute to hypovolaemia; adequate fluid replacement is mandatory. Blood is needed after two boluses of 20 ml/kg of intravenous crystalloid.

There is no place for radiological investigation until the circulatory status has been restored to normal, either by conservative management or by surgical intervention.

The secondary survey

The nature and mechanism of injury is a critical factor in assessing a child with suspected abdominal injury. Where possible, the direction and momentum of impact should be established and a full history must be taken, including a description of the scene from witnesses, as well as ambulance staff. It is important to distinguish between direct blunt trauma (for example, blows to the abdomen from people, cars or bicycles) and indirect or deceleration injuries (for example, falls or injuries to restrained passengers in vehicles).

MOVEMENT

Time is never wasted by looking carefully before touching the patient. The abdomen must be observed for movement, distension and for any surface injuries. Is the abdomen moving easily with respiration, or is it being held rigid? A rigid abdomen indicates internal injury but normal movement does *not* exclude organ damage.

DISTENSION

The normal abdomen of the supine child is flat or even scaphoid; in infants some convexity is normal. Distension may be due to air or fluid – if the stomach does not deflate after an orogastric or nasogastric tube (provided it is safe to do so) is passed, there may be intraperitoneal fluid, suggesting significant intra-abdominal injury. However, the absence of distension does *not* exclude other organ damage.

SURFACE INJURY

The surface of the abdomen (including the back and loins during the log-roll) must be carefully examined for signs of injury.

PALPATION OF THE ABDOMEN

This requires considerable skill, especially in the conscious child. It is vital to look at the face of the child and not the abdomen during the examination. A child should always be told what is about to happen before any examination is commenced. Reassurance will improve the validity of the examination findings. Gentleness is crucial in order to avoid spurious discomfort in the absence of injury.

The following should be sought and recorded:

- Areas of tenderness or pain.
- Rigidity of the abdomen suggesting peritonitis from blood or fluid (this may or may not be present even in unconscious children).
- Rebound tenderness suggesting peritoneal irritation; this is difficult to elicit reliably and is easy to elicit misleadingly by rough palpation.

AUSCULTATION

This is of very limited use in assessing children for intra-abdominal injury. Bowel sounds may be present when there is significant damage and absent when there is none, and in any case are difficult to hear in a noisy resuscitation room.

Investigations

Once the clinical examination is completed, consideration should be given to further investigations, especially if the mechanism of injury and/or clinical findings support the possibility of internal organ damage.

URINE EXAMINATION

Examination of the urine for blood is a useful tool in the assessment of abdominal injury, and a specimen should be obtained at the earliest possible opportunity. However, conscious children should not be catheterized for this purpose alone, and urinalysis may have to wait until a spontaneous sample is passed. In infants, a urine bag should be attached.

RADIOLOGY

Little information on the abdomen is gained from the standard chest and pelvic films taken during the resuscitation phase, but elevation of the diaphragm and pelvic fractures may be seen, and both may indicate intra-abdominal damage. Nothing is to be gained from plain abdominal X-rays, and these should not be performed.

ULTRASOUND

This is by far the most useful non-invasive tool, but it should only be undertaken by an experienced operator. Occasionally other clinicians may be proficient in rapid Focused Abdominal Sonography for Trauma (FAST).

The features of interest are:

- the presence or absence of free intraperitoneal fluid;
- evidence of solid-organ damage (contusion, laceration or rupture); and
- any retroperitoneal haematomas, especially round the duodenum, pancreas and kidneys or within the mesentery.

In most cases, any abnormality seen is an indication for CT scan unless the patient is haemodynamically unstable.

CT SCAN

This is the definitive investigation and should only be undertaken on a fully resuscitated child whose ABCs are normal and controlled. Ideally, both intravenous and enteral contrast should be given (the latter via the nasogastric tube).

Abdominal CT should be sequentially examined for:

- configuration and perfusion of solid organs: contusions, tears, rupture or areas of diminished perfusion in the liver, spleen, kidneys and pancreas and an intact pyelogram following i.v. contrast, indicating adequate renal function;
- integrity of the intestine, especially at fixed points such as the duodenum and duodenojejunal flexure;
- the presence and nature of any free intraperitoneal fluid; and
- integrity of the ureters and bladder.

DIAGNOSTIC PERITONEAL LAVAGE (DPL)

This is contraindicated in children as it does not influence management and may indeed confound it, since it will confuse any subsequent clinical examination or imaging which may be performed. DPL does not inform decisions about the need for operative intervention in children; such decisions should only ever be made on clinical or radiological grounds.

Definitive treatment of intra-abdominal injuries

The nature and extent of any internal organ damage should now have been defined. Details of the definitive management of abdominal injuries in children are too extensive for this manual, but the principles are outlined below. The vast majority of solid-organ injuries may be successfully treated conservatively; operative intervention is rarely required and is reserved for catastrophic or complex injuries. Hepatic and pancreatic injuries require specialist surgical attention. Intestinal perforations do require surgery, but are rare and often difficult to diagnose.

Any child with liver injuries, splenic injuries or other severe intra-abdominal injury should be nursed in a paediatric Intensive Care or High-Dependency Unit until it is clear that there is no risk of bleeding. Serial ultrasound is helpful in assessing the rate of healing of damaged organs such as hepatic or splenic haematomata.

LIVER INJURIES

Liver injuries are fairly common in children following blunt abdominal trauma, but the majority are simple contusions or small lacerations. The severity of a liver injury can usually be defined on CT scan, but occasionally angiography is required. Haemoglobin, haematocrit and liver function should be monitored regularly. Attention should be paid to blood and coagulation factor replacement. Rarely, severe complex laceration, stellate fracture or frank hepatic rupture is seen on CT scan; these injuries require the attention of a specialist hepatic surgeon, and partial hepatectomy may be required.

SPLENIC INJURY

Splenic injuries are common in children. Preservation of the spleen is paramount, and the vast majority of children do not require any surgical intervention. Haemorrhage usually stops with adequate fluid and blood replacement. The only indication for surgical intervention is catastrophic or continuing haemorrhage. Every effort should be made to preserve the spleen. Splenectomy is required in fewer than 5% of patients.

RENAL INJURIES

As with the other solid organs, the commonest injuries are contusions or minor lacerations, all of which heal without surgical intervention. Management is based on adequate fluid and blood replacement. Bed rest should be employed until haematuria ceases.

Rarely, complete avulsion of the renal pedicle occurs, causing complete non-function of the affected kidney and significant retroperitoneal bleeding. This is usually associated with severe deceleration injury (such as falls from a great height), and is evidenced by an absent pyelogram from a normal kidney on CT scan. In such cases, immediate revascularization of the kidney may be required; this should be performed by an experienced vascular or transplant surgeon.

INTESTINAL AND MESENTERIC INJURIES

These are rare in childhood, but are most frequently associated with deceleration trauma. Mesenteric tears result in free intraperitoneal bleeding with signs of peritoneal irritation; most settle with conservative treatment. Intestinal perforations occur most frequently at the points of intestinal fixation. Jejunal perforation may occur as part of the 'lap-belt complex' (due to ill-fitting car seat belts without shoulder restraints). Isolated intestinal perforation may not be evident immediately after injury; if the mechanism of injury suggests the possibility of intestinal damage, repeated clinical examination is required. Intestinal perforations require surgical repair.

PANCREATIC INJURIES

Significant injury to the pancreas is usually associated with severe compression injuries (such as handlebar or seat belt injury). Traumatic pancreatitis may complicate other injuries, and is probably more common than suspected. Pancreatic duct injuries are rare but serious, and difficult to diagnose; endoscopic retrograde pancreatography may be required. If the duct is severed, specialist surgical repair is indicated, and occasionally partial or complete pancreatectomy may be required.

URETER, BLADDER AND URETHRA

Severe injuries to these structures are rare in childhood and virtually never occur in isolation. Urethral damage is usually associated with severe external genital injury or complex pelvic fractures. There may be frank haematuria or blood at the external urinary meatus. Urethral catheterization should not be attempted; suprapubic catheterization is preferable, but should be carried out by a urologist.

DIAPHRAGMATIC RUPTURE

In severe compression injuries the diaphragm may be ruptured, allowing abdominal contents to herniate into the chest. This extremely rare injury is only seen in association with severe chest and abdominal injuries, and requires expert surgical intervention. A few diaphragmatic ruptures remain occult, particularly in ventilated children, and may only become apparent during weaning from ventilation.

Penetrating trauma

Fortunately, significant penetrating trauma is rare in children. The mainstay of management is prompt effective resuscitation, followed by early surgery.

BURNS

Several specific paediatric factors need to be appreciated, most of which can be accounted for by the differences in:

- size and body proportions; not only are children smaller, but they have a higher surface area to body weight ratio, and thus are more susceptible to fluid and heat loss.
- skin thickness; the thinner skin in a child is less resilient to injury and more prone to deeper burns.
- behavioural development; children are more prone to injury, and require greater emotional support during recovery.

Management

FIRST AID

If water has been used to control burning, it is essential to remember that there is an increased risk of hypothermia in children.

ADVANCED LIFE-SUPPORT MEASURES

A primary survey following the ABCDE approach, as outlined throughout this manual, should be followed. Commonsense must also prevail. An already petrified child will find being pinned down on a resuscitation trolley very distressing. Unless there is an indication of other injuries, the burned child can often have much of the assessment and interventions performed while on someone's lap, preferably that of a parent.

Gaining intravenous access may be difficult, and central line insertion and cut-downs on children require some expertise. The intraosseous route should be considered after two failed attempts at simple cannulation. Adequate analgesia should be administered early, and the conscious child be comforted as much as is possible.

BURN ASSESSMENT

The indicators of inhalation injury are the same as for adults. The variations in anatomy mean that the child's airway will tolerate less oedema before causing obstruction. The help of an experienced anaesthetist should be sought if there is any suspicion of inhalation injury.

With differing body proportions, calculating the percentage of total body surface area burned (% TBSA) is more difficult in the child. An accurate map of the burn should be made on a Lund and Browder chart, and then the % TBSA calculated.

The early assessment of burn depth is difficult in children with scalds, and unnecessary time should not be wasted on it. There is *no* indication for checking for sensation in the burn, particularly with a needle. This will scare the child and gives no useful information.

FLUID MANAGEMENT

Any child with a burn of 10% TBSA or over will require intravenous fluid administration. Use of Hartmann's according to the Parkland formula is the same as for adults. With a relatively greater surface area, the child will lose more fluid and the upper range of the formula should be used initially, i.e. 4 ml/kg/%TBSA.

The adequacy of the fluid resuscitation is best monitored by urine output. This needs to be a minimum of 1 ml/kg/h in children, and 2 ml/kg/h in infants. The good compensatory mechanisms in the child mean that there may be little warning of circulatory collapse, as blood pressure is maintained until there is considerable hypovolaemia. Frequent repeated assessment of the circulatory status of the child should be made, looking at heart rate, core–peripheral temperature gradients, capillary refill times and urine output.

BURN WOUND MANAGEMENT

As with adults, the burn wound should be interfered with as little as possible. Wrapping loosely in 'clingfilm' is normally all that is required before transfer.

Smaller burns which do not require transfer can be dressed with paraffin-based gauze. Flamazine bags are unlikely to be successful in small children.

Diaphragmatic breathing is more important in children, and extensive deep burns to the abdomen can compromise respiration. Escharotomies may be indicated, but this is a skilled surgical procedure and advice from the burns centre should be sought.

Transfer to definitive care

Any child with a burn of >5% TBSA should be referred to a burns centre. Other criteria are the same as for adults. The incidence of hypertrophic scarring is high in children. With the advent of modern techniques in wound management, all but the most superficial of burns should be referred for expert opinion early.

Children are more prone to gastric dilatation, and installation of a free-draining nasogastric tube is necessary before transfer. The higher metabolic demands and fluid loss in the child mean that maintenance fluids need to be given earlier. These should therefore be started before transfer and contain glucose in some form to maintain blood glucose within the normal range.

Burns are a common manifestation of NAI, and any suspicions should be clearly passed on to the burns team, and all facts documented. Initial investigations should not be allowed to delay transfer.

MUSCULOSKELETAL INJURIES

Characteristics of the musculoskeletal system in children

Injuries to the immature musculoskeletal system differ from those occurring in adulthood because of:

- Anatomical differences:
  - growth plates
  - epiphyses
  - thickness of periosteum.
- Biomechanical differences:
  - ligaments stronger than the growth plate
  - flexibility of immature bone.
- Physiological differences:
  - remodelling potential
  - increased speed of healing
  - potential for overgrowth.

Fracture patterns

Fractures can be described by anatomical location or fracture configuration. Particular fracture configurations in children include plastic deformation (bowing of a long bone), buckle or torus fractures (indicated by a 'bulge' in the metaphysis, usually occurring in the distal radius) and greenstick fractures with an intact cortex and periosteum on one side of the fracture.

The physeal injuries are usually classified by the Salter–Harris system (see Figure 13.1).[19]

Conventional adult classifications according to the relationships between the bony fragments and with surrounding structures also apply to paediatric fractures.

Management of musculoskeletal trauma in children

In young children a history is not always available, and the possibility that the accident described is not the cause of the presenting problem should be borne in mind. Thus, a careful search should be made for injuries elsewhere. In addition, it is common for children (and their parents) to ascribe to minor trauma a problem which could have another cause – the limp of Perthes' disease is a classic example.

Examination

The history may not reveal the site of the injury, and the main clue is likely to be pain. The more relaxed the child is, the more effective the examination will be. Swelling, deformity, abnormal posture, bruising and laceration should all be sought. Bony and soft-tissue tenderness should be elicited, and each joint isolated individually and its movement assessed. The neurological and circulatory status of the affected limb should be assessed and recorded, and the gait observed if appropriate.

Analgesia

Appropriate analgesia should always be given. In significant trauma, the intravenous route should be used with small aliquots of titrated intravenous opiate. Other methods of pain relief, including splintage, plaster of Paris immobilization and femoral nerve blocks, should not be forgotten.

Investigation

Biplanar X-rays, including the joint above and below the injury, are the first-line investigation.

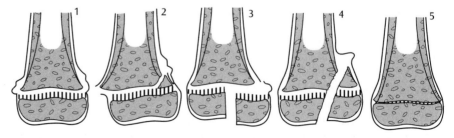

Figure 13.1 *Salter–Harris classification of physeal injuries.*

Treatment

The majority of fractures are treated conservatively. Operative intervention will be required if the fracture is displaced, compound or if there is associated soft-tissue injury. Displaced fractures and dislocations should be immobilized in a backslab in a position of comfort unless there is distal neurovascular compromise, when urgent realignment will be required.

Special situations

OPEN FRACTURES

A polaroid photograph should be taken of the open wound, large contaminants should be removed from the wound, and a sterile dressing should be applied which should not be removed until the patient is in the operating theatre. Profuse bleeding is controlled by local compression. Appropriate splintage and immobilization for the type of fracture is applied. Early intravenous antibiotics is the most important factor in reducing the rate of infection.[20] Cefuroxime or flucloxacillin are usually used with penicillin and metronidazole if there is soil or faecal contamination, and appropriate tetanus prophylaxis is essential. All such fractures require surgical débridement.

VASCULAR INJURY

The circulation can often be improved by reduction of the associated fracture or dislocation. This should be attempted in the A&E Department after suitable analgesia/anaesthesia has been given. The definitive management involves surgical stabilization of the fracture or dislocation, followed by assessment of the circulation and vascular exploration and repair if necessary.

NEUROLOGICAL INJURY

The extent of the deficit should be accurately assessed and documented, though this is often difficult in younger and uncooperative children. Not all neurological deficits associated with fractures or dislocations require active intervention, but all should be referred for specialist advice.

COMPARTMENT SYNDROME

Increased pressure within enclosed soft-tissue compartments of the extremities can cause irreversible muscle and nerve injury. The incidence of compartment syndrome is related to the severity of the trauma.

The lower leg and forearm are the commonest sites. Compartment syndrome can occur with open fractures, with pain that is either out of proportion to the injury and requires frequent strong analgesia, or is exaggerated by passive stretching of the distal joints, being the earliest indicator. Other important findings are swelling and tenseness of the compartment. Pallor, paralysis, paraesthesia and pulselessness are late findings, and the diagnosis should not be excluded if these are absent. Once the diagnosis is suspected, measurement of compartment pressures and/or fasciotomy should be performed.

Pitfalls in diagnosis

The history can be misleading – since falls are a common experience in childhood, serious problems such as septic arthritis may be falsely attributed to trauma.

In addition, ligaments are stronger than bone. In children, sprains or dislocations rarely occur; it is more likely for a fracture to occur through a growth plate.

Normal radiological variants can also be confused with injury. This occurs commonly with lateral cervical spine radiographs. For example:

- pseudosubluxation – physiological anterior displacement, usually of C2 on C3 (less commonly C3 on C4), occurs in up to 40% of children aged <8 years and in 20% of children aged <16 years.[21]
- Atlanto-dens interval – an increased distance (>3 mm) between the dens (odontoid) and anterior arch of C1 occurs in about 20% of young children.

PSYCHOLOGICAL ASPECTS

Children and adults involved in a traumatic episode, even in the absence of physical injury, are at risk of psychological injuries. The commonest psychological disorder associated with trauma is post-traumatic stress disorder (PTSD), which is seen in all ages. The horrific sounds, disturbing visual scenes and other sensory inputs of a catastrophe can invoke fear, terror and, above all, a sense of helplessness; these factors predispose to the development of PTSD. Between 15% and 30% of children involved in RTAs may develop PTSD or severe traffic-related fears.[22]

Unconsciousness with its consequent amnesia, while being a marker for possible brain injury, protects against PTSD as psychological mechanisms are not operational. PTSD may be preventable by protecting uninjured children from witnessing severe injuries, particularly if accompanying an injured parent, and by helping them to make sense of the event.

Other psychological sequelae, which occur after traumatic events, include:

- phobias (particularly of cars and roads);
- separation anxiety disorders (especially in young children);
- increased propensity to risk-taking (especially in adolescents, which renders them vulnerable to further accidents); and
- depression, especially if there is bereavement associated with the traumatic event.

Prevention of psychological injury

Practitioners treating children in the immediate aftermath of a traumatic event can contribute to the prevention of acute and long-term psychological problems[23] by:

- keeping young children with a familiar figure. If it is necessary to separate the children from this person (for example, due to the parents' own injuries) they must be cared for by one person until the arrival of a familiar figure.
- protecting the children from distressing sights, sounds, smells and other sensory inputs. Children should not see mutilating or bloody wounds, especially if these belong to a parent, and the cries of the injured should not be audible to children. The advent of audio-visually separated paediatric A&E areas from the general A&E areas may help in this respect.[24]
- ensuring that children have received adequate sedation and analgesia. This is especially important in those children who are clearly distressed or who need to have a potentially painful procedure carried out.
- taking time to explain to the child what is going to happen, and why. Careful explanation of one's actions directed towards the child's level of comprehension is imperative, irrespective of the underlying problem. It is important to avoid remarks such as 'You have been lucky, you could have been killed', as this increases death anxiety.
- giving advice and help to parents and other carers. Parents should be advised about the features to look out for, and told that further expert help is available. The Child Accident Prevention Trust publishes very useful literature including a helpful pamphlet, which should be given to parents, entitled 'Getting over an Accident. How to Help Your Child'.

> **Steps to diminish psychological injury:**
> - **Keep young children with a familiar figure**
> - **Protect them from distressing sights, sounds, smells and other sensory inputs**
> - **Ensure that children have received adequate sedation and analgesia**
> - **Take time to explain to the children what you are doing, and why**
> - **Give advice and help to parents and other carers**

Early treatment

Psychological sequelae are common – particularly in young children – and irrespective of the extent of injuries, as childrens' emotional immaturity can magnify their fears and concerns over the event. An assessment made six weeks after the incident should be made to look for symptoms of PTSD and other psychological disturbances. Referral can be made to expert help such as a clinical child psychologist or child psychiatrist accordingly.

NON-ACCIDENTAL INJURY

No precise information is available regarding the incidence of severe non-accidental paediatric trauma in the UK. However, a regional paediatric Intensive Care Unit serving a population of 1 million reported 15 cases of severe non-accidental trauma over a 3-year period.[25]

Patterns of injury

NAI involves a spectrum of trauma ranging from minor bruising to life-threatening injuries. This section deals mainly with life-threatening forms of NAI. Relatively minor injuries are, however, of great importance as assaults on the child may become more frequent and severe. The paediatric population is a heterogeneous one that extends from birth to 16 years; the mechanism of injury is usually age-related, with non-ambulant infants being more vulnerable to being shaken or thrown whereas older mobile children are more prone to being kicked or punched.[26] Bizarre forms of NAI can occur, however, in all age groups.[27,28] The role of shaking in non-accidental trauma is unclear. To attribute an injury to a particular cause requires a reliable history, which is generally lacking in NAI.

> **Head injury is the commonest form of severe non-accidental trauma**

Sudden deceleration of the head when striking a solid object has been proposed as the origin of most NAI-related brain damage seen in younger children.[29] Other reports suggest that severe brain injury is related to axonal shearing that occurs during shaking.[25] The spectrum of brain injury is extensive, but acute subdural haematoma is the commonest lesion.[29]

A deliberate direct blow to the abdomen may cause injury to the solid or hollow abdominal viscera. Liver, splenic, renal and pancreatic injuries have all been reported,[26] with one-third of cases in one series of pancreatitis in children being attributed to NAI.[30] The duodenum appears to be particularly vulnerable to non-accidental blunt trauma.[26]

The commonest non-accidental chest injury is rib fracture or fractures which are generally posterior and at the costovertebral junctions. These fractures are believed to result from gripping of the infant's chest during shaking, and may only become apparent as they heal. The rib injuries themselves do not contribute significantly to morbidity or mortality, and generally heal over three to four weeks without complications. Identification of these fractures is important, as the presence of posterior rib fractures in an infant is highly suggestive of NAI, and supplies strong evidence of an abusive mechanism for any associated injuries.

Presentation

One of the challenges of dealing with severe non-accidental trauma is that the history is likely to be unreliable. Deception and self-preservation are often the priorities of attending adults. Severe non-accidental trauma has a spectrum of presentations, and should be considered in any seriously unwell child where the diagnosis is unclear.

In young children severe non-accidental trauma may present as a medical emergency such as an apparent life-threatening event (ALTE). In a review of infants with severe non-accidental head injuries the three most common presentations were:

1. Convulsions
2. Drowsiness
3. Poor feeding.

Other presentations included unresponsiveness, lethargy, irritability, apnoeic attacks, diarrhoea and vomiting.[25]

Roughly one-third of severe non-accidental head injuries in infants are thought to be missed at the initial presentation.[25,31] Older children may be able to provide a history, but might be reluctant to do so out of fear.

The examination must be thorough, and any injury, whether old or new, should be documented meticulously. The commonest findings on examination of infants with a severe non-accidental head injury are a full fontanelle, irritability and coma.[25] Fundoscopy is particularly important since retinal haemorrhages, especially if bilateral, have a strong association with severe NAI.[25] Photography is an important adjunct to any future legal proceedings.

Bilateral retinal haemorrhages strongly suggest non-accidental injury

---

Management

Initial management should follow the 'ABC' prioritization described in earlier chapters. Further management will depend on the specific injuries sustained. The regional paediatric Intensive Care Unit should be involved in such cases of major trauma. Accurate and thorough documentation is essential, and clinical photographs should always be taken.

The child protection team or a senior paediatrician must be called at an early stage to investigate the circumstances of the child's injuries and to assess the need for protection of any 'at-risk' siblings.

No judgement should be made as to who the perpetrator is, but possible mechanisms should be considered by senior experienced medical opinion. The NAI child needs a multidisciplinary approach involving the general practitioner and social work services. Where appropriate, health visitors, school and the police may need to be involved in the later stages of the management of the child with NAI.

SUMMARY

Major trauma in children is fortunately rare and is a source of anxiety in carers, who find themselves dealing with unfamiliar problems in an emotionally charged environment. Attention to single protocols is therefore essential for optimum management. The same basic principles used in adults, tempered with a knowledge of the anatomical and physiological differences which apply to children, provide a firm base for good clinical care.

REFERENCES

1. The UK Trauma Audit and Research Network. The University of Manchester, Data 1994–1998.

2. Wyatt JP, McLeod L, Beard D, Busuttil A, Beattie TF, Robertson CE. Timing of paediatric deaths after trauma. *British Medical Journal* 1997; **314**: 868.

3. Jennett B. Epidemiology of head injury. *Journal of Neurology, Neurosurgery and Psychiatry* 1996; **60**: 362–9.

4. Sharples PM, Storey A, Aynsley-Green A, Eyre JA. Avoidable factors contributing to death of children with head injury. *British Medical Journal* 1990; **300**: 87–91.

5. *Advanced Trauma Life Support*. American College of Surgeons, Chicago, 1997.

6. The Advanced Life Support Group. *Advanced paediatric life support – the practical approach*. BMJ Publications, London, 1997.

7. Teasdale GM, Murray G, Anderson E, *et al*. Risks of acute traumatic intracranial haematoma in children and adults: implications for managing head injuries. *British Medical Journal* 1990; **300**: 363–7.

8. Lloyd DA, Carty H, Patterson M, Butcher C. Predictive value of skull radiography for intracranial injury in children with blunt injury. *Lancet* 1997; **349**: 821–4.

9. Royal College of Surgeons of England. *Report of the working party on the management of patient with head injuries*. Royal College of Surgeons of England, London, 1999.

10. Scottish Intercollegiate Guidelines Network 2000, in press.

11. Black TL, Snyder CL, Miller JP, Mann CM Jr., Copetas AC, Ellis DG. Significance of chest trauma in children. *Southern Medical Journal* 1996; **89**: 494–6.

12. Peclet MH, Newman KD, Eichelberger MR, *et al*. Patterns of injury in children. *Journal of Pediatric Surgery* 1990; **25**: 85–90.

13. Nakayama DK, Ramenofsky ML, Rowe MI. Chest injuries in childhood. *Annals of Surgery* 1989; **210**: 770–5.

14. Roux P, Fischer RM. Chest injuries in children: an analysis of 100 cases of blunt chest trauma from motor vehicle accidents. *Journal of Pediatric Surgery* 1992; **27**: 551–4.

15. Sivit CJ, Taylor GA, Eichelberger MR. Chest injury in children with blunt abdominal trauma: evaluation with CT. *Radiology* 1989; **171**: 815–18.

16. Beaver BL, Colombani PM, Buck JR, Dudgeon DL, Bohrer SL, Haller JA Jr. Efficacy of emergency room thoracotomy in paediatric trauma. *Journal of Pediatric Surgery* 1987; **22**: 19–23.

17. Stafford PW, Harmon CM. Thoracic trauma in children. *Current Opinion in Pediatrics* 1993; **5**: 325–32.

18. Eddy AC, Rusch VW, Fligner CL, Reay DT, Rice CL. The epidemiology of traumatic rupture of the thoracic aorta in children: a 13-year review. *Journal of Trauma* 1990; **30**: 989–91.

19. Salter RB, Harris WR. *Journal of Bone and Joint Surgery* **45A**: 587–622.

20. Patzakis MJ, Wilkins J. Factors in influencing infection rate in open fracture wounds. *Clinical Orthopedics* 1989; **243**: 36–40.

21. Cattell HS, Filtzer DL. Peudosubluxation and other normal variations in the cervical spine in children. A study of one hundred and sixty children. *Journal of Bone and Joint Surgery* 1965; **27A**: 1295–309.

22. Mirza KAH, Bhadrinath BR, Goodyer IM, Gilmour C. Post-traumatic stress disorder in children and adolescents following road traffic accidents. *British Journal of Psychiatry* 1998; **172**: 443–7.

23. Black D, Newman M, Harris-Hendriks J, Mezey G (eds). *Psychological Trauma: A Developmental Approach*. London: Gaskell, 1997.

24. Accident and emergency services for children. *Report of a multidisciplinary working party*. Royal College of Paediatrics and Child Health, London, 1999.

25. Haviland J, Ross Russell RI. Outcome after severe non-accidental head injury. *Archives of Disease in Childhood* 1997; **77**: 504–7.

26. Ng CS, Hall CM, Shaw DG. The range of visceral manifestations of non-accidental injury. *Archives of Disease in Childhood* 1997; **77**: 167–74.

27. Reece RM. Unusual manifestations of child abuse. *Pediatric Clinics of North America* 1990; **37**: 905–21.

28. Campbell-Hewson GL, D'Amore A, Busuttil A. Non-accidental injury inflicted on a child with an air weapon. *Medical Science and Law* 1998; **38**: 173–6.

29. Duhaime A-C, Christian CW, Rorke LB, Zimmerman RA. Non-accidental head injury in infants – the 'shaken baby syndrome'. *New England Journal of Medicine* 1998; **338**: 1822–9.

30. Ziegler DW, Long JA, Philuppart AI. Pancreatitis in childhood; experience with 49 children. *Annals of Surgery* 1988; **207**: 257–61.

31. Jenny C, Hymel KP, Ritken A, Reinert SE, Hay TC. Analysis of missed cases of abusive head trauma. *Journal of the American Medical Association* 1999; **281**: 621–6.

14

Trauma in women

OBJECTIVES

- To understand the anatomical and physiological changes which occur in pregnancy
- To recognize mechanisms of injury and injury patterns in the pregnant woman and the foetus
- To understand the principles of management of the pregnant woman and the foetus
- To recognize the implications of uterine trauma for the foetus
- To know the indications for early consultation with the obstetrician and gynaecologist and other specialists
- To be able to recognize and manage injuries associated with violence to women in general

INTRODUCTION

Trauma in women includes accidental injury to the pregnant woman and to the foetus, and to the gynaecological organs in association with major trauma to the abdomen and pelvis. Also included is deliberate injury, encompassing domestic violence, rape and ritual female circumcision (genital mutilation). Management of rape is outside the scope of this chapter; however, emergency medical attendants must be familiar with modern management approaches.[1] The major focus in this chapter is on trauma in pregnancy.

When managing trauma in any female patient aged between 10 and 60 years, the possibility of pregnancy must be considered. Not one, but two lives may be at risk and initial assessment and ongoing monitoring must include the foetus. Nevertheless, the outcome for the foetus is dependent upon successful management of the mother.

A multidisciplinary approach is demanded, with early involvement of an obstetrician and a neonatal paediatrician if appropriate, in addition to the usual members of the trauma response team. The need for emergency surgical intervention must be recognized.

EPIDEMIOLOGY

Accidental and non-accidental trauma in women is common, and is increasing.[2] Approximately 1 in 12 pregnant women will suffer injury at some stage during their pregnancy, and many require observation in hospital. In most cases these injuries are slight and are the result of falls or direct blows to the abdomen. However, even in cases of apparently minor trauma, complications associated with pregnancy occur in over 8% of women admitted to hospital.[3] In particular, the risk of foetomaternal transfusion must be considered in all cases beyond 11 weeks' gestation.[4] Isoimmunization is discussed below, but other complications associated with slight injury include premature labour, placental abruption and injury to the foetus.[3]

In a minority of cases, life-threatening maternal and foetal injury will occur. For example, trauma remains the most common cause of non-obstetric death. In the UK, between 1988 and 1990 and 1991 and 1993, 4% and 7% of deaths respectively were due to trauma.

ANATOMICAL CHANGES

The uterus

The pregnant uterus remains below the brim of the pelvis until the 12th week of pregnancy. During this time it is a thick-walled structure, and is well protected by the bony pelvis. However, during the second trimester the uterus rises out of the pelvis and becomes an abdominal organ which is increasingly easy to palpate. It remains thick-walled, and the small foetus remains mobile and cushioned by a relatively generous amount of amniotic fluid. By week 20 the uterus has reached the umbilicus. By 34/36 weeks the uterus becomes increasingly thin-walled and rises to reach the costal margin. During the last 2 weeks of gestation the uterus descends below the costal margin as the foetal head engages in the pelvis, while the amniotic fluid volume decreases. At term, amniotic fluid has a volume of between 550 and 1300 ml. The size and position of the pregnant uterus in weeks is illustrated in Figure 14.1.

The placenta

The fully formed placenta is a disc, approximately 2.5 cm in thickness, which tapers towards the edges. It is usually attached to the uterine wall anteriorly, well up in the area of the fundus. It is an inelastic structure, dark in colour and weighing approximately 500 g. Its lack of elastic tissue renders it vulnerable to shearing forces applied to the uterine wall – abruption of the placenta may occur and may be concealed, or result in vaginal bleeding.

The umbilical vessels are usually attached near its centre and immediately divide to form branches over its surface. The umbilical cord usually has two arteries and one vein, embedded in a protective myxomatous tissue known as Wharton's jelly.

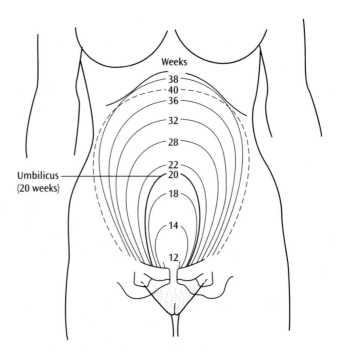

Figure 14.1. *Uterine height and gestational age.*

The foetus

Before the 12th week of pregnancy it is not possible to palpate the foetus per abdomen; however, by the 8th week, the presence of pregnancy can be determined by bi-manual palpation. At this stage the uterus is the size of a hen's egg. At 14 weeks, the foetus is the size of a grapefruit, and between 16 and 18 weeks the pregnant women is aware of foetal movements. However, cessation of foetal movement following injury is not a reliable sign of foetal injury or death. At 20 weeks, foetal movements may be palpated by the examining doctor, and by 24 weeks the foetus is large enough to be liable to injury by blunt or penetrating injuries to the overlying abdominal wall. At this date, foetal heart sounds are audible – the rate varies between 120 and 140 beats/minute, and should be regular. From the 26th week, foetal parts become palpable.

Maternal anatomy

In late pregnancy the uterus progressively displaces the abdominal viscera upwards and to the sides, forming a protective cushion or shield, and providing a relative degree of maternal protection against penetrating injury in particular. However, a further effect is to cause elevation of the diaphragm by up to 4 cm, which has implications for the insertion of chest drains. There is also an increased risk of hiatus hernia, with reflux of gastric contents. Pregnancy also results in increased vascularity in the pelvis with the enlargement of thin-walled pelvic veins and a more dynamic circulation.

PHYSIOLOGICAL CHANGES

Airway (A)

Airway compromise may result from an increased tendency for reflux of gastric contents, in particular when dealing with a supine pregnant woman with an altered conscious level.

Breathing and ventilation (B)

There is an increased oxygen demand during pregnancy, and high-flow oxygen administration during resuscitation of the injured pregnant woman is a high priority.

A normal rise in tidal volume of 40% with a 25% fall in residual capacity results in a physiological hyperventilation and leads to a $PaCO_2$ of 4.0 kPa (30 mmHg) at term. It is important that this degree of pregnancy-related hypocapnia is recognized as a normal feature of late pregnancy. Consequently, a finding of a $PaCO_2$ of 5.3 kPa or higher is associated with maternal and foetal acidosis and impending respiratory failure.

Circulation (C)

During pregnancy, cardiac output increases by 1.0–1.5 l/min, and blood volume increases by up to 50% to maintain adequate circulation in both mother and foetus. Haemoglobin levels do not increase in proportion to the increase in circulating blood volume and a physiological anaemia results. This may be exacerbated by genuine anaemia due to iron or other deficiency. Systolic and diastolic blood pressures fall by 5–15 mmHg during the second trimester, returning to normal values in later pregnancy. In the third trimester, the resting pulse rises by 15–20 beats/minute.

Because of these changes, shock assessment in the injured pregnant woman can be difficult. In an otherwise healthy pregnant woman, losses of up to 1.5 l may occur without clinical signs of shock. Shunting of uterine and placental blood into the maternal circulation causes this masking of maternal shock. Therefore, hypovolaemic shock in the foetus may be present for a time, while the mother appears normovolaemic.

> **Maternal blood loss of up to 1.5 l may occur without visible signs of shock**

Despite these increases in blood volume and cardiac output, episodes of benign maternal hypotension are common. Supine maternal hypotension is a well-recognized feature of later pregnancy and is due to compression of the vena cava by the gravid uterus, resulting in marked reduction in venous return from the lower body. Cardiac output may fall by one-third. In the non-injured patient the condition is easily by managed by repositioning the torso. Although the condition is benign in the healthy pregnant women, it may be lethal in the presence of haemorrhagic shock (see below).

While the circulating volume rises, alterations in blood composition occur and need to be recognized. These are, in addition to the anaemia discussed above:

- a rise in white blood cell count (WBC) in later pregnancy, peaking during labour;
- slight elevation in clotting factor levels;
- a fall in plasma proteins; and
- shortening of prothrombin and partial thromboplastin times.

Central nervous system (dysfunction) (D)

Severe pre-eclampsia and eclampsia are serious complications of late pregnancy, and threaten the life of both the mother and foetus (note that these conditions may mimic head injury). Alteration in conscious level or fitting in the presence of hypertension, oedema and proteinuria should raise suspicion, and expert obstetric help must be summoned.

Other systems

GASTROINTESTINAL

Relaxation of the gastro-oesophageal sphincter and delayed gastric emptying is a feature of pregnancy. Since an unconscious, supine patient may aspirate gastric contents, it is important always to assume the presence of a full stomach. A nasogastric or orogastric tube should be passed, and the airway must be secured as a matter of urgency.

MUSCULOSKELETAL

The pelvic joints and ligaments are relaxed in pregnancy. The symphisis pubis may separate in late pregnancy, and in the third trimester the gap may be up to 1 cm. This needs to be considered when interpreting pelvic X-rays.

ENDOCRINE

The pituitary gland is vulnerable during pregnancy, and may increase in mass and weight by up to 50%. Both traumatic haemorrhagic shock and postpartum haemorrhage may lead to necrosis of the pituitary, resulting in Sheehan's syndrome.

MECHANISMS OF INJURY

The patterns of injury common to all trauma victims apply in equal measure to the pregnant woman. These include:

- Road traffic accidents – driver or passenger
- Road traffic accidents – pedestrian impact
- Motorcycle and bicycle accidents
- Burn injury
- Intentional injury

- Falls
- Exposure to blast.

There are risks specific to pregnancy which will be discussed in later sections.

Knowledge of the mechanism of injury (MOI) is increasingly recognized as important in successful management of the multiply injured, and the pregnant woman is no exception to this. Knowledge of the mechanics of blunt injury, wound ballistics and environmental conditions are invaluable in patient assessment, and reduce the chances of missing occult injury.[5]

The vast majority of pregnant women suffer blunt or penetrating trauma; indeed, in European and North American practice, blunt injury is the predominating mechanism.[6,7] Intentional injury caused by partners accounts for a significant minority, in one series reaching over 31%.[2] Penetrating injury in pregnancy is still rare in United Kingdom practice, while burn injury, though uncommon in pregnancy, is associated with high foetal mortality rates.[8] In a climate of terrorism there is a risk of exposure to the effects of blast injury.

Blunt impact

Road traffic accidents (RTAs) still predominate among blunt impact trauma cases, and deaths from head and intra-abdominal injury are the leading cause of non-obstetric mortality. Invariably this also results in foetal death; maternal death remains the most common cause of foetal death, followed by placental abruption. Domestic violence involving pregnant women is increasing, and is typically characterized by direct blows to the abdomen. Falls are another common cause of maternal and foetal injury.

Seat belts have been shown to reduce maternal mortality, though poorly applied or designed restraints may increase foetal mortality.[9] Correctly worn seat belt restraints, comprising three-point harnesses with lap belts across the upper thighs and the diagonal belt placed above the pregnant uterus reduce the risk of injury to the foetus, particularly due to placental abruption.[10]

The abdominal wall musculature, the pregnant uterus and amniotic fluid all afford some protection to both mother and foetus by absorbing applied forces. However, acceleration, deceleration and shearing forces or direct blows applied to the abdominal wall in later pregnancy may result in placental abruption, with or without disseminated intravascular coagulation, ruptured uterus and direct injury to the foetus.[11]

There is increasing recognition that apparently trivial degrees of direct abdominal wall impact may have serious consequences for the foetus. Farmer *et al.*[12] have shown that the extent of maternal injury does not necessarily correlate with the degree of foetal injury. Lethal foetal injury associated with placental disruption or direct injury may occur in the face or minimal maternal injury. The message for the medical attendant is to have a high index of suspicion in all cases, even when injury appears to be trivial.

Penetrating injury

There is potential for a wide variety of injury mechanisms and injury patterns. These include:

- penetration by vehicular parts or debris from the environment (fences or railings);
- stab injury by knives or related objects;
- low-energy-transfer missiles (bullets or fragments); and
- high-energy-transfer missiles (bullets or fragments).

In the UK, the usual pattern of injury is by stabbing or penetration by objects in RTAs, or following falls.

Stab wounds and low-energy-transfer missile wounds result in laceration and crushing in the direct path of the missile or penetrating blade. The outcome is determined by the nature of the structures penetrated. During the first trimester, patterns of injury in the pregnant and non-pregnant woman are similar, provided that the injury track does not extend into the pelvis. In later pregnancy the uterus acts a shield for the mother, but the foetus is at particular hazard. Injury to maternal organs has been reported as low as 20% in one series.[13] In addition, the uterine musculature and the amniotic fluid effectively retard missile velocity, reducing energy transfer and wounding potential, with outcome for the foetus being determined by the structures injured. Penetration of the umbilical cord or placenta may result in abruption and haemorrhage, which may be catastrophic for both foetus and mother.

High-energy-transfer missile injury is rare in peacetime, but is a noted feature of war, terrorism and armed conflict.[14] Although this form of injury in pregnancy is fortunately extremely rare, intra-abdominal high-energy-transfer in late pregnancy is likely to be lethal for both mother and foetus.

Operative intervention is recommended in all cases of penetrating injury in the pregnant woman.[15] At laparotomy, the uterus must be carefully assessed for evidence of penetration and the viability of the foetus assessed. Evidence of uterine penetration is widely regarded as an indication for immediate Caesarean section. In early pregnancy (less than 28 weeks), operative delivery of the foetus is associated with risk of foetal death, and it may be appropriate in carefully selected cases to preserve the pregnancy, though this decision must be made by an obstetrician.

Burn injury

Burn injury caused by flame or hot liquid in the first trimester differs little from a similar injury in the non-pregnant patient. Beyond the first trimester an increasing percentage of maternal cardiac output is diverted to the uterine and placental circulation, reducing maternal compensation in the face of sudden loss of circulating volume. Maternal mortality rises sharply with the extent of the surface area burn. Burn injuries of less than 30% body surface area (BSA) appear to have little effect on maternal or foetal survival, provided that management is optimal and is delivered with assistance from teams from both obstetric and burn units working teams. When injury exceeds 50% of the BSA, maternal death is certain unless the foetus is delivered.[16] Delay not only poses grave risk to the mother but also exposes the foetus to increasing risk due to maternal hypoxia and hypovolaemia.

Electrical burn injury is rare in pregnancy, but poses a unique risk of foetal electrocution because of the low resistance offered by uterus and amniotic fluid. Electrical burn injury in pregnancy should prompt emergency admission to a critical care environment for continuous foetal monitoring by Doppler ultrasound. Even if the foetus survives electrocution, long-term monitoring is required to detect foetal growth retardation and oligohydramnios.

INITIAL ASSESSMENT AND MANAGEMENT

Initial assessment and management strategies for the pregnant woman do not differ from the approach outlined in Chapter 3, and optimal care of the mother is the best immediate management possible for the foetus. The following management pathway is recommended.

If advanced notification is given, the following information should be obtained:

- The number of weeks' gestation
- Mechanism of injury
- Obvious injuries sustained
- Vital signs at scene
- Treatment given.

This information should provide the emergency room personnel with an early indication of the severity of injury, and the need to summon additional help. Laboratory, radiology, operating theatre and Critical Care Units should be alerted if appropriate. The injured pregnant woman should be managed in an environment capable of providing optimal care for her and the foetus.

Initial assessment and resuscitation: maternal

Here, a logical and sequential approach is vital. While the general approach should not differ, pregnancy dictates some modifications.

AIRWAY AND CERVICAL SPINE CONTROL

The increased risk of airway compromise in the face of altered conscious level which may result from silent regurgitation of gastric contents should be recognized. Facial and oral swelling may make intubation technically difficult. In particular, neck swelling may mask normal landmarks, including the cricothyroid membrane. The need to secure and protect the airway must be anticipated. Intubation must be performed by a skilled anaesthetist using a rapid sequence induction technique if the patient is other than deeply unconscious. Cricothyroid pressure is essential until the airway is definitively protected, and collar sandbags and tape should be replaced by manual in-line stabilization for the duration of the procedure.

BREATHING AND VENTILATION

The normal physiological hyperventilation associated with advanced pregnancy should be recognized; it may be necessary to hyperventilate artificially if ventilatory support is required. Swelling of the soft tissues of the neck and upper chest may mask tracheal deviation. If a chest drain is required, the presence of a high diaphragm should be considered.

CIRCULATION AND HAEMORRHAGE CONTROL

Inferior vena caval compression must be avoided from the outset by one of the following:

- elevation of the right hip with a wedge;
- log-rolling into the left lateral position; or
- manual displacement of the uterus to the left.

> **Always relieve inferior vena caval compression**

Following vascular access, blood should be taken for a Kleihauer–Betke test. Vigorous shock therapy, instituted early, is particularly required in late pregnancy due to enhanced maternal compensatory mechanisms.

> **In the pregnant patient, the end-point of fluid resuscitation should be the maintenance of a normal or near-normal systolic blood pressure**

If surgical intervention is judged necessary in order to control maternal haemorrhage in any cavity, this should not be deferred because of the pregnancy. Ongoing maternal haemorrhage will lead to foetal hypoxia and foetal death. Controlling maternal haemorrhage is the best means of ensuring foetal survival.

DISABILITY

If the level of consciousness is altered, the possibility of eclampsia or severe pre-eclampsia must be considered.

EXPOSURE AND ENVIRONMENT

Neither the mother nor foetus can be properly assessed without full exposure. The patient must be undressed in a warm environment, and hypothermia avoided.

Following initial assessment and stabilization of the mother, attention should now be turned to an initial assessment of the foetus. Although best performed by an obstetrician, this assessment should be within the competence of any member of the attending trauma team.

Initial assessment and resuscitation: the foetus

A detailed obstetric assessment of the maternal abdomen and pelvis should only commence following stabilization of the mother, and should include the following stages.

ASSESSMENT OF FOETAL MATURITY AND PLACENTAL INTEGRITY/POSITION

A detailed obstetric history (if available) and a clinical assessment of fundal height should give an accurate estimate of foetal viability (over 24 weeks' gestation). Gestational age, foetal viability and placental position can also be confirmed using pelvic ultrasound. This investigation may also be used to diagnose placental abruption and intrauterine haemorrhage.

ASSESSMENT OF UTERINE INTEGRITY

The uterus should be examined per abdomen. Signs of premature contractions, tenderness or rigidity, or extrauterine foetal parts are sought and their presence demands immediate obstetric consultation and consideration of urgent surgical intervention. Digital or speculum examination of the vagina requires special expertise and should be performed by an obstetrician. Vaginal examination may reveal bleeding or amniotic fluid loss. Additional findings include the condition of the cervical os and the presence of pelvic fracture. Vaginal examination in the injured pregnant woman is fraught with hazard, and injudicious or clumsy examination may precipitate catastrophic bleeding from unsuspected placenta praevia or may reveal a previously concealed placental abruption. Consequently, such examinations are usually best performed by an obstetrician – this having the additional benefit that it avoids repeated examinations.

ASSESSMENT OF FOETAL DISTRESS

The normal foetal heart rate is 120–160 beats/min and is best assessed using Doppler ultrasound. This examination is only useful once the uterus has risen above the pelvic brim (after the 12th week). Bradycardia of less than 100 beats/min is a clear sign of foetal distress. If the mother is conscious and able to report foetal movements, a cardiotocogram can be utilized to monitor foetal heart rate during uterine contractions. The presence of any of the signs of foetal distress or decompensation summarized in Table 14.1 should prompt immediate skilled assessment by an obstetrician.

Table 14.1 *Signs of foetal distress or decompensation*

- Bradycardia of <100 beats/min or abnormal foetal baseline heart rate
- Repeated decelerations in response to uterine contractions
- Absence of acceleration in response to foetal movements
- Increasing uterine activity
- Positive Kleihauer–Betke test

Traumatic foetomaternal haemorrhage can be detected by the Kleihauer–Betke test, which identifies the presence of foetal red blood cells in the maternal circulation.[17] In rhesus-negative women with a positive Kleihauer–Betke test, anti-D immunoglobulin should be administered to prevent rhesus isoimmunization.

There is unnecessary controversy surrounding maternal abdominal radiography. If X-rays are required, they should be performed, as their benefit outweighs the associated risks to mother and foetus.

> **Perform X-rays if you have to**

Secondary assessment: mother and foetus

This assessment is conducted in precisely the same manner as a secondary assessment in the non-pregnant patient. It is a head-to-toe examination of the stabilized mother and foetus, and is conducted in a systematic manner. The head, neck and chest examinations are identical, apart from taking into account the anatomical and physiological changes alluded to earlier. However, assessment of the abdomen and pelvis deserves special consideration, and pelvic and vaginal assessments are best performed by the attending obstetrician. The following findings are significant and demand immediate obstetric consultation:

- uterine contractions;
- tetanic contractions with vaginal bleeding;
- asymptomatic vaginal bleeding;
- leakage of amniotic fluid;
- abdominal pain and/or tenderness;
- abnormal foetal heart activity;
- dilation of the os; and
- cervical effacement.

The indications for Focused Abdominal Sonography for Trauma (FAST) and diagnostic peritoneal lavage (DPL) are the same as in the non-pregnant patient. However, performing DPL in the heavily pregnant patient is fraught with difficulty and probably best avoided. If it is carried out in the pregnant patient, an alternative insertion site must be used.

CRITICAL DECISION-MAKING

Throughout the assessment of both mother and foetus, decisions must be made concerning emergency surgical intervention. Emergency laparotomy may be indicated as part of the maternal primary survey. Common indications in this phase are hypovolaemic shock as a result of uncontrolled intra-abdominal haemorrhage, evidence of solid-organ injury including uterine rupture, or the presence of penetrating abdominal injury. Emergency Caesarean section may be indicated if there is evidence of uncontrolled foetal distress, placental abruption, or where burn injury greater than 50% is present. In late pregnancy it may be necessary to deliver the foetus by Caesarean section in order to gain access to other injured organs or structures.

The decision to perform a peri-mortem or post-mortem Caesarean section will be discussed later in the chapter.

Surgical intervention may also be indicated during the secondary assessment and beyond. It may take time for signs of foetal or maternal distress to emerge or intervention may be necessary in light of the investigation results. The important point is the need for continuous assessment of both mother and foetus throughout all assessment phases.

Surgical intervention: specific indications

PLACENTAL ABRUPTION

Placental abruption is the most common cause of foetal death following blunt trauma, the reported incidence varying from 6.6% to 66%.[18] Onset is typically within 48 h of injury. Diagnosis can be subtle, particularly if abruption is concealed (no vaginal bleeding) for a time. Overt signs include:

- vaginal bleeding;
- uterine irritability;

- uterine tenderness;
- uterine rigidity with tenderness;
- tetanic contractions;
- rising fundal height; and
- unexpected maternal shock.

Early diagnosis is important, and a high index of suspicion is recommended. Delayed diagnosis – particularly if it is associated with abruption associated with more than 50% separation – may result in catastrophic disseminated intravascular coagulation (DIC) in the mother. The diagnosis can be confirmed in most cases by ultrasound, and liberal use of the technique is recommended. Definitive management is by emergency Caesarean section.

UTERINE RUPTURE

This condition is usually associated with blunt trauma, which may be trivial in those previously exposed to a classical section. In the absence of previous surgery, it is rare for rupture to occur without injury to other structures or organs.[19] Typical signs include one or more of the following:[20]

- loss of foetal movement;
- loss of, or abnormal foetal heart sounds;
- extrauterine foetal parts palpable on abdominal examination;
- abdominal guarding or rigidity;
- vaginal bleeding;
- X-ray evidence of free intraperitoneal air; and
- unexpected maternal shock.

Immediate laparotomy is indicated. Evacuation of the uterine contents with primary repair is best, but emergency Caesarean hysterectomy may be required if laceration is extensive with involvement of parametrial vessels and structures.

UTERINE PENETRATION

Gunshot and stab wounds may extend to involve the uterus. Signs may be subtle, as lethal maternal injury is rare. Consequently, injury to the foetus may not be evident until maternal initial assessment has been completed and a primary survey of the foetus is conducted. The signs of foetal distress have already been considered. Suspicion of uterine or foetal injury mandates a laparotomy and careful intraoperative assessment by an obstetrician.

Peri-mortem and post-mortem Caesarean section

Peri-mortem or post-mortem section may be indicated in carefully selected cases, but it is unlikely to deliver a live foetus when performed following maternal cardiopulmonary arrest due to traumatic haemorrhagic shock. At the time of arrest flowing trauma, the foetus has usually suffered prolonged hypoxia and hypovolaemia. Time is of the essence – delay beyond 4–5 min generally results in foetal death.[15]

ACCIDENTAL NON-OBSTETRIC TRAUMA

Non-obstetric trauma, while uncommon, has been reported.[21] Common causes include falls astride, consensual sexual intercourse, sexual assault, and injudicious insertion of a wide variety of objects into the genital tract. The genital tract may also be injured in association with penetrating and blunt high-energy pelvic trauma. Some injury patterns are recognized.

Vulval injury

Falls astride may result in contusion or laceration. Closed injuries can usually be managed conservatively, but it may be necessary to drain extensive haematomas. Lacerations are managed in the usual way, with control of haemorrhage being by direct pressure, followed by direct repair in an operating theatre.

Vaginal injury

Tears to the hymen may occur following first coitus, resulting in brisk bleeding. Rarely, tears to the hymen extend posteriorly into the perineum and anal sphincter. These injuries require assessment under general anaesthesia in an operating theatre.

Vaginal lacerations result from the insertion of a variety of objects, and may be situated in any part of the vaginal tract. Careful examination under anaesthesia is usually indicated to determine accurately the extent of injury. On rare occasions, injury may extend into the peritoneal cavity, necessitating laparotomy. Clinical decision-making is in no way different from other cases where the peritoneum has been breached.

Injury to the non-pregnant uterus

Blunt uterine injury in this context is rare, and almost never occurs in isolation. The most common mechanism is high-energy pelvic disruption. Penetrating injury is rare in European practice, and may result from stab injury or penetration by bullets or fragments.

INTENTIONAL VIOLENCE

Domestic violence can be defined as 'physical, psychological, economic or sexual abuse inflicted by one partner on another, in an intimate relationship'. It may involve verbal abuse, threats, and accusation, deprivation of freedom, or physical or sexual assault. Women are more likely (90% of cases) to be injured than men in the domestic environment, but men may not be the initial aggressors. Although known as domestic violence, it may not necessarily take place at home. Violence between adult partners occurs in all social classes, all ethnic groups and cultures, all age groups, in disabled people as well as able-bodied, and in both homosexual and heterosexual relationships.

Scope of the problem

According to the British Crime Survey in 1992:

- One in ten women reported some degree of physical violence in their relationship.
- Those most at risk were divorced or separated women.

The British Crime Survey in 1996 reported that:

- 60% of incidents involved current partners.
- 20% of incidents involved former partners.
- Four out of five incidents took place in the home.

Nearly one-third of incidents resulted in the need for medical intervention, with 3% defined as serious. Intentional violence in the domestic setting carries a risk of death. Heath[22] reported that 40–45% of female homicide victims in England and Wales are killed by their partner or ex-partner, while further findings from Heath's report revealed that:

- one in five of all murder victims is a woman killed by a partner or ex-partner;
- one-third of all crimes reported against women results from domestic violence;
- one-quarter of all reported assaults occur in the domestic environment; and
- domestic violence is more common than violence in the street or public house.

Intentional violence in pregnancy

Domestic violence often begins or escalates during pregnancy, its incidence during pregnancy varying from 0.9% to 20%. Indeed, domestic violence is more common than serious pregnancy problems such as pre-eclampsia, gestational diabetes and placenta praevia.[23]

Barriers for detection of intentional violence

Perhaps the main reason for the non-recognition of intentional violence is lack of awareness of its prevalence. Often, medical personnel are of the opinion that it is not the physician's role to intervene, and even if medical attendants recognize the problem, few know how to help. There are patient-related barriers to the identification of abuse, and many of the victims are held captive in their homes. Victims may believe that their injuries are not severe enough to seek help, and after a while they may even fail to recognize that they are being abused. Other reasons may be religious or cultural barriers, fear of safety, shame or humiliation. Arrest and prosecution of the perpetrators may result in more severe violence from an angry assailant on release.[24]

Diagnosis and clinical findings

If you do not look, you do not find. In 81% of cases the explanation of the mechanism for injury is inconsistent with the extent of physical injury. Substantial delay exists between the time of injury and presentation for treatment. Injuries in pregnancy and injuries that are hidden by clothing must be viewed with suspicion. These patients are often accompanied by partners who insist on staying with the patient and answer all the questions. Abused women suffer a high incidence of psychiatric disorders (particularly depression), and various self-damaging behaviours, including drug and alcohol abuse, suicide and para-suicide. Frequent visits to hospitals with vague complaints, chronic abdominal pains, and atypical chest pains may be pointers to the presence of domestic violence. Familiarity with injury patterns associated with domestic intentional violence is essential for all those working in the emergency and obstetric services. Bilateral multiple bruises and lacerations in various stages of healing are common.

Table 14.2 *Injury patterns in the abused*[25]

- Patterned injuries (injuries that show the imprint of objects used)
- Injuries to the arms, especially defensive bruises along the ulnar border
- Injuries to the genitals and breasts
- Injury to the abdomen during pregnancy, vaginal bleeding and threatened abortion
- Periorbital haematoma
- Nasal fracture
- Perforated tympanic membrane
- Fractured mandible
- Burns from cigarettes, electrical appliances, friction and arson
- Occult presentations (masked by drug/alcohol abuse or psychiatric problems)

Victims are highly represented among A&E department users, as most assaults take place out of routine working hours when general practitioners and obstetricians are relatively inaccessible.

How to help

Injuries should be carefully documented, preferably photographically, or by means of drawings and diagrams. The victim's statements regarding circumstances of abuse should be recorded, and detailed records must be maintained in case of subsequent legal action. The patient should be offered appropriate help and guidance.

RITUAL GENITAL MUTILATION

The United Kingdom is a multi-cultural society, and female genital mutilation – previously confined to other areas of the world – is now almost certainly practised. The term female circumcision is widely used, but actually encompasses a wide variety of mutilating genital procedures, ranging from minimalist cutting to extensive surgical excision of large portions of the female external genitalia.[26] As many of these procedures are practised in a clandestine way, patients with complications may present to A&E Departments. In managing such conditions, the possibility of injury must first be considered. Early complications are haemorrhage and damage to adjacent organs such as the bladder and bowel. Short-term complications include acute urinary retention, secondary haemorrhage and other manifestations of sepsis. Longer-term complications include scarring with resulting stenosis of the introitus, dysuria and menstrual problems. The patient is likely to be a young girl or adolescent.

SUMMARY

Pregnancy results in significant physiological and anatomical changes that may confuse the initial assessment and resuscitation of the injured pregnant woman. Evaluation of the injured pregnant woman and her foetus therefore requires a multidisciplinary approach, involving all those normally involved with the management of trauma, together with support from obstetricians and neonatal paediatricians. Nevertheless, the general approach is the same as for the non-pregnant patient, but recognizing the unique impacting factors mentioned above.

Attention must first be directed towards the mother, and this offers the best prospect for the foetus. Doctors and other health professionals must be aware of conditions unique to pregnancy such as placental abruption, uterine rupture, DIC, rhesus isoimmunization and a variety of indicators of foetal distress.

Time is of the essence!

REFERENCES

1. Knight B. *Legal Aspects of Medical Practice* (5th edn). London: Churchill Livingstone, 1992.
2. Poole GV, Martin JN, Perry KG, Griswold JA, Lambert CJ, Rhodes RS. Trauma in pregnancy: the role of interpersonal violence. *American Journal of Obstetrics and Gynecology* 1996; **174**: 1873–7, discussion 1877–8.
3. Goodwin TM, Breen MT. Pregnancy outcome and foetomaternal haemorrhage after non-catastrophic trauma. *American Journal of Obstetrics and Gynecology* 1990; **162**: 665–71.
4. Pearlmann MD, Tintinalli JE, Lorenz RP. A prospective controlled study of outcome after trauma during pregnancy. *American Journal of Obstetrics and Gynecology* 1990; **162**: 1502–10.
5. Collicott PE. Concepts of trauma management – epidemiology, mechanisms and prevention. In: Skinner D, *et al.* (eds). *Cambridge Textbook of Emergency Medicine*. Cambridge: Cambridge University Press, 1997.
6. Vaizey CJ, Jacobsen MT, Cross FW. Trauma in pregnancy. *British Journal of Surgery* 1994; **81**: 1406–15.
7. Shah KH, Simons RK, Holbrook T, Fortlage D, Winchell RJ, Hoyt DB. Trauma in pregnancy: maternal death and foetal outcomes. *Journal of Trauma* 1998; **45**: 83–6.
8. Schneider H. Trauma and pregnancy. *Archives of Gynecology and Obstetrics*, 1993; **253** (Suppl.): S4–S14.
9. Schonfield A, Ziv E, Stein L, *et al.* Seat belts in pregnancy and the obstetrician. *Obstetrical and Gynecological Survey* 1987; **42**: 275–82.
10. Pearce M. Seat belts in pregnancy. *British Medical Journal* 1992; **304**: 586–7.

11. Ali J, Yeo A, Gana TJ, McLellan BA. Predictors of foetal mortality in pregnant trauma patients. *Journal of Trauma* 1997; **42**: 782–5.

12. Farmer DL, Adzick NS, Cromblehome WR, Cromblehome TM, Longaker MT, Harrison MR. Fetal trauma: relation to maternal injury. *Journal of Pediatric Surgery* 1990; **25**: 711–14.

13. Lavin JP, Scott Polsky S. Abdominal trauma during pregnancy. *Clinical Perinatology* 1983; **10**: 423–37.

14. Ryan JM, Rich NM, Dale RF, Morgans BT, Cooper GJ (eds). *Ballistic Trauma – Clinical Relevance in Peace and War*. London: Arnold, 1997.

15. Higgins SD. Trauma in pregnancy. *Journal of Perinatology* 1988; **8**: 288–92.

16. Matthews RN. Obstetric implications of burns in pregnancy. *British Journal of Obstetrics and Gynaecology* 1982; **89**: 603–9.

17. Rose PG, Strohm MT, Zuspan FP. Fetomaternal haemorrhage following trauma. *American Journal of Obstetrics and Gynecology* 1986; **153**: 844–7.

18. Higgins SD, Gairite TJ. Late abruptio placenta in trauma patients: implications for monitoring. *Obstetrics and Gynecology* 1984; **63**: 10S–12S.

19. Stauffer DM. The trauma patient who is pregnant. *Journal of Emergency Nursing* 1986; **12**: 89–93.

20. Auerbach PS. Trauma in the pregnant patient. *Topics in Emergency Medicine* 1979; **1**: 133–47.

21. Sill PR. Non-obstetric genital tract trauma in Port Moresby, Papua New Guinea. *Australia and New Zealand Journal of Obstetrics and Gynaecology* 1987; **27**: 164–5.

22. Heath I. Domestic violence and the general practitioner. *Maternal and Child Health* 1994; pp 316–20.

23. Cunningham FG, *et al*. *Williams Obstetrics* (19th edn). Norwalk, Connecticut: Appleton and Lange, 1993.

24. Morley R, Mullender A. *Preventing domestic violence to women*. London: Home Office Police Department, 1994. (Police Research Group, Crime Prevention Unit, series paper number 48.)

25. Gruntfield A, Mackay K. Diagnosing domestic violence. *Canadian Journal of Diagnosis* 1997; **September**: 61–9.

26. Khaled MA, Cox C. Female genital mutilation. *Trauma* 2000; **2**: 161–7.

15

Injuries due to burns and cold

OBJECTIVES

- To explain the basic pathophysiology of burn injury
- To highlight the role of the ABCDE approach in managing initial life-threatening manifestations of burns
- To describe a system of assessing burn injuries
- To describe the essential interventions required in the Emergency Department
- To identify those burn injuries that require referral for definitive care

INTRODUCTION

The burn victim presents healthcare professionals with difficult challenges. The unpleasant nature of the injury is exacerbated by high levels of distress in the victim, their relatives and often in staff. While minor burns are a common part of Emergency Department activity, the major burn is an infrequent event. Of the 175 000 or so burns cases seen each year in UK hospitals, approximately 13 000 are admitted. Of these, only about 800 require intravenous resuscitation.

Burns are potentially life-threatening injuries. As with all victims of trauma, appropriate and timely assessment, resuscitation and transfer to definitive care offers the best chance for optimal recovery.

PATHOPHYSIOLOGY

Cutaneous injury

Temperatures little over 40°C denature proteins and cause cellular dysfunction. Above 45°C, cellular repair mechanisms are overwhelmed and cell death occurs in about 1 h. A temperature over 60°C causes necrosis and vessel thrombosis almost immediately.[1] The extent of injury is dependent on the heat and duration of the burn. Heat is dissipated away from the area of contact and surrounding tissues may sustain a less severe injury.

Those tissues that survive but have sustained heat damage are subject to an inflammatory process. This evolves for several hours after the burn and can cause further injury both locally and systemically. Appropriate management of a burn can minimize this process and result in an improved outcome.

The magnitude of the inflammatory response is related to the extent of the tissue injury. This is most easily expressed as the percentage of the total body surface area (TBSA) that is burnt; this is recorded as %TBSA.

Part of the inflammatory response increases capillary permeability, and there is a loss of fluid from the intravascular space. The most superficial burns cause only erythema and there is no significant capillary leakage. Areas so affected should not, therefore, be considered as part of the burn. In burns of greater than approximately 20% TBSA, the inflammatory mediators affect the whole body and patients develop a Systemic Inflammatory Response Syndrome (SIRS).[2] There is a massive intravascular fluid loss and burn shock develops.[3] This is a progressive process that develops for many hours after the injury, and appearance of the clinical signs of SIRS can be delayed. If there is hypovolaemic shock early after a burn, other causes need to be excluded.

Burns greater than 20% TBSA cause a life-threatening systemic injury

---

A goal of the initial management of the major burn is to prevent the development of burn shock. Historical experience has shown that any adult with a burn greater than 15% TBSA and any child with a burn greater than 10% TBSA benefits from the prophylactic administration of intravenous fluids.

Intravenous fluid resuscitation is required for all burns greater than:
- **15% TBSA in adults**
- **10% TBSA in children**

Burn depth

The depth of a burn will dictate wound management, but has little bearing on initial resuscitative measures. The wound is dynamic and its appearance can change over the first couple of days. It is not appropriate to spend a long period of time trying to assess burn depth in the Emergency Department.

The classification of burn depth is purely descriptive.[4] Burns involve either the full thickness, or only part of the thickness of the skin. Partial thickness burns are subclassified depending on which parts of the skin are involved; epidermal, superficial dermal and deep dermal.

- *Superficial (epidermal) burns*: these cause erythema alone and are most commonly seen as sunburn. They are not included when calculating %TBSA.
- *Superficial dermal burns*: superficial dermal burns cause blistering, but leave the deep dermal vasculature and epidermal appendages intact. These burns are associated with erythema which blanches with pressure. Capillary refill is preserved.
- *Deep dermal burns*: in these burns there is damage to the deeper blood vessels and haemoglobin is sequestered in the tissue. The redness associated with these burns does not blanch; hence this is sometimes referred to as 'fixed staining'.
- *Full thickness burns*: these destroy the normal dermis and leave a firm, leathery layer of necrotic tissue known as eschar. This necrotic tissue can be waxy white or red. Soot or charred tissue may mask the underlying appearance.

It is important to remember that burn wounds are not homogeneous, and a mixed pattern may be seen. For example, surrounding full-thickness burns which are characteristically painless, there is usually a border of intensely painful partial thickness burn.

Inhalation injury

Inhalation injury is not a homogeneous entity, but consists broadly of three variable components.

THE TRUE AIRWAY BURN

This is caused by inhalation of hot gases in the form of flame, smoke or steam. The upper airways are efficient at dissipating heat, and the larynx closes quickly. The resulting injury is thermal in nature and affects the supraglottic airway. The initial manifestation is upper-airway oedema which develops over a period of hours and is maximal between 12 and 36 h.

THE LUNG INJURY

If the products of combustion are inhaled, they dissolve in the fluid lining the bronchial tree and alveoli. The result is a chemical injury to the lower airways which produces various manifestations of pulmonary failure, often delayed by many hours or days.

SYSTEMIC INTOXICATION

Absorption of the products of combustion into the circulation through the alveoli can lead to systemic toxicity. The most commonly encountered intoxications are from carbon monoxide and cyanide. These account for the majority of deaths from fires, and normally occur at the scene. Carbon monoxide competes with oxygen for binding to haemoglobin, having 240 times its affinity. It therefore displaces oxygen, effectively causing hypoxaemia. It also binds to the intracellular cytochrome system, causing abnormal cellular function. A low level of carboxyhaemoglobin (<10%) causes no symptoms and can be found in heavy smokers. Above 20%, feelings of fatigue and nausea can start and higher mental functions are impaired. Levels above 40% lead to progressive loss of neurological function, and death occurs with levels over 60%. It should be noted that in the presence of carboxyhaemoglobin, pulse oximeter readings are unreliable indicators of oxygen saturation (%SaO$_2$).

Inhalation injury can consist of any combination of the above, and its presence significantly worsens the prognosis following a burn.

INITIAL ADVANCED LIFE SUPPORT

Burn victims are trauma victims and the initial assessment is the same as for any other seriously injured patient. There may be injuries other than the burn and these must be treated or excluded. As a general principle though, any burn involving greater than 10% TBSA should be regarded as significant and assessed and treated in a resuscitation bay.

Although effective first aid is likely to have been performed in the pre-hospital setting, it is essential to ensure that the burning process has been stopped. Smouldering clothes or those soaked in scalding fluids, jewellery and watches (which will act as a reservoir of heat) should be removed without delay. Dousing the affected area in cold water will stop the burning process. Chemical powders should be brushed off.

Immediate cooling of the burn wound modifies local inflammation and reduces progressive cell necrosis.[5] This is best achieved by the topical application of cool water, preferably flowing water, though proprietary wet gels may be used as an alternative. Cooling the wound also has a beneficial analgesic effect. Very cold water and ice are to be avoided, as they cause local vasoconstriction and worsen the situation.

Ideally the cooling should be started immediately and continued for about 20 min. It is uncertain if there is any benefit beyond this time. Protracted cooling will lead to systemic hypothermia, particularly in small children.

A full primary survey must be performed using the ABCDE approach as described throughout this manual. Resuscitative interventions should be carried out as indicated. The full manifestations of the burn injury will evolve over a few hours. This first assessment is to identify any injuries that may compromise survival while a more thorough assessment of the burn is undertaken.

Airway and breathing

In the initial assessment of the airway and breathing the most important aspect is to diagnose any degree of inhalation injury. Potential complications can therefore be anticipated and appropriate interventions instigated.

The development of signs and symptoms from airway oedema and pulmonary injury occurs progressively over several hours. The key to diagnosis is therefore a high index of suspicion with the frequent re-evaluation of those considered to be at risk.

> **A high index of suspicion is the key to diagnosing inhalation injury**

The presence of any of the following indicate the possibility of an inhalation injury (Table 15.1).

Table 15.1 *Indicators of possible inhalational injury*

- A history of exposure to fire and/or smoke in an enclosed space such as a building or vehicle
- Collapse, confusion or restlessness at any time
- Hoarseness, cough or any change in voice
- Stridor
- Burns to the face including singed nasal hairs
- Soot in saliva or sputum
- An inflamed oropharynx
- Raised carboxyhaemoglobin levels
- Exposure to a blast
- Deteriorating pulmonary function

In all cases a high concentration of humidified oxygen must be administered.

If any degree of upper airway obstruction is present, endotracheal intubation is mandatory. In severe cases this may require the use of a surgical airway. The presence of stridor indicates that some degree of obstruction already exists. If there is a strong suspicion of inhalation injury but obstruction is not evident, an experienced anaesthetist should be called urgently to assess the patient. Upper-airway oedema will continue to develop over the first few hours. If there is any doubt, the patient should be intubated.

> **If inhalation injury is suspected, experienced anaesthetic expertise is required promptly.**
> **If in doubt, intubate**

MANAGEMENT OF INHALATIONAL INJURY

Treatment of inhalational injury is through application of supportive measures. All patients should receive high-flow humidified oxygen. The most likely problem with an upper-airway burn is obstruction, while a lower-airway injury will result in difficulty in ventilation and gas exchange. Both processes evolve over several hours, and this should be anticipated. The management of lower-airway injury is highly specialized. Even in the absence of a cutaneous burn, inhalational lung injury should be referred to a burns centre.

Management of systemic intoxication is aimed at maximizing oxygen delivery. The most significant intoxicant is carbon monoxide. Carboxyhaemoglobin has a half-life of 250 min in a patient breathing room air, but this reduces to 40 min when breathing 100% oxygen. Administration of the highest oxygen concentration feasible should therefore be used, and this may necessitate intubation and ventilation. Dissociation of carbon monoxide from intracellular cytochromes is slower and can lead to a secondary rise in carboxyhaemoglobin levels. Oxygen administration should therefore continue for at least 24 h. Hyperbaric oxygen treatment speeds up carbon monoxide clearance, but is not easily available and is associated with certain risks. Its use is controversial and it has not been shown to improve outcome in properly conducted trials.[6] Specific treatments for other types of systemic intoxicants are not in routine use.

Circulation

It should be noted that hypovolaemic shock secondary to a burn takes some time to produce measurable physical signs. If the burn victim is shocked early, other causes should be excluded. A history of a blast, vehicle collision or a fall while escaping the fire should raise suspicion of other injuries. If the patient has hypovolaemic shock, this should be treated as outlined elsewhere in this manual, independent of the severity of burn.

Early hypovolaemic shock is rarely due to the burn

Intravenous access should be established, ideally with two large-bore cannuli. It is possible to cannulate through burnt skin, but this should be avoided if possible. Alternatives include intravenous cut-down, intra-osseous infusion in children or central routes including the femoral vein. Blood must be sent for laboratory baseline investigations (including carboxyhaemoglobin levels if an inhalation injury is suspected).

Several formulae have been developed empirically over the years to allow the requirements for intravenous fluid to be calculated.[3,7] Which fluid to use is contentious, and there is still much debate over colloid versus crystalloid regimes. The concept of replacing like with like, although attractive, is an over-simplification. The current recommendation in the UK is to use crystalloid resuscitation fluid in the first 24 h based on the Parkland formula.

ESTIMATING INTRAVENOUS FLUID REQUIREMENTS

The Parkland formula provides the total volume of intravenous crystalloid that is likely to be required to prevent burns shock in the first 24 h from the time of injury. It is calculated as follows:

Fluid requirement in the first 24 h
= (2 – 4 x %TBSA burn x kg body weight) ml crystalloid

The weight of a child can be determined by asking the parents, or by the use of a Broselaw tape.

Half the calculated volume is required over the first 8 h after the burn, and the second half is administered in the next 16 h.

In the Emergency Department the higher starting volume based on 4 ml/%burn/kg should be used. Corrections can be made once the patient is in the burns centre. The fluid requirement starts at the time of injury and the administration rate should reflect this; as a consequence, there may be a period of catch-up.

The calculated volume required commences at the time of injury

---

It should be noted that the formula calculates the volume required to make up for fluid loss due to the burn. It does not allow for other losses such as haemorrhage from other injuries, nor for maintenance requirements.

The Parkland formula provides an estimate of the likely requirements. Burns are not homogeneous, and patients respond in different ways. It is essential that the adequacy of the resuscitation is monitored, as both over- and under-resuscitation can be detrimental. Urinary output reliably reflects the circulatory state of the patient and is easy to measure. Indeed, it is the mainstay of monitoring burns patients. Heart rate and non-invasive blood pressure readings are poor indicators of resuscitation in burns.

Minimum urine output should be:

- 0.5 ml/kg/h in adults
- 1.0 ml/kg/h in children
- 2.0 ml/kg/h in infants

These are minimum rates, and an output of 1 ml/kg/h should be aimed for in adults. Accurate measurement of urinary output requires the insertion of a urethral catheter.

Deep burns, particularly those following electrocution, cause the release of breakdown products of myoglobin and haemoglobin. These are excreted in the urine and turn it a dark red colour. In addition, the deposition of these compounds in the renal tubules can lead to renal failure. The initial treatment is to increase fluid resuscitation, aiming at achieving a urinary output of 2 ml/kg/h. Alkalinization of the urine and the use of mannitol can help, but should be started only after consultation with the local burns centre. As with all trauma cases, regular re-evaluation is essential.

Disability

A reduced level of consciousness, confusion and restlessness normally indicate intoxication and/or hypoxia secondary to an inhalation injury. The possibility of alcohol or drug ingestion and the presence of other injuries must not be overlooked.

Exposure

All clothing, including underwear, jewellery, watches and any other restricting items must be removed. The risk of hypothermia is often overlooked. The removal of clothing and liberal use of cold water at the scene, during transfer and in the Emergency Department leads to the not uncommon event of the burns centre receiving a hypothermic patient. Judicious local cooling of the burn should be accompanied by covering uninvolved areas and aiming to get the ambient temperature to 30°C.

> **Hypothermia is a significant risk during the management of burns**

Other initial interventions

Immunity against tetanus should be ensured. In the absence of any specific indications, such as associated contaminated wounds, there is no requirement for antibiotic prophylaxis. Insertion of a urinary catheter will be required in all patients with significant burns. Insertion of a nasogastric tube should also be considered.

> **Antibiotics are not indicated in the early management of burns**

Burns are painful, and their victims are often terrified. Adequate intravenous opiate analgesia should be administered early together with an anti-emetic.

> **Adequate intravenous opiates should be administered early**

Before progressing to the specific management of the burn and a full secondary survey, the initial assessment should be rapidly but thoroughly repeated.

MANAGEMENT OF THE BURN

Inhalational injury

There is little else that can be done in the Emergency Department beyond intubation and ventilation. Any patient with a suspected inhalation injury should be closely observed in an area equipped for intubation. If there is an inhalation injury then the patient should be managed by an experienced anaesthetist until arrival at the receiving burns centre. Pulse oximetry readings must be interpreted with caution. Arterial blood gas analysis and a chest X-ray should be performed, but these may be normal initially. There is no evidence that administration of steroids is beneficial (although pre-injury users should continue their steroids).[8]

> **The use of steroids is not indicated in inhalation injury**

Patients with an inhalational injury, or who are suspected of having an inhalational injury and who are to be transferred to another hospital, should be anaesthetized and intubated before transfer.

The cutaneous burn

Whatever the cause of the burn, the severity of the injury is proportional to the volume of tissue damage. In terms of survival, the %TBSA involved is the most important factor. Functional outcome is more often dependent on the depth and site of the burn.

CALCULATING %TBSA BURN

Use of the 'rule of nines' will give an effective rough initial assessment of the area of the body which has been burnt, as long as simple erythema is excluded (Figure 15.1).

The palmar surface of the patient's hand (including the fingers) equates to approximately 1% TBSA and can be used to estimate small areas of burn.

As an alternative, a more detailed assessment can be made using a Lund and Browder burns chart (Figure 15.2).

When using this chart it is important to be clear and accurate. The burnt areas should be carefully recorded on the chart and the %TBSA burnt calculated once again, ignoring simple erythema. In very large burns it can be easier to calculate the size of area not burnt. Differentiating between full- and partial thickness burns is not essential.

Initial treatment

If the patient's only injuries are burns, and there is to be no undue delay in transfer to a burns centre, the only requirement for most burns is to reduce heat and water loss and to make the wound less painful. This can be achieved by loosely covering the burn with clingfilm, though this must not be wrapped around limbs but rather laid on in sheets in order to avoid constriction due to swelling. The patient should then be kept warm with dry blankets. Accurate assessment of the wound will take place at the burns centre, and there should be as little interference with the lesion as possible. There is no indication for applying any form of topical antiseptic solution or cream.

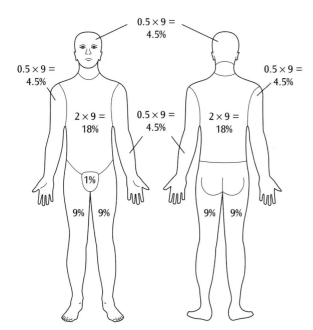

Figure 15.1 – *The 'Rule of Nines'.*

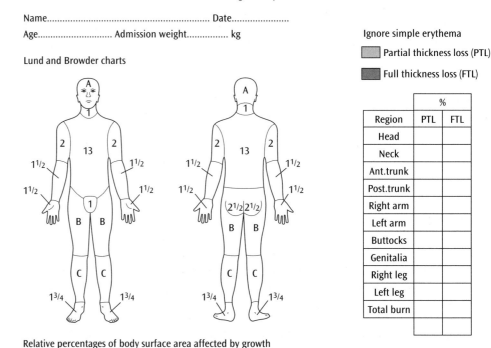

Figure 15.2 *Lund and Browder burns chart.*

The chart image contains the following:

Chart for estimating severity of burn wound

Name.. Date.....................
Age........................... Admission weight............... kg

Lund and Browder charts

Ignore simple erythema

Partial thickness loss (PTL)

Full thickness loss (FTL)

Region	PTL	FTL
Head		
Neck		
Ant.trunk		
Post.trunk		
Right arm		
Left arm		
Buttocks		
Genitalia		
Right leg		
Left leg		
Total burn		

Relative percentages of body surface area affected by growth

Area	Age 0	1	5	10	15	Adult
A = 1/2 of head	9 1/2	8 1/2	6 1/2	5 1/2	4 1/2	3 1/2
B = 1/2 of one thigh	2 3/4	3 1/4	4	4 1/2	4 1/2	4 3/4
C = 1/2 of one leg	2 1/2	2 1/2	2 3/4	3 1/4	3 1/4	3 1/2

> **Do not apply ointments or creams**

Circumferential full-thickness burns can act like a tourniquet and compromise circulation. Division of the constriction is known as escharotomy. This is not a straightforward undertaking, and is only rarely required in the resuscitation room. Full-thickness burns of the entire trunk preventing respiration is an indication for urgent life-saving escharotomy.

Burns which do not require transfer to a burns unit are best treated by dressing with a petroleum jelly-based dressing such as Jelonet®. There is no advantage to antibiotic-impregnated dressings. Significant hand burns, which cannot be dressed with Jelonet can be placed in Flamazine® (silver sulphadiazine) bags.

SPECIAL BURNS

Chemical burns

The severity of a chemical burn is related to:

- the product causing the burn;
- the concentration of the chemical;
- the amount of the chemical; and
- the duration of contact.

Although a knowledge of the chemical which has produced the burn is helpful, in many cases, this information will unfortunately not be available. However, with modern health and safety legislation, there is a requirement for companies to keep safety data on dangerous products they use. Victims of chemical burns from industrial sites will often arrive at hospital with information exceeding that which is readily available in medical texts. Whether the burning substance can be identified or not, the initial management of the burn process should continue along conventional lines.

DOMESTIC CHEMICAL BURNS

In domestic incidents, the trade-name of a household product is frequently all that is available. Poisons units are able to provide details of the contents of domestic products, and their help should be sought.

Some compounds may cause systemic toxicity and some induce an inhalation injury. Unless the product is totally familiar, it is worth contacting a Poisons unit, even for what appear to be minor chemical burns.

Treatment

In all cases the mainstay of treatment is continuous copious irrigation with water.[9] If powder or lumps of the product are visible, these should be removed first. All of the patient's clothes should be removed, including underwear. Applying soaks is inadequate – there needs to be continuous irrigation.

Contamination and injury to others is a serious risk when dealing with chemical burns, and all those involved should wear appropriate protective equipment. Any clothes or materials from the victim, together with used irrigation fluid, must be treated as being contaminated.

Irrigation should continue for about 20–30 min. Acids produce coagulative necrosis, and the eschar helps to reduce penetration. Alkalis cause liquefaction, and penetration into deeper tissues is more significant. Irrigation for alkali burns should therefore continue for longer, ideally for at least an hour. Indicator paper can be placed intermittently on the wound to see if the pH is returning to neutral. Once again, risk of hypothermia with prolonged irrigation should not be forgotten.

The use of neutralizing agents can cause exothermic reactions and worsen the burn; hence, they should not be used.

Very serious injury can develop following what appears to be an innocuous exposure. There is sometimes a requirement to administer specific antidotes. All chemical burns should be discussed with a burns centre for details of specific treatments, and most such patients will need to be transferred. Chemical burns of the eye require prolonged irrigation, and early consultation with ophthalmic expertise is mandatory.

Specific burns

PHOSPHORUS BURNS

Phosphorus burns are uncommon, and most experience has been gained from conflict where it is used as a weapon. Phosphorus is a translucent, fat-soluble and water-insoluble solid, which melts at 44ºC and ignites at 34ºC. It fumes in air and ignites spontaneously. With skin contact it causes chemical and thermal injury, and there is a risk of systemic absorption due to its high fat-solubility, producing hypocalcaemia, CNS depression and liver failure.

Treatment involves thorough and constant water irrigation and removal of phosphorus particles (sometimes requiring excision). Copper sulphate solutions have been used to convert the phosphorus into a cupric phosphide, which is easily identified as it is black. This also prevents absorption of the phosphorus, although copper itself is systemically toxic and little benefit has been shown.[10]

HYDROFLUORIC ACID BURNS

Hydrofluoric acid (HF) is commonly used in the manufacture of fluorocarbons, PTFE (Teflon) and high-octane fuel. It is also used to clean glass and remove rust.

HF causes coagulative necrosis at its point of contact, and a liquefaction necrosis occurs in the deeper tissues causing the formation of deep ulcers. The fluoride ion is absorbed locally and systemically and binds to intracellular calcium and magnesium, arresting cell functions and causing cell death with the consequent release of potassium. The potassium irritates the nerve endings and causes extreme pain.

Even with small TBSA burns there can be a rapid fall in serum calcium and sodium, and a rise in potassium and fluoride; therefore specific therapy is required in addition to general advice about irrigation. Calcium gluconate gel can be applied locally to the area and massaged in until the pain is abating. Local infiltration with calcium gluconate should also be carried out. Serum calcium and potassium levels should be monitored and intravenous supplementation may be required.[11–13]

Electrical burns

Passage of electricity through the body produces heat which can cause burns. The type of injury seen depends on voltage, and two groups are generally recognized:

1. Low-voltage (under 1000 V): this includes the normal domestic mains supply of 240 V and the common industrial supply of 415 V. Electrocution leads to cutaneous contact burns at the sites of entry and exit. The tissue damage extends through the full thickness of the skin, and deep structures immediately under the wounds can be damaged.
2. High-voltage (over 1000 V): in high-voltage burns, the entry and exit wounds may be associated with massive local damage. There may be multiple entry and exit wounds. As current flows through the tissues, extensive deep damage occurs. Entire compartments can be destroyed, sometimes without involving the overlying skin. Fasciotomies are frequently required. A flashover can occur, causing secondary ignition of clothes and a large cutaneous burn.

In both types of burn, the obvious cutaneous injury is an under-representation of the true extent of the tissue damage. In appropriate cases close attention must be paid to monitoring the fluid balance and urine output. Urinary excretion of the breakdown products of haemoglobin and myoglobin is common in extensive electrical burns. Renal failure is a significant risk in this situation, and is best prevented by the administration of additional intravenous fluids, aiming for a urinary output of 2 ml/kg/h. The receiving burns centre may advise alkalinization of the urine and administration of mannitol.

Many electrocutions result in falls, and there can also be violent tetanic muscle spasms. There is therefore a high risk of associated injuries. A thorough secondary survey with comprehensive and accurate documentation is essential. Cardiac dysrythmias can occur following passage of current across the thorax. Cardiorespiratory arrest is often reversible and prolonged efforts at resuscitation are justified. In all cases of electrocution, a 12-lead ECG should be performed; if this is abnormal, continued monitoring and a cardiac opinion should be sought. If the ECG is normal and there is no cardiac history, there is no evidence to suggest that continued cardiac monitoring is beneficial.

Electrical burns are complex and challenging to manage, and all cases should be referred to a burns centre. If there is an undue delay in transfer, then consideration needs to be given to early fasciotomies. These should be done only following discussion with the burns centre.

Pitfalls in electrical burns
- **there may be significant deep tissue damage**
- **associated injuries are common**
- **the standard formula will under-predict fluid requirements**
- **electrical burns are complex injuries and require referral**

TRANSFER TO DEFINITIVE CARE

Referral criteria

The following injuries should be referred to a burn centre:

- burns greater than 10% TBSA in an adult;
- burns greater than 5% TBSA in a child;
- full-thickness burns greater than 1% TBSA;
- burns of special areas; face, hands, feet, genitalia, major joints;
- complex electrical burns;
- presence of an inhalational injury;
- circumferential burns;
- burns in the very young and very old; and
- significant chemical burns.

In all cases, early contact with the nearest burn centre should be made. Advice on initial management and transfer will be given. In addition, there may be specific local guidelines that need to be followed.

Preparation for transfer

By this stage, all patients will have had a primary survey with appropriate resuscitative interventions, a full assessment of the burn, and initial burn management as outlined. Before transfer it is important to ensure that:

- a thorough secondary survey has been performed and any associated injuries have been identified and appropriately managed;
- maximum inspired oxygen is being administered;
- if there is any suspicion of an inhalational injury, the patient has been assessed by an experienced anaesthetist and intubated if necessary;
- adequate intravenous access is secured and appropriate fluid resuscitation has started;
- the burn wound is covered with clingfilm and the patient is being kept warm;
- the patient has been given adequate analgesia;
- there is a urinary catheter in place;
- there is a free-draining nasogastric tube in place; and
- all findings and interventions, including fluid balance, are clearly and accurately documented.

All patients should be transferred with an appropriately trained escort.

If it is likely that a delay in transfer will exceed 6h, then the patient will require management in an appropriate environment with regular discussion taking place with the burns unit. In this situation escharotomies, cleaning and dressing of the burn wound and the commencement of maintenance intravenous fluids and/or nasogastric feeding may be necessary.

INJURIES DUE TO COLD

In the UK, injuries due to cold are uncommon, and when seen are normally associated with social deprivation or neglect. They are manifested as:

- hypothermia, the systemic effects of a reduced core temperature; and
- local tissue damage.

Hypothermia

Hypothermia is defined as a reduction in the core temperature to <35°C, below which cognitive ability is reduced. Below 32°C, hypothermia is described as severe and there is cardiac irritability and progressive loss of consciousness. The normal measurable parameters of cardiac and respiratory function vary and may be difficult to elicit. The pathophysiological changes are normally reversible with rewarming.[14]

Unfortunately, hypothermia is seen as a result of poor care of the severely injured trauma victim. The exposed unconscious patient in a cold resuscitation bay being administered unwarmed intravenous fluids has little chance of maintaining a normal core temperature. Hypothermia is an additional pathophysiological insult that impacts unfavourably on outcome.

Special low-reading thermometers need to be used when diagnosing hypothermia, while in severe cases an oesophageal probe is required.

In mild cases the patient should be kept in a warm room (30°C if possible) and all cold and wet clothes removed and replaced by warm blankets. Warmed fluids can be given by mouth or intravenously.

In severe hypothermia an initial assessment following the ABCDE approach should be performed. Invasive monitoring will be required, and the patient may be best managed in an Intensive Care environment. Unconscious cases require active core re-warming, and this may entail peritoneal lavage, haemodialysis or cardiopulmonary bypass – all of which should only be performed by experienced clinicians.

With a core temperature below about 27°C there may be no external signs of life, yet full recovery from this situation is possible. The patient will require intubation and ventilation, and active core re-warming must be commenced. Because of cardiac irritability, unnecessary movements may trigger ventricular fibrillation, but cardiac massage must be continued in the absence of spontaneous cardiac output until the patient is warm enough for spontaneous output to return or for defibrillation to be effective. Expert management in an Intensive Care setting is essential.

Diagnosing death in this situation is difficult. The axiom 'not dead until warm and dead' is still valid, although due account of the circumstances surrounding the hypothermia must be taken. Resuscitative measures should continue until the core temperature is at least above 32°C or there is no rise in core temperature, despite active re-warming.

Local tissue damage

Extremities such as fingers, toes, nose and ears may freeze when exposed to severe cold. The damage caused during freezing is exacerbated by a re-perfusion injury on thawing, and tissue necrosis may follow. Typically, frozen skin is white and then becomes blue or purple on thawing. This is accompanied by swelling and can be extremely painful. Blistering of the skin may follow, and days later a thick carapace forms which blackens. Eventually, sometimes after months, the carapace is shed to reveal new healthy skin underneath. In severe cases significant amounts of tissue are lost in this process and this can include auto-amputation of entire digits.[15]

Frostnip is a minor form of frostbite in which the skin turns white and numb and which reverses on re-warming. Short-term pain and hyperaemia are the only sequelae.

If a body part is frozen, re-warming should be started as soon as possible. This is best achieved by immersion in circulating water heated to 40°C. This should continue for at least 30 min or until thawing is complete. This process can be extremely painful, and strong analgesia will be required.[16]

The subsequent management of the affected parts requires specialist care and referral should be made to a burn centre or plastic surgery unit. Avoidance of secondary infection is important, but antibiotics should be reserved for treatment rather than prophylaxis.

SUMMARY

The principles of burn management can be summarized as follows:
- First aid
  - Stop the burning process
  - Cool the burn
  - Be aware of hypothermia
- Initial assessment
  - Use the ABCDE approach
  - Identify and treat life-threatening injuries
  - Provide adequate analgesia
- Inhalation injury
  - Maintain a high index of suspicion
  - Seek experienced anaesthetic help
  - If in doubt, intubate
- Cutaneous burn
  - Calculate %TBSA burn
  - Calculate fluid requirements using Parkland formula
  - Fluid requirements start from the time of injury
  - Monitor urine output
- Transfer to definitive care
  - Refer all appropriate cases
  - Ensure full documentation
  - Ensure safe transfer.

REFERENCES

1. Moritz AR, Henriquez FC. Studies of thermal injury II. The relative importance of time and surface temperature in the causation of cutaneous burns. *American Journal of Pathology* 1947; **23**: 695–720.
2. Arturson G. The pathophysiology of severe thermal injury. *Journal of Burn Care and Rehabilitation* 1985; **6**: 129–46.
3. Baxter CR. Fluid volume and electrolyte changes in the early post-burn period. *Clinical Plastic Surgery* 1974; **1**: 693–703.
4. Jackson DM. The diagnosis of the depth of burning. *British Journal of Surgery* 1953; **40**: 588–96.
5. Jandera V, Hudson DA, deWet PM, Innes PM, Rode H. Cooling the burn wound: evaluation of different modalities. *Burns* 2000; **26**: 265–70.
6. Scheinkestel CD, Bailey M, Myles PS, *et al.* Hyperbaric or normobaric oxygen for acute carbon monoxide poisoning: a randomised controlled clinical trial. *Medical Journal of Australia* 1999; **170**: 203–10.
7. Pruitt BA Jr. Fluid resuscitation of extensively burned patients. *Journal of Trauma* 1981; **21**(Suppl): 690–2.
8. Levine BA, Petroff PA, Slade CL. Prospective trials of dexamethasone and aerosolized gentamicin in the treatment of inhalational injury in the burned patient. *Journal of Trauma* 1978; **18**: 188–93.
9. Leonard LG, Scheulen JJ, Munster AM. Chemical burns: effect of prompt first aid. *Journal of Trauma* 1982; **22**: 420–3.
10. Eldad A, Simon GA. The phosphorous burn – a preliminary comparative experimental study of various forms of treatment. *Burns* 1991; **17**: 198–200.
11. Goodfellow RC. Hydrofluoric acid burns. *British Medical Journal* 1985; **290**: 237.
12. Baxter CR, Shires GT. Physiological response to crystalloid resuscitation of severe burns. *Annals of the New York Academy of Sciences* 1968; **150**: 874–94.

13. Baxter CR, Crystalloid resuscitation of burn shock. In: Polk HC, Stone HH (eds). *Contemporary Burn Management*. Boston: Little, Brown & Co, 1971; pp. 7–32.

14. Riddell DI. A practical guide to cold injuries. *Journal of the Royal Naval Medical Service* 1986; **72**: 20–5.

15. Mills WJ. Frostbite. *Alaska Medicine* 1983; **25**: 33–8.

16. Smith DJ, Robson MC, Heggers JP. Frostbite and other cold induced injuries. In: Auerbach PS, Geehr EC (eds). *Management of Wilderness and Environmental Emergencies*. St Louis: CV Mosby, 1989, pp.101–18.

16

Blast and gunshot injuries

OBJECTIVES

- To understand the ballistic aspects of wounds due to firearms
- To appreciate the scientific basis and classification of blast injury
- To outline basic protocols for the treatment of blast and gunshot wounds

INTRODUCTION

Ballistic trauma, be it from gunshot wounding or explosive blast, occurs throughout the world. In the developed world, criminal acts increasingly involve the use of firearms,[1] and terrorist attacks in the form of urban bombing campaigns have resulted in major incidents characterized by multiple severely injured casualties.[2]

Many of the clinicians responsible for treating ballistic injury will have had little previous experience of these types of wounds. As such, some knowledge of the mechanism of wounding can assist in formulating treatment strategies for the wounds encountered. It is also important to have some knowledge of the standard treatment protocols relating to these injuries.

BALLISTIC FEATURES OF GUNSHOT WOUNDING

The science of ballistics addresses the aspects of missile and bullet flight and relates these to the potential for injury. When a bullet strikes tissue it will impart some of its kinetic energy into it. This will cause the tissue to accelerate away from the track of the projectile resulting in a *temporary cavity* around the track of the missile. Once the bullet has passed, the inherent elasticity of the tissues will cause the temporary cavity to collapse, leaving some degree of *permanent cavity* along the missile track.

The extent to which cavitation occurs is, in part, governed by the amount of kinetic energy imparted to the tissues by the projectile. The size of a temporary cavity is also related to the elasticity of the tissue being penetrated and the wound track length. The equation governing this is:

kinetic energy = $\frac{1}{2} m (V_1^2 - V_2^2)$

where m is the mass of the projectile, V_1 the velocity on entering the tissues and V_2 the velocity on exiting.

The degree to which the projectile's velocity is attenuated in transiting the tissues is dependent upon the diameter of the bullet, its orientation and flight characteristics on impact, and the nature of the tissue itself.

In practice, the masses of most commonly used bullets are similar and thus the injurous potential is largely defined by the velocity of the projectile. In this regard gunshot wounds can largely be broken down into three categories depending on the nature of the weapon used as handguns, shotguns and military rifles.

Handguns

The commonest types of these weapons fire a bullet with a diameter of 9 mm and a muzzle velocity of around 1000 feet per second. As such there is only a small temporary cavity, and the injury is essentially confined to the bullet track. Provided that the bullet has not transected any major structures the degree of injury may only be slight, unless essential organs are damaged. Some of the bullets for these types of weapon are designed to deform on impact.[3] These are the hollow or soft (lead)-tipped bullets, which, on impact, tend to flatten, presenting a greater surface area to the direction of travel, and thus resulting in an increased transfer of energy and greater wounding effect.

Shotguns

A shotgun cartridge contains multiple pellets of a specified diameter. This diameter can be from 1 mm ('birdshot') to 10 mm ('buckshot'). Once fired, the pellets disperse in a cone-shaped pattern. The degree and rapidity of dispersion is proportional to the size and number of pellets as well as the diameter of the shotgun barrel at the muzzle. Due to their aerodynamics the velocity of individual pellets will attenuate over short distances, even in air. Furthermore, the conical dispersion leads to a rapid decline in the number of pellets which will hit a particular target as range increases. These two factors lead to the weapon being virtually ineffective at ranges over 50 metres. At close range, however, the shotgun can create very severe patterns of injury. Although each pellet may only be travelling at low velocity, the combined effect of multiple pellets is a formidable destructive force, shredding tissues and causing massive disruption.

Military 'assault' rifles

One of the commonest of these weapons worldwide is the AK47 (an estimated 125 million such rifles are in circulation), with a bullet of 7.62 mm diameter and 39 mm in length which leaves the weapon at a speed of around 900 m/s (3000 feet/s). In all assault weapons rifling of the barrel sets the bullet spinning, which, combined with the increased velocity, leads to greater accuracy at long range. Rather than follow a uniform flight path the bullet has a periodic motion, oscillating around its flight axis. Weapons of this kind are in widespread use among terrorist organizations.

The very much greater kinetic energy of these bullets leads to a much bigger temporary cavity than seen in low-velocity weapons. The subatmospheric pressure in the cavity will suck in clothing and other debris from outside the wound, causing contamination. The shock front of accelerating tissue, propagating away from the point of impact, causes stretching and tearing of the tissues, cellular disruption and microvascular injury. The margin of tissue around the cavity, termed the *zone of extravasation*,[3] is full of haemorrhage, has little tendency to further bleeding and, if muscle, shows no tendency to contract when stimulated. This tissue is non-viable and will become a culture medium for infection if left in place. The shock wave itself can cause fracture of bone and intimal disruption of major vessels.

The oscillating nature of the bullet trajectory can cause it to 'tumble' on impact. When this occurs, due to the non-uniform motion and greater presenting area, even greater proportions of the kinetic energy are transmitted. The resulting tissue acceleration can lead to the exit wound of such a bullet being very much larger than the entry.

The nature of the tissue being transited has a great impact on the extent of damage occurring. Relatively elastic compressible tissue such as lung propagates the shock wave to a much lesser extent than dense, fluid-filled tissue such as liver. Hence a high-velocity bullet may transit lung causing only contusion, while causing gross disruption to solid organs – particularly those surrounded by an inelastic capsule.

BLAST INJURY

Explosive injury occurs as a result of the blast wave. At the time of detonation of an explosive charge, a small volume of explosive is converted into a large volume of hot gas.

There is a resultant rise in pressure to above atmospheric, termed the *blast overpressure*, which rapidly moves away from the point of detonation. The leading edge of this blast wave, where air molecules are being heated and accelerated, is the shock front.

A blast event occurring outdoors has a simple pressure–time profile. In contrast, explosions occurring in confined spaces have complex propagation patterns. When the blast wave hits an obstacle such as a wall, a proportion of the energy is transmitted through the obstacle and a proportion is reflected. Interference patterns from the interaction of the reflected waves and the oncoming blast wave can lead to the blast overpressure being magnified several fold at certain locations. This effect is a major factor in the number and severity of casualties which result following the bombing of public houses and similar buildings.[4] A study from Israel,[5] which compared the injury patterns from terrorist bombings in closed versus open air environments, confirms the marked increase in injuries related to primary blast effects when the explosion occurs in a confined space, but notes no difference in other injury patterns. This effect also explains the mortality associated with the Guildford (five deaths) and the Birmingham (21 deaths) public house bombings in the UK in the early 1970s.[6]

Blast injuries are classified as follows

- Primary: injuries due to the blast wave.
- Secondary: injuries due to fragments.
- Tertiary: injuries due to displacement.
- Burns.
- Crush injury.
- Psychological effects.

Primary blast injury

Primary blast injury arises directly from the interaction of the blast wave with the body. As the blast wave hits the body wall, the tissues are displaced and accelerated. Homogeneous tissues are accelerated uniformly, but considerable strains are produced at the interfaces between different media (for example, air and fluid). It is these strains which lead to the injury patterns seen in primary blast injury. The commonest manifestation is tympanic barotrauma, with around 50% of exposed drums being ruptured at overpressures of 100 kPa for 10 ms or more.[7] Also vulnerable from this mechanism of injury are the lung and bowel. Tympanic injury is very dependent on the incidence of the damaging blast wave; patients standing side-on to the origin of a blast are much more likely to suffer tympanic rupture than those facing the blast. Thus, although tympanic rupture is a marker of significant blast exposure, its absence is of no significance.

When the blast wave hits the thorax, sudden movement of the chest wall causes parts of the lung to be compressed between the chest wall and other structures such as the liver or mediastinum. This compression results in contusions at these sites. Furthermore, the diaphragm rises violently as the pressure wave compresses the abdominal contents. Pressure differentials thus created within the lung may induce further haemorrhage and cause air emboli to enter the circulation. Alveolar septae are torn, lung parenchyma shears away from the vascular tree, and the alveolar epithelium is shredded. In a study from Northern Ireland such primary blast lung injury was seen in 45% of the victims who died at the scene of the explosion.[8]

Damage to the gastrointestinal tract is more common with underwater explosions than in air blast.[9] Severe damage and evisceration are seen at post-mortem examination for cases within the 'lethal zone' in the immediate vicinity of an explosion. At greater distances from the blast perforation of the gut wall, mesenteric tears or haemorrhages can result.

Secondary blast injury

Secondary blast injury is due to the impact of fragment material included in the explosive device or from other surrounding objects accelerated by the explosion. Examples of the former include preformed fragments from military munitions or nails packed around improvised explosive devices. In terms of surrounding objects causing secondary blast injury, one of the commonest sources of this is glass fragments from windows broken by the blast. In contrast to bullets, fragments from bombs or explosive munitions are non-aerodynamic. This causes the fragment velocity to attenuate rapidly in flight. As a result, secondary blast injury is not associated with cavitation or large volumes of non-viable tissue surrounding the wound track.[10] Furthermore, penetration is often limited to superficial areas only. Nevertheless, because these wounds are invariably multiple, they can present a major management problem.

Tertiary blast injury

Tertiary blast injury is due to displacement, either of the body as a whole or of one part relative to another. An example of the former would be the injury caused by the blast wind propelling the whole body against a fixed structure such as a wall. Relative displacement gives rise to amputations or subtotal amputations. A survey of blast casualties from Northern Ireland revealed that amputations through joints were very uncommon, the principal site being through the shafts of long bones.[11]

Burns

Burns result either from the initial flash of the explosion or from the secondary combustion of the environment, or if the victim's clothes catch fire.

Crush injury

Crush injury from falling masonry as a consequence of the structure of the building being weakened by the explosion is a common cause of injury and death, especially in terrorist incidents.

Psychological effects

Because of the disfiguring nature of many of the injuries and the circumstances in which many explosions occur, psychological effects, among both victims and carers, are common and can be severe.

TREATMENT OF BALLISTIC INJURY

There are a number of common themes in the management of all ballistic injuries. Most of the wounds encountered will be to the limbs, as gunshots to the head, chest and abdomen have a high rate of on-scene mortality.[12]

Protocols for treating gunshot wounds and blast injury have been adopted and publicized by the International Committee of the Red Cross (ICRC),[13] who have extensive experience of treating such injuries as part of their war surgery programmes.

Initial measures

The initial measures in the treatment of blast injury or gunshot wounds are similar to those for any severe injury. Firstly, a primary survey is carried out with resuscitation of the patient, addressing life-threatening conditions according to ABC... priorities. Fluids should be administered according to the principles described in Chapter 3. Dressings should be applied to open wounds. All victims of blast or bullets are likely to be the subject of some form of police investigation, and as a consequence clothes should be removed carefully and never cut through holes made by bullets or other projectiles. Property should be carefully labelled and bagged individually.

For the conscious patient intravenous opiate analgesia should be administered, with the dose titrated against the level of discomfort. Antibiotics should also be given at the first opportunity. For an adult patient, the ICRC recommend benzyl penicillin (6 million units, i.v.).

It should be remembered that the patient may not have been immunized against tetanus. As the wounds from blast or high-energy-transfer bullets are often grossly contaminated and contain de-vitalized tissue, such wounds are at risk of infection with *Clostridium tetani*. In view of this risk, administration of anti-tetanus serum and tetanus toxoid should be available.[14]

Where possible, X-rays of the injured areas should be taken, as these may show evidence of injury such as a haemopneumothorax as well as the presence and severity of any fractures. If any delay in surgical treatment is anticipated, some form of fracture splintage should be utilized where appropriate.

Wound assessment

Before proceeding to surgical treatment, certain aspects of the wound need to be assessed. Already from the history there may be some knowledge of the nature of the weapon used, and from this the degree of tissue damage can be estimated. However, inspection of the wound(s) may provide further information relevant to the treatment protocol to be followed. The wound assessment should therefore include:

- site of the entrance wound (and exit, if present);
- sizes of entrance and exit wounds;
- cavity formation;
- the anatomical structures which may have been transited;
- distal perfusion;
- presence of fractures; and
- degree of contamination.

This information should be recorded carefully, and appropriate photographs taken.

For some ballistic injuries to the limbs the severity of injury will be such that the limb is deemed *unreconstructable*, and in these cases primary amputation will be required.

Surgical management

The majority of bullet wounds will require surgical exploration and débridement, as will wounds due to fragments and blast amputation and tissue lacerations. Prompt discussion with a surgeon is therefore a vital part of the management of these patients.

Wound débridement and excision is a surgical procedure involving removal from the wound of any dead and contaminated tissue which, if left, would become a medium for infection. It is most relevant to high-energy-transfer bullet wounds which feature large cavities and considerable amounts of dead tissue and contamination. In wound excision all dead and contaminated tissue as well as foreign material should be excised. Some low-energy-transfer (velocity) wounds such as those from most handguns, because of the minimal cavitation and zone of extravasation, do not need the extensive débridement and excision outlined above. These wounds can, in certain circumstances, be managed without surgery.

The optimal management of the multiple small-fragment wounds seen as a result of secondary blast injury can be difficult, as the often large numbers of these wounds precludes the above approach being applied to each one. Because there is no cavitation associated with such injury and, due to the poor aerodynamic qualities of random fragments, the degree of penetration is usually not great. A reasonable approach is to clean all the wounds as thoroughly as possible by irrigation under general anaesthesia and then surgically to débride/excise only those major wounds associated with gross, deep contamination and tissue damage.[10]

Amputations

In some circumstances the severity of ballistic injury to a limb will be such that amputation is warranted. The decision to amputate is often difficult, and in such cases a second opinion from another surgeon may be valuable. Amputations due to blast are rarely, if ever, suitable for re-implantation procedures and such prolonged procedures should therefore not be attempted. The correct management is the formation of a suitable stump using viable tissue proximal to the wound.

Regional injuries

Lung is a relatively elastic and compressible tissue. As a result of these features there is relatively little cavitation and zone of extravasation, even when lung is transited by a high-energy-transfer bullet. As such there is no need for extensive débridement and excision of the bullet track. Penetration within 5 cm of the midline of the thorax is associated with a risk of injury to the great vessels or heart, but otherwise the most significant risks associated with ballistic penetration of the chest are of haemo- and pneumothorax. Both of these conditions can usually be treated with tube thoracostomy alone.

Gunshot wounds to the head which transit the cranial cavity carry a very poor prognosis, especially if from a high-energy-transfer weapon.

In the UK, gunshot wounds to the abdomen are managed by laparotomy. Blast exposure may lead to the development of intestinal perforation, and careful observation and early resort to surgery is therefore appropriate.

Ear injuries vary from mild tympanic perforation to complete disruption of the ossicles.

SUMMARY

Blast and gunshot wounds are a potential source of severe injury. Some understanding of ballistics can help in the assessment of these injuries, and also help to determine the surgical strategy necessary for their care. Treatment according to basic principles following the pattern described for all the victims of trauma will lead to the best possible clinical outcome.

REFERENCES

1. Bowyer GW, Payne L, Mellor SS, *et al*. Historical overview and epidemiology. In: Ryan JM, *et al* (eds). *Ballistic Trauma: Clinical Relevance in Peace and War*. London: Arnold, 1997.
2. Hill JF. Blast injury with particular reference to recent terrorist bombing incidents. *Annals of the Royal College of Surgeons of England* 1979, Vol. 61, pp. 4–11.
3. Hutton JE, Rich NM. Wounding and wound ballistics. In: McArinch JW, *et al*. (eds). *Traumatic and Reconstructive Urology*. Philadelphia: W.B. Saunders 1996, pp. 3–26.
4. Mannion SJ *et al*. The 1999 London bombings: The St Thomas' Hospital experience. *Injury* 1999.
5. Leibovici D, Gorfiton M, Stein M, *et al*. Blast injuries: bus versus open-air bombings – a comparative study of injuries in survivors of open-air versus confined space explosions. *The Journal of Trauma: Injury, Infection and Critical Care* 1996; **41**(6): 1030–5.
6. Waterworth TA, Carr MJT. An analysis of the post-mortem findings in the 21 victims of the Birmingham pub bombings. *Injury* 1975; **7**: 89–95.
7. Mellor SG, Dodd KT, Harmon JW, Cooper GJ. Ballistic and other implications of blast. In: Ryan JM, *et al* (eds). *Ballistic Trauma: Clinical Relevance in Peace and War*. London: Arnold 1997, pp. 47–59.
8. Hadden MA, Rutherford WH, Merrett JD. The injuries of terrorist bombing: a study of 1532 patients. *British Journal of Surgery* 1978; **65**: 525–31.
9. Owen-Smith MS. Explosive blast injury. *Journal of the Royal Army Medical Corps* 1979; **125**: 4–16.

10. Bowyer GW, Cooper GJ, Rice P. Small fragment wounds: biophysics and pathophysiology. *The Journal of Trauma: Injury, Infection and Critical Care* 1996; **40**: S159–S164.
11. Hull JB, Cooper GJ. Pattern and mechanism of traumatic amputation by explosive blast. *The Journal of Trauma: Injury, Infection and Critical Care.* 1996; **40**: 198–205.
12. Spalding TJW, Stewart MP, Tulloch DN, Stephens KM. Penetrating missile injuries in the Gulf War 1991. *British Journal of Surgery* 1991; **78**: 1102–4.
13. Coupland RM. *War Wounds of Limbs.* Oxford: Butterworth-Heinemann, 1993.
14. Advanced trauma life support manual. *Resource document 6: Tetanus immunisation.* Chicago: American College of Surgeons, 1993.

17

Psychological reactions to trauma

OBJECTIVES

- To understand normal reactions to trauma
- To describe the acute psychiatric reactions to trauma
- To outline the general principles of 'breaking bad news'
- To understand psychological first aid
- To appreciate the impact of trauma care on staff

INTRODUCTION

Following trauma, formal psychiatric intervention normally becomes a realistic prospect only when the patient's physical condition has been stabilized. Only occasionally would specialist psychiatric involvement be required at the most immediate phase of care. Such cases are likely to involve: pre-existent psychiatric illness; psychotic disorders (which are rare), serious suicidal risk; and psychiatric complications of head injuries.

There are, however, certain psychiatric symptoms and acute reactions which emerge in the early stages after trauma, and these may have to be addressed. Otherwise, they are likely to compromise medical care. It is also important to be able to distinguish normal from pathological reactions to trauma, or the former may be misdiagnosed and handled inappropriately.

NORMAL REACTIONS TO TRAUMA

Clinically, normal and abnormal reactions are usually distinguished by the severity and duration of the latter and by the extent to which they render the patient dysfunctional. Apart from psychotic symptoms (such as delusions and hallucinations), reactions to trauma are on a continuum from 'normal' to 'abnormal'. Common normal reactions to trauma are described below, and these have been detailed elsewhere.[1] It is important to recognize the management implications of these reactions for the effective clinical care of patients.

Numbness, shock and denial

This is Nature's way of temporarily shielding us from potentially overwhelming stress.

The implication is that patients in this phase will find it difficult to absorb information and instructions. Patience and repetition of information are likely to be required. Information should be given in small 'doses'.

Fear

Fear is an essential trigger to the 'fight/flight' mechanism, and therefore it is biologically adaptive.

The implication is that as a result of fear patients may resist treatment, particularly if it is administered at the scene or close to the scene of the incident. Every effort must be made to reassure them that this is a normal reaction (and not a sign of weakness), and to confirm that they are now safe. A confident, professional approach to the patient helps to dispel fear.

Depression, apathy and helplessness

Trauma nearly always involves loss, and loss commonly leads to low mood and apathy. This reaction is particularly obvious after extreme or prolonged trauma (for example, after being trapped) when patients have had the chance to realize how serious is their condition and circumstances.

The implication is that because of their low mood, loss of drive and their sense of helplessness patients may find it difficult to cooperate with rescuers and medical personnel. Again, patience, encouragement and reassurance are essential.

Elation

This is similar to what the military describe as 'combat rush'. It may be associated with the relief of being rescued, and/or it may be the effect of major neuroendocrinal changes which represent the body's biological response to major trauma.

The implications are first, that patients may fail to realize how serious their injuries are, particularly because in this state the pain threshold is raised. Compliance with medical instructions may be compromised. The second implication is that calm and authoritative reassurance is required to ensure compliance. Sedation is unlikely to be useful, and it could obfuscate diagnosis.

Irritation and anger

Trauma victims are often angry at what has happened once they recognize the serious consequences, but a legitimate target may not present itself. Thus, rescuers and medical personnel may become the target, as patients criticise what they (mis)perceive to be inadequate care or efforts to help.

The implication is that tolerance is required. Confrontation and defensive justifications ('I'm only doing what I have to') do not help. The patients' grievances should not be taken personally, even if their attitude does cause resentment when everyone is doing their best to help.

Guilt

Some survivors, particularly when there have been fatalities and when children have been involved, may feel guilty even when in reality they have not been responsible. Paradoxically, they may even describe guilt at having survived when others have died.

The implication is that where legitimate, appropriate reassurance that they were not responsible should be given, but it is important to beware of pre-judging circumstances on scant information and giving false reassurance. If in doubt, it is best to listen empathically and not to make judgements or 'take sides'.

Flashbacks

These are involuntary, dramatic replays of the trauma or elements thereof, accompanied by intense emotion and autonomic changes. Flashbacks are commonly visual, but they may involve any or all sensory modalities.

The implication is that it is essential to reassure the victim that these are normal reactions and that, however disturbing, they tend to remit over time.

Cognitive and perceptual disturbances

Survivors of trauma commonly report that events occurred as though in a slow-motion film. Less commonly, they describe them as having occurred in a 'blur'. Commonly, there will be gaps in their recall due to, for example, temporary unconsciousness and 'tunnel vision'. The latter occurs when the individual focuses on one particular feature of the environment – usually the main source of threat – to the exclusion of other peripheral details. Also, survivors commonly report the passage of events in the wrong order.

The implications are that where possible, corroboration of the patient's account should be obtained, particularly if that information is relevant to medical care. Patients should also be reassured that this is a normal reaction and that they are not at fault. (Many feel guilty or silly for not being able to recall what has happened.) In addition, if the facts are known with certainty, it can be helpful to fill in some gaps – particularly with regard to what has happened. Many victims arrive at Accident and Emergency Departments without knowing what has taken place. Explaining the circumstances to them helps to counteract the feeling of being out of control and helpless.

Autonomic hyperarousal and hypervigilance

Trauma overstimulates the autonomic nervous system, this effect being reflected in an exaggerated acoustic startle response and hyperacusis. Patients are also overly sensitive to what they perceive as further threat, and this may include efforts to rescue or to help them.

The implications are that it is useful to explain what lies behind these effects. The routine use of medication is not indicated (although it may be required in extreme cases; see below). An understanding and patient approach is also crucial.

Bereavement reactions

It should be remembered that many victims of trauma have not just been traumatized; they have also been bereaved. Thus, in addition to some of the features above, they may also display the features of an acute grief reaction.

> **While grief is most commonly precipitated by the death of a loved one, trauma may give rise to other 'losses', including loss of function, loss of looks (as occurs after serious burn injuries), or a loss of a limb through amputation (surgical or traumatic)**

Typical acute grief reactions include:

- denial and disbelief ('I can't believe he's dead');
- apathy ('I don't care whether I live or die');
- pining and searching (despairing efforts to find evidence the tragedy has not occurred); and
- acute distress (often in waves and episodes of irresistible tearfulness).

Management of acute grief reactions

The management of the grieving patient inevitably overlaps with that of the traumatized patient. However, the following points should be noted.

1. Our *listening* can be more effective and less intrusive than is our *talking*. (Often, we talk because we are anxious at the silences created by the bereaved.) Listening to the distress of others is not easy, but it helps the bereaved more than talking at them.
2. Moreover, unintentionally, certain clichés and platitudes can be hurtful. ('Don't forget, you're a young man and you've still a lot ahead of you', said to a young man who lost his leg in a motorcycle accident.)

3. Reassurance that the reactions are normal is an important component; the patients are not being silly or 'neurotic', and they are not showing signs of losing their minds. Grief and distress are not illnesses.

4. Tolerance of the patient's irritability and apparent lack of appreciation and gratitude, however hard, is essential. In their suffering they may not display the normal courtesies of life.

In a survey of patients with severe burn injuries the nursing staff found it most difficult to deal with the regular stream of complaints about 'inept' débridement, altered theatre lists and changes in nursing personnel.[2]

Critical retaliation does not help; it only serves to exacerbate the overall level of stress and foster iatrogenic anxiety and guilt.

ACUTE PSYCHIATRIC REACTIONS

This section will consider the acute stress reaction, panic attack, dissociation, alcohol withdrawal syndrome and the DTs (delirium tremens), and violent behaviour.

Acute stress reaction

As defined in the tenth edition of the *International Classification of Mental and Behavioural Disorders* (ICD-10),[3] this condition is a '. . . transient disorder of significant severity which develops in an individual without any other apparent mental disorder in response to exceptional physical and/or mental stress and which usually subsides within hours or days. . . . The risk of this disorder developing is increased if physical exhaustion or organic factors (for example in the elderly) are also present'.

Patients will characteristically display an initial state of shock, constricted field of consciousness, impaired concentration and disorientation, followed by a fluctuating picture which may include depression, agitation, anxiety, social withdrawal and autonomic overreactivity.

This condition may interfere with medical care, and it may represent a very distressing experience for patients (and sometimes their relatives).

Panic attack

Panic attacks are associated with sudden and severe anxiety, unpredictable onset, palpitations, profuse sweating, an inexplicable sense of impending doom, tremor, dyspnoea, an almost irresistible urge to flee, chest pain, paraesthesiae, and choking or smothering sensations.

These attacks usually peak within 10 min. They are usually short-lived, but may endure for several hours. They are often aborted whenever the patient feels safe and secure. They may also be associated with hyperventilation, though it is not clear whether hyperventilation causes the panic attack or vice versa.

Hyperventilation may also lead to the hyperventilation syndrome, a syndrome characterized by its protean clinical features. Physical causes should also be considered, including pulmonary embolism, acute or chronic pulmonary disease, asthma and the excessive ingestion of aspirin.[4]

Dissociation

This is a psychogenic condition of acute onset induced by trauma and severe stress. It involves a partial and incomplete integration of cognitive processes such that the patient may display amnesia, stupor and disturbances of physical function, such as a paralysis or loss of sensation in the absence of any physical aetiology. There is usually a sudden and complete recovery within a few days after the source of stress has been removed or reduced.

MANAGEMENT OF ACUTE REACTIONS

The general principles of the management of these acute symptoms are as follows.

- Patients should be reassured that their condition is benign, and it should be explained that the symptoms are usually short-lived and self-limiting.
- Benzodiazepines may be used for short-term relief if the symptoms are overwhelming and are likely to jeopardize medical care. Usually lorazepam (2–4 mg) given intramuscularly is sufficient to bring these symptoms under control. A beta-blocker (for example propanolol 40–60 mg daily) may reduce autonomic overreactivity, but it has little effect on anxious thoughts or on panic symptoms. Neuroleptics have no role unless there is also markedly aggressive or self-destructive behaviour.
- Hyperventilation may be aborted by re-breathing into a paper bag for a few minutes (but it is necessary to exclude cardiorespiratory causes of anxiety.) Patients should also be instructed to take slow, measured breaths. These symptoms will recede as the CO_2 levels return to normal.

- **Caution must be exercised in the use of benzodiazepines with patients with head injury or a history of benzodiazepine dependence**
- **Short-term use is the guiding principle in benzodiazepine therapy**

Violent behaviour

Perhaps reflecting societal changes, medical and emergency personnel are increasingly likely to encounter violent or potentially violent situations.[5] Violent or threatening behaviour can be very distressing and alarming, and it may jeopardize patient care. Thus, it is important to be able to anticipate and to abort potentially violent situations, by conducting rapid assessment, containment and resolution.[6]

This section offers some guidelines for achieving such aims.

WARNING SIGNS

Obviously, it is best to anticipate a potentially violent scenario. However, it is often not possible in a clinical emergency to assess a situation thoroughly or to obtain historical data which would help to identify the prodromal signs of a violent outbreak. However, caution should be exercised if the patient:

- has a history of violence;
- displays threatening, challenging or abusive behaviour;
- reports some irreconcilable grievance against authority including medical, nursing and emergency personnel; or
- has an identifiable psychiatric condition (especially schizophrenia, depression, alcohol/substance abuse, paranoia, antisocial or explosive personality disorder, or an organic cerebral disorder, including epilepsy and frontal lobe damage).

MANAGEMENT OF VIOLENT EPISODES

To some extent how a violent situation is dealt with depends on its cause. However, the following are useful general pointers for the inexperienced. It is worth noting, moreover, that much violence is precipitated by fear and misunderstanding on the part of those who become aggressive.

1. Try not to deal with the situation alone. It is not a time for false or 'macho' heroics.
2. You should always try to explain throughout what is happening, particularly since it is likely to be necessary to approach closely and to touch the patient. The patient may be very defensive of his/her 'psychological space'. Try not to approach unexpectedly from behind.
3. It may be helpful (if otherwise acceptable) to leave a door or screen open. This avoids a patient feeling trapped.

4. It is vital to maintain a calm, reassuring and confident manner. Being challenging, threatening and confrontational will not help; indeed, it is likely to inflame the situation. While it may not come easily in such situations, politeness is more likely to calm a potentially violent situation than an abrasive or authoritarian attitude.

5. Slow movements and regular forewarning of what is going to happen are less likely to precipitate a violent reaction than are sudden, dramatic and unexpected movements.

6. Excessive eye contact should be avoided, as this can be regarded as confrontational and challenging.

7. Physical restraints should obviously be avoided unless they are absolutely necessary. It is vital not to attempt to restrain someone unless there are sufficient staff to ensure that the exercise can be conducted safely and successfully. (It is helpful to identify staff who are trained in safe and appropriate restraint techniques.) A 'free for all' in which staff are injured must be avoided. Before beginning to restrain the patient, a carefully prepared plan in which everybody knows what they are supposed to do and when, must be in place.

> **Do not underestimate how strong a disturbed individual can be, even if they have a low body weight and are of slight stature**

8. Occasionally, sedation may be required, but injections should be avoided unless the patient is immobilized and restrained sufficiently.

The neuroleptics and haloperidol have commonly been used as sedatives, but there are concerns about their long half-lives and their tendency to reduce the convulsive threshold. Droperidol (20 mg intramuscularly) is the neuroleptic of choice as it is well absorbed and has a short half-life. If the patient is severely and acutely disturbed and the background to their disturbance has not been clarified, droperidol and lorazepam may be used adjunctively. The latter has an anticonvulsant effect which counters any problems that might be induced by droperidol, particularly in patients who may be withdrawing from alcohol. They both have short half-lives and thus avoid extended oversedation (see Figure 17.1). In the case of drug-induced psychosis, neuroleptics should be avoided; a benzodiazepine (for example, diazepam, 10 mg intravenously) is more suitable.

> - **When restraining a patient, ensure that their airway is maintained and that he/she can breathe freely**
> - **Restraints should be removed slowly only when you are certain that the risk of violent behaviour has been sufficiently reduced**
> - **When psychotropic medication looks as though it is inevitable, it may be helpful to seek a psychiatric opinion**
> - **Because of the risk of sudden death in violent patients, the Royal College of Psychiatrists' Consensus Report advises against the prolonged use of very heavy doses of antipsychotics**

ALCOHOL-RELATED PROBLEMS

Alcohol is a regular visitor to Accident and Emergency Departments, and is commonly associated with traumatic events. Some 25% of emergency admissions to hospitals in England and Wales are due to excessive alcohol consumption, and 80% of fatal road traffic accidents (RTAs) involve alcohol.[7]

Thus, high blood-alcohol levels may complicate the management of the trauma victim. There are well-established principles underlying the emergency management of alcohol-related problems.[8]

Those patients with problems of acute intoxication may display problems of violence (see above). Such incidents tend to be transient, and their effects are generally dose-related.

The following is for guidance only. It may be appropriate to adhere to this guidance. Discussion with a senior colleague is recommended at any stage.

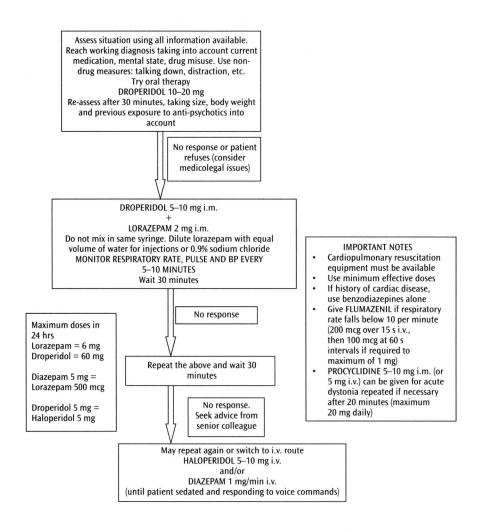

Assess situation using all information available. Reach working diagnosis taking into account current medication, mental state, drug misuse. Use non-drug measures: talking down, distraction, etc.
Try oral therapy
DROPERIDOL 10–20 mg
Re-assess after 30 minutes, taking size, body weight and previous exposure to anti-psychotics into account

No response or patient refuses (consider medicolegal issues)

DROPERIDOL 5–10 mg i.m.
+
LORAZEPAM 2 mg i.m.
Do not mix in same syringe. Dilute lorazepam with equal volume of water for injections or 0.9% sodium chloride
MONITOR RESPIRATORY RATE, PULSE AND BP EVERY 5–10 MINUTES
Wait 30 minutes

No response

Maximum doses in 24 hrs
Lorazepam = 6 mg
Droperidol = 60 mg

Diazepam 5 mg = Lorazepam 500 mcg

Droperidol 5 mg = Haloperidol 5 mg

Repeat the above and wait 30 minutes

No response. Seek advice from senior colleague

IMPORTANT NOTES
• Cardiopulmonary resuscitation equipment must be available
• Use minimum effective doses
• If history of cardiac disease, use benzodiazepines alone
• Give FLUMAZENIL if respiratory rate falls below 10 per minute (200 mcg over 15 s i.v., then 100 mcg at 60 s intervals if required to maximum of 1 mg)
• PROCYCLIDINE 5–10 mg i.m. (or 5 mg i.v.) can be given for acute dystonia repeated if necessary after 20 minutes (maximum 20 mg daily)

May repeat again or switch to i.v. route
HALOPERIDOL 5–10 mg i.v.
and/or
DIAZEPAM 1 mg/min i.v.
(until patient sedated and responding to voice commands)

* 5 mg (oral and i.m.) for the elderly.

Figure 17.1 *Algorithm for drug treatment of psychiatric emergencies. (Reproduced with the kind permission of Grampian Primary Care NHS Trust.)*

However, alcohol-dependent patients may pose additional difficulties because of the impact of withdrawal symptoms (Table 17.1). These begin 6–24 h after cessation of drinking, they are extensive, and they may be life-threatening.

Table 17.1 *Alcohol withdrawal symptoms*

• Tremor (fine and rapid)
• Nausea (or retching)
• Excessive sweating (especially in the morning)
• Tinnitus
• Hyperacusis
• Muscle cramps
• Impaired sleep (often with nightmares)
• Variable mood (including irritability and anxiety)
• Perceptual disturbances (including visual hallucinations)
• Convulsions (these tend to appear about 24 h after withdrawal)

Delirium tremens

In extreme cases, withdrawal may lead to the condition called 'delirium tremens' (the DTs). This affects about 5% of physically addicted drinkers, and is a florid acute confusional state which should be regarded as a medical emergency. It occurs 1–4 days after withdrawal from alcohol, although there may be prodromal signs such as insomnia, fleeting and fragmentary delusions, tremulousness and fear.

Delirium tremens is associated with vivid and visual hallucinations and delusions, ataxia, autonomic hyperarousal, insomnia, agitation, impaired concentration, profound confusion, low-grade pyrexia and fear.

> **Ultimately, if untreated, delirium tremens can result in cerebral obtundity, convulsions and death**

MANAGEMENT OF WITHDRAWAL SYMPTOMS

Rehydration and restoration of electrolyte imbalance, and thiamine injections are needed when there is a risk of acute encephalopathy.

A balanced diet is required to avoid carbohydrate overload, since this can further deplete thiamine levels and precipitate the Wernicke–Korsakoff syndrome. This syndrome is characterized by confusion, clouding of consciousness, ocular palsies and nystagmus, disturbance of gait, peripheral neuropathy, marked impairment of memory and retrograde amnesia. To fill the gaps in their memory, patients 'confabulate', i.e., they 'recollect' imaginary events and details.

If there is evidence of hypoglycaemia, oral or parenteral glucose replacement should be provided slowly and with thiamine in order to avoid precipitating Wernicke's encephalopathy.

Long-half-life benzodiazepines (e.g. diazepam or chlordiazepoxide) are the medications of choice, especially when there is a risk of fitting. (Longer-half-life benzodiazepines lead to fewer fluctuations in blood levels and prevent the patient going in and out of withdrawal symptoms.) However, care must be taken in cases of head injury and respiratory disorder. Diazepam (20 mg) or its equivalent can be given at 6 h intervals, the dose being reduced step-wise, usually over a period of 5–7 days. Beta-blockers can be useful, but they have no impact on insomnia or dysphoria.

Generally, it is wise to provide routine and/or parenteral administration of a vitamin supplement.

PSYCHOLOGICAL FIRST AID

How we react to victims of trauma in the early stages after their traumatic experience may influence to a considerable extent how they adjust to it. 'Psychological first aid' is particularly relevant after major incidents, and was first described in detail by Raphael.[9] Below is a modified version of her framework, developed later by Alexander.[10]

1. Comfort and protect

In their bewildered and shocked state, survivors of trauma need to be comforted and to be protected from their own unintended further risks to their own safety. (One lady after a multiple and fatal RTA on a motorway tried to cross over three lanes of busy traffic – unaware of the risk – because she saw an ambulance on the other side.)

Comfort can be conveyed by words, but sometimes a compassionate touch may be more eloquent than a carefully prepared script.

2. Counteract helplessness

A sense of helplessness is a poor prognostic indicator after trauma. Thus, in the case of those who are at least 'walking wounded' or uninjured, they can be invited to help at the scene of the accident. This may counter the experience of helplessness and subsequent guilt commonly reported by victims. They may, for example, help to comfort the injured, warn others of the site of the accident and relay important messages.

3. Reunion with friends or relations

Attempts should be made to help victims to establish contact with other relevant persons, for example, family members, friends and other survivors.

4. Re-establish order

Characteristically, trauma results in victims feeling out of control and vulnerable; their world has been turned upside-down. Victims of trauma will therefore welcome indications that order and control have been re-established. Information about what is going to happen, the availability of contact with family and friends and even the humble cup of tea help to convey the impression that chaos and uncertainty have ended.

5. Expression of feelings

In the early stages of trauma in particular, it is unlikely to be helpful to do more than to allow victims of trauma to express spontaneously how they feel. 'Emotional mining', that is to say forcing individuals to describe their feelings is not helpful.[10]

It is important to avoid 'taking sides' with regard to culpability. It is possible that one's opinions (albeit well-meaning) may be quoted to others at a later stage. Also, it is sometimes the case that victims change their own views later. With the increasing likelihood of legal and compensation proceedings, it is wise to be cautious about passing an opinion.

6. Provision of *accurate* information

In some ways this relates to point (4) above about inducing a sense of order and control. However, concessions must be made. In the earliest phase after trauma, because of their stunned, numbed state victims will find it difficult to absorb much information, and they may tend to hear only what they want to hear. Slow delivery and the patient repetition of information are likely to be necessary (see 'Breaking bad news', p. 235).

7. Psychological triage

While the majority of individuals will eventually adjust to even the most horrific events, a number will go on to develop chronic or severe problems of post-traumatic adjustment. It is helpful to be alert to 'at-risk' factors. These factors can be categorized in relation to those which relate to the trauma and the patient (Tables 17.2 and 17.3).

Table 17.2 *Trauma-related prognostic indicators*

- Extended exposure to the trauma (for example, those who are trapped)
- (Perceived) threat to life, even if there is subsequently proved to be no objective risk
- Multiple deaths/and mutilation
- Sudden and unexpected events
- Man-made (rather than an 'act of Nature')

Table 17.3 *Patient-related prognostic indicators*

- Serious physical injury (bear in mind how 'serious' an injury appears to the patient may not necessarily reflect the severity in medical or surgical terms; it may be the personal meaning and implications of the injury to the patient)
- Previous psychiatric history
- Severe acute stress reaction
- Particularly anxious personality
- Lack of support
- Concurrent life stresses (there may be major problems in the patient's life which compromise his/her ability to cope with the most recent trauma)

THE GENERAL PRINCIPLES OF BREAKING BAD NEWS

Giving bad news to patients and relatives will never be an easy task, and there can never be a standard script. What is said, to whom, and when and where must always be tailored to suit individual circumstances. However, the following guidelines may provide a helpful framework. (See also references 11–13.)

These guidelines will be presented under three subheadings: preparation; delivery of information; and follow-up.

Preparation

Ideally, you should prepare yourself by:

- ensuring that you know who you are going to speak to;
- establishing as much information as possible about the circumstances, socioeconomic level and occupation of those involved, as these will give some idea of the level at which what is said should be pitched;
- finding out what they have already been told (beware, they may have been misinformed or may have heard wrongly or selectively);
- anticipating what they may wish to know;
- covering up or removing any clothing which is stained with blood or other body fluids; and
- finding a suitable room or site which offers as much privacy as possible and a minimum risk of interruption (pagers and telephones can be distressing intrusions on such occasions, and are guaranteed to go off at the least opportune time).

Delivery of information

This should be made in step-wise fashion.

INTRODUCTION

Initially, the approach should be to:

- give your name, status and involvement in the proceedings;
- confirm the identities of those present; and
- adopt a suitable posture (standing over somebody who is seated or lying down is not ideal).

ASSESSMENT

Here, the approach is to:

- find out what they already know;
- find out what they want to know ('Total' and unsolicited truths can be as hurtful and as distressing as a total veil of secrecy and obfuscation); and

- listen (even if you are anxious and find silences uncomfortable). Listening helps us to find out what others want to hear; it gives them a chance to digest unpalatable news, to compose themselves, and to identify further questions.

COMMUNICATION STYLE AND LEVEL

The following approach should be used.

- Pitch what needs to be said at a level most likely to be understood. Clear, plain English, and a slowish delivery with pauses will help. (When we are anxious we tend to speak too quickly.)
- Diagrams and notes can facilitate communication and understanding.
- Avoid clichés and platitudes ('I know how you feel' – *No, we don't!*).
- Titrate the dose of information in relation to what patients and relatives seem able to absorb. Avoid overwhelming them with too many facts.
- Shocked and distressed individuals cannot think as quickly or as clearly as normal. (Every now and again, it is helpful to check that you are explaining things clearly.)
- Be honest. There is no shame in admitting that you do not know the answer to a question. Tell the patient or relative if and when the required information can be found.

Follow-up

The delivery of bad news is the first step towards adjustment for patients and relatives, and it can be facilitated in the following ways.

- Allow some privacy while they come to terms with the news and have a chance to compose themselves. (However, it is wise to ask if they wish someone to accompany them, such as a nurse or chaplain.)
- Ensure they know what will happen next in relation to, for example, medical care and the return of any possessions and clothing. (If the clothing has been damaged either in the trauma or due to medical intervention, or if the police have retained items, this should be explained as sensitively as possible.)
- Forewarn them if there are likely to be legal proceedings – the involvement of the Office of the Procurator Fiscal (in Scotland) or the Coroner (in England and Wales).
- Explain if there is to be a post-mortem examination. (Bear in mind personal, religious and cultural sensitivities to such an event.)
- The possibility of organ donation needs to be raised most sensitively. (Again, bear in mind the above sources of sensitivity about the post-mortem care of a body.)
- Provide any information about sources of help in the community (leaflets or handwritten notes help). There are a number of organizations which deal with survivors of trauma and the bereaved. These lists are available usually from the Local Reference Library, and it helps to be familiar with them.
- Ensure they know how to obtain further information if required.

VIEWING THE BODY

This is an emotive and contentious issue, particularly if the body has been badly mutilated or burned, and it has been discussed in other literature.[14] The advantages of allowing relatives to view the body (if they genuinely wish so to do) are as follows:

1. It helps to dispel any denial or uncertainty about the reality of the death.
2. It helps to dispel fantasies about how the deceased looks in death. Usually, relatives report that what they have seen was not as bad as they had feared, but, beware, sometimes it is worse (see 'Preparation', p. 235).
3. It allows relatives the chance to say 'Goodbye' or 'Sorry'. They may also wish to have the opportunity to take, for example, a lock of hair.

To increase the likelihood of relatives finding this to be a positive experience, the following guidelines should be considered:

1. Prepare them for what they will see, smell, and feel.
2. Describe and explain any damage to the body, including resuscitation marks and other signs of medical intervention.
3. Offer them time to be alone with the body (although some may wish to have a member of staff with them).
4. Have a member of staff meet with them after they have viewed the body to ensure that they are alright, and to answer any questions which this experience may have generated.

RELATIVES IN THE RESUSCITATION ROOM

This question too has generated much debate.[15] To have relatives in the resuscitation room can be threatening to staff, particularly to less experienced ones,[16] and if it is to be the policy that relatives are invited to be present during resuscitation, then staff training should include learning how to deal with distressed relatives before, during and after resuscitation efforts.

Most relatives appear to want to be offered the chance to be present, although not all will take up this offer.[17] The advantages of their being present may be to:

- demonstrate that all reasonable efforts have been made to save the life of their loved one;
- dispel the mystery of what takes place during a resuscitation;
- create a greater bond and mutual understanding between relatives and staff; and
- foster a sense of being part of a signal event in their lives rather than feeling peripheral and excluded from it.

If the relatives are allowed to view the proceedings in the resuscitation room, then the following steps should be taken:

1. Prepare them for what they will see and hear.
2. Provide them with an informed chaperone.
3. Ensure that all staff in the resuscitation room are aware that relatives will be present.
4. Provide follow-up after the relatives have left the resuscitation room, as they may need some support and they may have questions to raise.

IMPACT OF TRAUMA CARE ON STAFF

Training and careful selection of staff are powerful antidotes to the potentially disturbing effects of dealing regularly with severely injured and dying patients and their relatives. Extended experience of such work may also contribute to trauma care personnel developing their own successful methods of coping with the rigours of their work.

However, despite the protective effect of these factors, it has been shown that not even senior staff are impervious to the emotional impact of their work.[18] The prevalence of 'compassion fatigue' has also been identified among those who provide dedicated care to the victims of trauma.[19] Those who are involved in such work must not fail to acknowledge that, however rewarding their work is, it is capable of exacting a substantial emotional toll.

Most staff will cope with unpleasant incidents. However, there are warning signs which suggest when individuals may be struggling and require some extra help:

- Excessive use of substances – alcohol, tobacco and food
- Unusually poor time-keeping and work record
- Unexpected overwork and underwork
- Excessive irritability and moodiness
- Unusual carelessness and/or proneness to accidents
- Inability to attain a realistic view of an incident; unable to stop talking about it and re-living it.

MINIMIZING THE EMOTIONAL IMPACT OF WORK ON STAFF

Peer support

Good and supportive relationships with colleagues are probably the most potent antidote to the deleterious effects of trauma work. Unfortunately, peer support is sometimes not available because there are concerns about confidentiality and about being seen to be 'weak' in the eyes of one's colleagues.

Also, some colleagues are reluctant to approach their peers who have had a 'hard' time for fear of saying the wrong thing, or of being seen as being interfering.

Organizational and managerial practices

Carefully conducted research has shown that the way an organization reacts to its employees has a major impact on their ability to adapt to unpleasant tasks.[20,21]
Valuable features include:

- having opportunities to discuss openly their feelings and reactions;
- mutual support among colleagues (including senior as well as junior ones);
- a clear definition of purposeful duties;
- 'black' or 'gallows' humour (although this does not seem to be appropriate when children are the casualties); and
- attention by management to the physical needs of trauma care staff, and good leadership.

Psychological debriefing

Psychological debriefing after unpleasant events is not a new concept; it has been used for many years by the military. More recently, however, its use among the emergency services has been developed by Mitchell and Everly[22] and Dyregrov.[23] A number of models of debriefing exist, but their essential features are:

- normalization of emotional and other psychological reactions;
- enabling (not 'forcing') the natural expressions of emotions;
- identifying successes in terms of how the incident was dealt with;
- identifying any problems (rather than 'failures') and solutions;
- enabling staff to 'let go' of the incident in order that they can disengage before they go home or move on to other duties; and
- carrying out triage to identify staff who may need further help and back-up.

> **Debriefing should be a positive personal and professional learning experience; it should not be an opportunity for blame and recrimination**

If debriefing is used, it is recommended that:

- debriefers are familiar with the particular incident.
- debriefers are familiar with normal and pathological reactions to traumatic events.
- debriefers are familiar with group dynamics (a group is more than a sum of the individuals therein).
- the proceedings are confidential (managers sometimes ask to be 'flies on the wall').
- individual differences are recognized; some individuals find it naturally easy to speak about painful issues and their emotional reactions, but others do not. There is nothing to be gained in coercing or embarrassing participants into 'confessing' how they feel.
- debriefing usually takes place about 24–72 h after an incident. However, this needs to be implemented sensitively. There is no value in forcing individuals to take part

prematurely in a debriefing when they are too emotionally vulnerable or too shocked to contribute or to benefit from it. Indeed, to do so might be harmful.

- it is not viewed as a psychiatric 'treatment' for sick people; it is an effort to help normal individuals who have endured an abnormal event to come to terms with it.
- it should not be regarded as a cosmetic exercise to protect organizations against subsequent litigation.
- mandatory debriefing should probably be avoided as it assumes that all staff are equally ready for such a procedure. This is unlikely to be the case. Some individuals may have their ability to cope with an unpleasant incident compromised by, for example, concurrent life stresses including physical and emotional ill-health.

As with premature debriefing (see above), there is a risk of making certain individuals worse if they are not ready to talk about their experiences. Such individuals may be 're-traumatized'.

While debriefing (conducted at the right time by competent individuals) is generally regarded favourably by participants, independent, empirical evidence to justify its use is currently lacking. Further research is urgently required to identify its effectiveness

---

SUMMARY

Historically, the psychological care of trauma victims, at least in the early phases, has been viewed as either irrelevant or as the soft underbelly of surgical and medical care. Such mistaken views have compromised the total care of trauma victims.

It has now been clearly demonstrated that even in well-adjusted individuals trauma triggers powerful emotional reactions, most of which are normal reactions to abnormal events. These have to be recognized and addressed to ensure the proper care of trauma patients.

Breaking bad news and viewing human remains are emotive and challenging issues, even for experienced clinicians. How best to conduct such matters requires further empirical enquiry, but there are now some guidelines which allow staff to help patients and relatives in relation to the delivery of distressing news and viewing the deceased.

Challenging and rewarding trauma care most certainly is, but it is also emotionally demanding, and it takes its toll of even senior staff. Identifying staff who are under pressure and responding to their emotional needs is a neglected, but important, aspect of trauma care.

ACKNOWLEDGEMENTS

Particular thanks are due to Dr J.M. Eagles, consultant psychiatrist, Royal Cornhill Hospital, Aberdeen, for his specialist advice on certain issues relating to medication.

REFERENCES

1. Alexander DA. Psychological aspects of trauma. In: Greaves I, Porter K, Burke D (eds). *Key Topics in Trauma*. Oxford: Bios Scientific Publishers, 1997.
2. Alexander DA. Burn victims after a major disaster: reactions of patients and their caregivers. *Burns* 1993; **19**: 105–9.

3. World Health Organization. The ICD-10 Classification of Mental and Behavioural Disorders: *Clinical Descriptions and Diagnostic Guidelines*. Geneva: WHO, 1992.
4. Smith C, Sell L, Sudbury P. *Key Topics in Psychiatry*. Oxford: Bios Scientific Publishers, 1996.
5. Ireland A, McNaughton GW. Violence against staff in Accident and Emergency – an under-reported problem. *Health Bulletin* 1997; **55**: 359–61.
6. Gill D. Violent patients. In: Smith C, Sell L, Sudbury P (eds). *Key Topics in Psychiatry*. Oxford: Bios Scientific Publishers, 1996.
7. Buckley P, Bird J, Harrison G. *Examination Notes in Psychiatry* (3rd ed) Oxford: Butterworth-Heineman, 1996.
8. Merson S, Baldwin D. *Psychiatric Emergencies*. Oxford: Oxford University Press, 1995.
9. Raphael B. *When Disaster Strikes: How Individuals and Communities Cope with Catastrophe*. New York: Basic Books, 1986.
10. Alexander DA. Psychological intervention for victims and helpers after disasters. *British Journal of General Practice* 1990; **40**: 345–48.
11. Buckman R. Communication in palliative care: a practical guide. In: Doyle D, Hanks GWC, MacDonald N (eds). *Oxford Textbook of Palliative Medicine*. Oxford: Oxford University Press, 1993.
12. McLauchlan CAJ. Handling distressed relatives and breaking bad news. In: Skinner D, Driscoll P, Earlam R (eds). *ABC of Trauma* (2nd ed.). London: BMJ Publishing Group, 1996, pp. 103–8.
13. Hind CRK. *Communication Skills in Medicine*. London: BMJ Publishing Group, 1997.
14. Joseph S, Williams R, Yule W. *Understanding Post-traumatic Stress*. Chichester: Wiley and Sons, 1997.
15. van der Woning M. Should relatives be invited to witness a resuscitation attempt? A review of the literature. *Accident and Emergency Nursing* 1997; **5**: 215–18.
16. Mitchell MH, Lynch MB. Should relatives be allowed in the resuscitation room? *Journal of Accident and Emergency Medicine* 1997 **14**: 366–9.
17. Barratt F, Wallis DN. Relatives in the resuscitation room: their point of view. *Journal of Accident and Emergency Medicine* 1998; **15**: 109–11.
18. Alexander DA, Atcheson SF. Psychiatric aspects of trauma care: a survey of nurses and doctors. *Psychiatric Bulletin* 1998; **22**: 132–6.
19. Figley CR. *Compassion fatigue. Coping with secondary traumatic stress disorder in those who treat the traumatized*. New York: Brunner/Mazel, 1995.
20. Alexander DA, Wells A. Reactions of police officers to body-handling after a major disaster: a before-and-after comparison. *British Journal of Psychiatry* 1991; **159**: 547–55.
21. Alexander DA. Stress among police body handlers. *British Journal of Psychiatry* 1993; **163**: 806–8.
22. Mitchell JT, Everly GS. *Critical Incident Stress Debriefing*: CISD. Ellicot City: Chevron Publishing, 1995.
23. Dyregrov A. The process of psychological debriefings. *Journal of Traumatic Stress* 1997; **10**: 589–605.

18

Analgesia and anaesthesia for the trauma patient

OBJECTIVES

- To understand the different modalities available for the management of pain
- To outline the most appropriate agents available for the relief of pain in trauma
- To identify the techniques available for the provision of local, regional and general anaesthesia
- To appreciate the need to seek anaesthetic assistance in the management of emergency general anaesthesia

INTRODUCTION

The International Association for the Study of Pain defined pain as 'An unpleasant sensory and emotional experience associated with actual or potential tissue damage or described in terms of such tissue damage'.[1]

Trauma patients will all suffer different degrees of pain, and the severity of this pain will not depend only on the nature of the injuries. It has long been recognized that the patients' perception of the injuries and events surrounding them as well as their emotional and psychological states will all influence the severity of the pain,[2] and this must be taken into consideration when attempting to relieve pain. In addition, pain should be relieved for physiological as well as compassionate reasons.

PATHOPHYSIOLOGY

Pain results in sympathetic stimulation and increases the level of circulating catecholamines. This causes peripheral vasoconstriction and tachycardia, increasing both myocardial work and afterload. As a result, cardiac ischaemia may be precipitated, especially in patients with ischaemic heart disease. Peripheral vasoconstriction results in blood being diverted to central compartments, and hence vascular beds such as the splanchnic circulation may suffer ischaemia. This may add to ischaemia already occurring in a patient who has lost circulating volume.

Patients with painful chest and abdominal injuries are less likely to cough and clear secretions from their lungs, resulting in secretion retention. As a consequence, hypostatic pneumonia may complicate their clinical course.[3] However, it must be remembered that analgesia itself may exacerbate these potential problems by causing respiratory depression. It is essential, therefore, to titrate analgesia carefully in patients.[4]

PAIN RELIEF IN THE 'RESTLESS' TRAUMA PATIENT

Many trauma patients are restless and distressed after their injuries, and it is important to recognize the cause of such restlessness before administering analgesia. There are important causes of restlessness that must be excluded and treated before administering analgesia, including:

- hypoxaemia;
- head injury;
- the effects of drugs or alcohol; and
- a full bladder.

> **Avoid analgesics in a restless patient until other treatable causes have been identified and corrected**

GENERAL CONSIDERATIONS

Patients with multiple trauma (including head injury), will require analgesia, and this must not be withheld because of inappropriate concern regarding its effect in confusing patient assessment. Local anaesthetic blocks are useful in this situation, though opioid analgesics may be required. When administering opioids to patients with head injuries it is necessary always to:

- titrate the drug intravenously;[2]
- note the dose and time of administration;
- monitor the patient carefully;
- have naloxone available; and
- have appropriate facilities for the artificial support of respiration.

> **Do give analgesia to patients with head injuries if required, but do so carefully and with appropriate patient monitoring**

ANALGESIA FOR THE TRAUMA PATIENT

When considering the administration of analgesia to trauma patients, three factors should be considered:

1. The patient; their clinical condition, existence of any allergies, and concomitant medications.
2. The route of drug administration; this will dictate the speed of onset and duration of action of the analgesic drug.
3. The drug; its effect, side effects, adverse reactions, potential antagonists and possible drug interactions.

Routes of drug administration

INTRAVENOUS ROUTE

Intravenous administration allows the drug to reach its site of action rapidly, and this is a particularly effective and controllable way of administering analgesia in the trauma patient. The optimal method of administering intravenous opiates is to administer small, titrated doses. It is important to remember that because a hypovolaemic patient has a reduced circulating volume, the onset of action may be delayed and the total dose required is often reduced.

Administration by the intravenous route increases the risk of serious anaphylactic reactions. In addition, extravasation of the drug into the tissues may cause a painful reaction and with some drugs, cause tissue necrosis.

INTRAMUSCULAR ROUTE

As a result of poor peripheral circulation in the shocked trauma patient, absorption of the administered analgesic may be delayed or reduced.[5] This results in ineffective analgesia, and a second dose of drug may be given. When the circulation is restored, a large depot of drug is rapidly absorbed, but this has a potential for overdosage. Intramuscular injections may also cause discomfort. Similar considerations are true for the subcutaneous route of drug administration.

ORAL ADMINISTRATION

The principal disadvantage of this route is its slow absorption, leading to delayed onset of action, which may be up to 1 h after administration. This is exacerbated in trauma patients where gastric emptying may be delayed. Drugs absorbed from the gut enter the portal circulation and may be partly metabolized in the liver, reducing their efficacy. Oral administration of drugs in trauma patients has limited use, and is reserved for minor uncomplicated trauma.

RECTAL AND SUBLINGUAL ADMINISTRATION

These routes of administration allow more rapid absorption of the drug. The portal circulation is also bypassed, and thus more drug reaches the site of action.

Non-steroidal drugs such as diclofenac 100 mg per rectum and piroxicam 20 mg sublingual are useful drugs for relieving mild to moderate pain in trauma patients.

INTRA-OSSEOUS ADMINISTRATION

Drugs and fluids administered by the intra-osseous route reach the circulation almost as rapidly as by the intravenous route. All drugs used for resuscitation, analgesia and anaesthesia intravenously may also be administered by this route.[6]

INHALATION

See Nitrous oxide (p. 246).

INFILTRATION

See Local anaesthesia (p. 247).

> **Intravenous opioid, titrated to effect is the optimum method of administering analgesia to trauma patients**

SYSTEMIC ANALGESIC DRUGS

An analgesic is a drug which relieves pain without depressing consciousness (as an anaesthetic drug would). Examples include opioids; non-steroidal anti-inflammatory drugs; nitrous oxide; and ketamine.

Opioids

These are drugs that are structurally related to morphine and are either naturally occurring or synthetic.[7] They are classified by their actions on receptors for endogenous peptide neurotransmitters, enkephalins, endorphins and dynorphins. 'Opiates' is the term reserved for drugs derived from the opium poppy, *Papaver somniferum*.

Several classes of opioid receptors exist, and best known are the μ, κ and δ subtypes. The various opioid analgesics act as either agonists, partial agonists or antagonists at these various receptors (Table 18.1).

Table 18.1 *Classification of opioid drugs, receptor types and clinical effects*

	Receptor		
	μ	κ	δ
Agonists	Morphine Diamorphine Pethidine Fentanyl Alfentanil Codeine Methadone	Pentazocine	Pentazocine
Partial agonists	Buprenorphine	Nalbuphine	
Antagonists	Naloxone Pentazocine Nalbuphine	Naloxone	
Effects	Analgesia	Analgesia	Anti-analgesia, reversal of overdose
Adverse effects	Respiratory depression Sedation Cough suppression Dependency Miosis Bradycardia Nausea, vomiting	Dysphoria Miosis	Dysphoria Mydriasis Respiratory stimulation Tachycardia

Many opioids are poorly absorbed orally due to extensive hepatic 'first-pass' metabolism. In trauma patients they are best administered intravenously and titrated to effect. The principal adverse effect is respiratory depression, and opioids should be avoided in patients with a respiratory rate of less than 10 per minute; they must also be administered with caution in patients with a depressed level of consciousness. Nausea, vomiting and sedation may also be troublesome. Patients do not become dependent on opioids when these are used to relieve pain acutely.

The dose of morphine required to produce analgesia varies considerably in different patients, with up to 30 mg being needed in fit, healthy young patients. Histamine release may occur after i.v. administration. Pethidine has similar side effects to morphine, and euphoria, hypotension and tachycardia may also occur. Diamorphine is a potent alternative to morphine.

Fentanyl is a lipid-soluble, highly potent synthetic opioid which is a useful, rapidly-acting analgesic, but it too has similar side effects to morphine. Fentanyl is commonly used with anaesthetic induction agents to help reduce the hypertensive response to intubation, especially in patients with head injury. Large doses can cause chest wall rigidity and make artificial ventilation difficult.

Alfentanil and remifentanil are similar to fentanyl, but much more rapidly acting, especially remifentanil. They have a very limited place as analgesics in the trauma patient, especially as remifentanil is extremely short acting and can produce profound respiratory depression.

Nalbuphine is a partial κ agonist and μ antagonist, its advantage being that it has a ceiling level of effect. With doses over 30 mg there is no increase in analgesic effect and, more importantly, no increased risk of respiratory depression.

Nalbuphine may be administered by pre-hospital personnel, though in the Emergency Department the antagonist and partial agonist effects of the drugs may make subsequent doses of morphine less effective in controlling pain.

Nalbuphine is not recommended as an analgesic for use in hospitals.

Codeine is a weak opioid which is better absorbed after oral administration than morphine, and 10–20% of it is metabolized to morphine. It is less sedating than morphine, and has minimal effects on pupillary responses and in the past has been the opioid of choice in patients with head injury.

Table 18.2 *Pharmacokinetic characteristics of common opioid analgesics*

Drug	Dosage	Route	Time to onset	Duration of action
Morphine	0.1–0.2 mg/kg	i.v.	10 min	2–4 h
Diamorphine		i.v.		
Pethidine	1 mg/kg	i.v.	10 min	1–2 h
Fentanyl	1–2 µg/kg	i.v.	2–5 min	30–60 min
Nalbuphine	10–30 mg	i.v.	2–3 min	3–4 h
Codeine	30–60 mg	i.m or p.o.	20–30 min	4 h
Tramadol	100 mg bolus, followed by 50 mg every 20 min to a maximum of 3 mg/kg	i.m or p.o.		

Tramadol is a µ receptor agonist, and also inhibits neuronal re-uptake of noradrenaline and 5-hydroxytryptamine in the spinal cord. It is a useful analgesic for moderate pain, and causes less respiratory depression than other opioids.[8] It may be given intravenously or orally, but may cause seizures and should not be used in patients with epilepsy.

OPIOID REVERSAL

Naloxone is an antagonist of opioid analgesics and must be available whenever opioid analgesia is being used.

If naloxone is being used to confirm or eliminate overdosage as a cause of a reduced conscious level in a patient who may have taken illicit opiates, a large enough dose should be given to ensure that failure to respond is not due to inadequate dosage. A dose of 2 mg is a useful guide in adults, administered slowly over a few minutes. Bolus doses should be administered with care, since reversal of opioids may precipitate severe pain, hypertension and seizures. The onset of effect is 2–3 min, and the duration of effect is 20–30 min. The patient should therefore be closely observed, as the effects of the opioid may re-occur once the effect of naloxone has worn off and repeated doses or even an infusion may be necessary.

Anti-emetics

Nausea and vomiting are common side effects of opioids, and effective anti-emetics to be administered with opioids include:

- Prochlorperazine 12.5 mg i.m. every 8 h
- Cyclizine (an antihistamine) 50 mg i.v. or i.m. every 8 h
- Metoclopramide 10 mg i.v. or i.m every 8 h.
- Ondansetron [a 5-hydroxytryptamine-3 (5-HT$_3$) antagonist] 4–8 mg given i.v. or i.m.

Cyclizine may cause mild sedation and tachycardia. Side effects include extrapyramidal effects. Intravenous use is to be avoided as severe hypotension may occur. Ondansetron has a duration of action of about 8 h, though bradycardia, hypotension and hypersensitivity reactions may occur.

Non-steroidal anti-inflammatory drugs (NSAIDs)

These drugs act by inhibiting the cyclo-oxygenase enzyme system, thus reducing prostaglandin synthesis. Prostaglandins are involved in the central modulation of pain and in the periphery sensitize nerve endings to the action of histamine and bradykinin; they are also involved in the inflammatory response, and act as free radical scavengers and membrane stabilizers. They are useful analgesics for mild to moderate pain, and in higher doses act as anti-inflammatory and antipyretic drugs.[9] Most NSAIDs may be administered orally, intramuscularly or rectally, though a few are available for intravenous use.

A wide range of NSAIDs is available, and each doctor should be familiar with, and use, a limited number, perhaps one or two. Commonly used alternatives include ibuprofen (400 mg 8-hourly), diclofenac (orally 50 mg 8-hourly or rectally 100 mg every 8 h), piroxicam (sublingually, 20 mg daily) and ketorolac (10 mg given slowly initially followed by 10–30 mg every 4 h). Intramuscular injections of diclofenac, although available, are painful and should not be given.

The side effects of NSAIDs vary with the individual drugs and doses, and may include:

- acute renal failure;
- fluid retention;
- gastrointestinal discomfort, peptic ulceration and bleeding;
- antiplatelet effects causing bleeding;
- hypersensitivity; and
- acute bronchospasm (10% of asthmatics may develop this condition).

NSAIDs are therefore contraindicated if there is a definite history of renal impairment, cardiac failure, peptic ulceration and asthma. The incidence of complications is significantly increased in the elderly, in whom the use of these drugs should be avoided.

Paracetamol

Paracetamol is an effective analgesia for mild to moderate pain, and may be given either orally or rectally in a dose of up to 1 g every 6 h. It acts as a central inhibitor of cyclo-oxygenase, reducing prostaglandin synthesis, and is also an effective antipyretic.

NSAIDs and paracetamol are useful for relieving mild to moderate pain by a variety of routes

---

Nitrous oxide

Nitrous oxide is a colourless, sweet-smelling, non-irritant gas. It is insoluble in the blood, and when inhaled has a rapid onset of effect. It is not metabolized and is excreted rapidly from the body via the lungs. By itself, nitrous oxide is not sufficiently potent to produce anaesthesia; however, it is usually mixed with oxygen as a 70:30 carrier gas mix administered through a Boyle's machine (through which volatile anaesthetic agents are administered), thus reducing the dose of volatile anaesthetic needed to produce anaesthesia. Nitrous oxide is a very potent analgesic and has a potency similar to that of 15 mg of morphine administered subcutaneously.[10]

A mixture of 50% nitrous oxide with oxygen is called 'Entonox'. Cylinders of this mixture are coloured French blue, with white shoulders. Entonox is usually delivered via a demand valve, either through a facemask or a mouthpiece. The onset of the analgesic effect is 45–60 s, and the effect is maximal after 3–4 min. Entonox is very useful for pain relief in short emergency procedures such as reduction of fractures and application of splints.[11]

Nitrous oxide is 15 times more soluble in the plasma than nitrogen, and therefore it diffuses into air-filled body cavities more rapidly than nitrogen diffuses out. This means that enclosed airspaces such as the middle ear, gut, intracranial air or pneumothoraces may expand in size, causing either an increase in pressure or volume, depending on the compliance of the space involved. Thus Entonox should be avoided in patients with an undrained pneumothorax, bowel obstruction or recent craniotomy. Nitrous oxide is also a potent cerebral vasodilator, and may increase intracranial pressure in patients with head injuries.[12] Entonox is also contraindicated if the patient gives a recent history of diving.

> **Entonox is an excellent analgesic for short painful procedures carried out on trauma patients**

Ketamine

Ketamine is useful as a sole analgesic and anaesthetic agent, particularly in the pre-hospital setting. It is also useful in the Accident and Emergency Department.[13]

Ketamine is a derivative of phencyclidine and is unlike other anaesthetic agents. It produces a dissociative state where the patient's eyes may remain open, they may vocalize and move, but have no recall of events. In subanaesthetic doses ketamine is a profound analgesic, causing sympathetic stimulation that results in tachycardia and hypertension. In a patient who is hypovolaemic this is a useful effect, as ketamine will not result in the profound hypotension and cardiovascular depression often seen with other anaesthetic agents. However, ketamine has a direct myocardial depressant effect, and may cause hypotension in a patient who is profoundly shocked and already maximally sympathetically stimulated. Similarly, patients with high spinal cord injuries may develop hypotension when ketamine is administered.

> **Ketamine should not be used in the profoundly hypotensive patient**

Ketamine is a mild respiratory stimulant and does not depress respiration in the way opiates can. It also preserves the airway reflexes to some extent, and is a bronchodilator.

Its adverse effects include an increase in cerebral blood flow that results in raised intracranial pressure in patients with head injuries.[14] Nausea and vomiting may occur, and excessive salivation which can compromise the airway. Patients recovering from ketamine anaesthesia may also experience disturbing hallucinations, which may be prevented by using a benzodiazepine and allowing the patient to recover in a darkened, quiet environment.

For anaesthesia, a dose of 1–2 mg/kg i.v. or 5–10 mg/kg i.m. is required. The onset of effect may take several minutes if given i.m.

For an analgesic dose, 0.25–0.5 mg/kg i.v. or 1–4 mg/kg i.m. should be given. The onset is much slower, and duration of action is 10–20 min.

LOCAL ANAESTHESIA

Local anaesthetic techniques are extremely useful for pain relief in trauma patients.[15] Appropriately placed injections of local anaesthetics can produce excellent analgesia, without the side effects of systemic analgesic agents. Local anaesthetic drugs do have their own side effects and must be used with care, by experienced personnel.

Local anaesthetic agents may be used in the following ways:

- Topical
- Subcutaneous infiltration
- Peripheral nerve block
- Nerve plexus block
- Intravenous regional analgesia (Bier's block).

The intrathecal and epidural routes are not suitable in the Emergency Department.

Local anaesthetic agents

A local anaesthetic is a drug which reversibly blocks the transmission of peripheral nerve impulses[16] by inhibiting the increase in sodium permeability in excitable cells that gives rise to the action potential, thereby preventing membrane depolarization. Local anaesthetic agents have this stabilizing effect on the plasma membranes of all types of excitable cells, not only on neurons.

When administering local anaesthetic agents, three important factors need to be considered:

1. Potency, which is directly related to lipid solubility.
2. Speed of onset.
3. Duration of action, which depends on the extent of protein binding and intrinsic vasoconstriction which limits the dissipation of the drug away from the site of action.

Most local anaesthetic agents are intrinsic vasodilators, though vasoconstrictor agents may be co-administered with them to prolong the duration of the drug and limit its toxicity. Preparations of local anaesthetics with adrenaline are available for this purpose. The speed of onset and duration of the local anaesthetic are also influenced by the type of local anaesthetic block being used.

Small unmyelinated nerves are blocked before larger myelinated ones; thus, sympathetic fibres and pain fibres are blocked before sensory and motor nerves.

Local anaesthetics deposited directly onto a nerve (for example, in a femoral nerve block) act more quickly than when the anaesthetic has to diffuse towards the nerves, such as a plexus block or subcutaneous infiltration. The vascular supply to the area being blocked also determines the duration of action and the toxicity of the agents being used. Where there is a good blood supply the local anaesthetic agent is more rapidly removed by the blood, and more of the agent is likely to be absorbed systemically, thus making toxicity more likely.

Side effects of local anaesthetics

These can be divided into four groups: (i) toxicity reactions; (ii) hypersensitivity; (iii) reactions to adjuncts (adrenaline or preservatives); and (iv) nerve damage.

LOCAL ANAESTHETIC TOXICITY

Local anaesthetics act non-specifically on excitable plasma membranes, their toxic reactions being seen predominantly in the cardiovascular and central nervous systems.

The toxic doses for each agent are widely available; however, if a local anaesthetic is injected directly into the vascular system or the central nervous system, only a tiny dose may be enough to precipitate toxicity. Intravascular and intrathecal injection therefore must be carefully avoided.

Toxic reactions tend to follow the following progression of symptoms and signs:

- perioral numbness and tingling and complaint of a metallic taste;
- visual disturbances, tinnitus, dizziness;
- slurred speech;
- tachycardia, hypertension;
- muscular twitching;
- convulsions;
- hypotension, bradycardia;
- ventricular arrhythmias; and
- cardiac arrest.

Patients undergoing any local anaesthetic block should have intravenous access established before the injection of local anaesthetic and basic cardiovascular monitoring, ECG, pulse oximeter and blood pressure monitoring should be available.

As with all anaesthetic and analgesic administration, the operator should be aware of the diagnosis and treatment of toxicity reactions (Table 18.3).

Table 18.3 *Management of local anaesthetics toxicity*

Basic Advanced Life Support protocols should be followed.[17]
• Secure the airway
• Administer high-flow oxygen
• Ensure adequate ventilation
• Resuscitate the circulation
Convulsions may be treated with diazepam (0.1 mg/kg) or i.v. midazolam
Cardiac arrythmias, particularly those caused by bupivicaine, may be difficult to treat
Cardiac massage should be continued
Cardiac pacing may be required

HYPERSENSITIVITY

Anaphylactic and anaphylactoid reactions are uncommon, but are more likely to occur with the ester-based agents, as well as to the preservative, methylhydroxybenzoate.

REACTIONS TO ADJUNCTS

Adrenaline may be used with local anaesthetic agents to cause vasoconstriction and prolong the action of the local block. Adrenaline and other vasoconstrictors must be avoided in areas where there are end arteries, for example the digits, nose, ears and penis.

In patients with cardiac disease, adrenaline-containing local anaesthetic solutions must be used with care, as systemic absorption of adrenaline may cause tachycardias, cardiac arrythmias and may precipitate cardiac ischaemia.

NERVE DAMAGE

Direct trauma to peripheral nerves with a needle and injection of local anaesthetic directly into a nerve can cause permanent nerve damage. Short, bevelled needles designed specifically for local anaesthesia should be used where possible. A conscious patient will complain of pain and paraesthesia if the nerve is penetrated while attempting a nerve block, and the needle should be withdrawn immediately.

Commonly used local anaesthetics

LIGNOCAINE (AMIDE)

- Very commonly used
- Onset of action is 5 min for peripheral use, 20 min for plexus blocks
- Duration of action is 60–90 min
- Dose 3 mg/kg
- Dose with adrenaline 7 mg/kg.

A eutectic mixture of local anaesthetic (EMLA) is a white cream containing lignocaine 2.5% and prilocaine 2.5% applied under an occlusive dressing which provides topical analgesia to the skin. It is effective within 30–60 min.

PRILOCAINE (AMIDE)

- Onset of action is similar to that of lignocaine
- Duration of action is 60–90 min
- Dose 5 mg/kg
- Dose with adrenaline 8 mg/kg.

Prilocaine doses over 600 mg may cause methaemaglobinaemia, but this may be treated with methylene blue (2 mg/kg). Prilocaine is commonly used for intravenous regional anaesthesia.

BUPIVICAINE (AMIDE)

- Onset of action is 20 min peripherally, and 45 min for plexus block
- Duration of action is up to 24 h in plexus blocks
- Dose 2 mg/kg (with or without adrenaline).

Bupivicaine is more toxic than other agents, and has a great affinity for cardiac muscle, thus making resuscitation more difficult.

AMETHOCAINE

Amethocaine is used as a topical preparation for conjunctival and corneal anaesthesia (see Chapter 11).

Local anaesthetic blocks

There are a large number of local anaesthetic blocks,[16] and those described below are suitable for use in the Emergency Department.

The following general principles should always be followed when a local anaesthetic block is being used:

- The patient should be informed about the block and its side effects.
- Consent for the procedure should be obtained.
- A history of local anaesthetic allergy should be sought, and the procedure abandoned if necessary.
- Intravenous access must be established.
- Standard monitoring should be established.
- Resuscitation equipment must be readily available.
- The skin over the area where the block is to be performed should be cleaned, and an aseptic technique used.

FEMORAL NERVE BLOCK

This block is particularly useful for providing analgesia in patients with a fracture of the femoral shaft.

Anatomy

The femoral artery and vein and femoral nerve all pass behind the inguinal ligament deep to the fascia lata. The artery and vein are enclosed in a facial sheath, with the vein being more medial. The femoral nerve lies behind and lateral to this sheath. Its position may vary between individuals, sometimes being very close to the sheath, sometimes several centimetres lateral to it. (Remember NAVY: Nerve – Artery – Vein – Y fronts.) Just below the inguinal ligament the femoral nerve divides into several branches (Figure 18.1).

Techniques

A line drawn from the pubic tubercle to the anterior superior iliac spine marks the position of the inguinal ligament. The femoral artery can be palpated in the centre of this line, and the femoral nerve is located about 1 cm lateral to the artery just below the inguinal ligament. The needle is directed posteriorly and distally at a 45º angle. A 'click' may be felt as the needle pierces the fascia lata, and paraesthesia or pain may occur if the needle has penetrated the nerve. If paraesthesia or pain are obtained the needle should be withdrawn slightly before injection in order to prevent neuronal damage. The total depth should be no more than 2.0–3.5 cm.

Characteristics of femoral nerve-blocking agents include:

- Dose: 10–20 ml 1% lignocaine, or 0.25% bupivicaine
- Onset time: 10–30 min
- Duration: 4–6 h, longer if using bupivicaine.

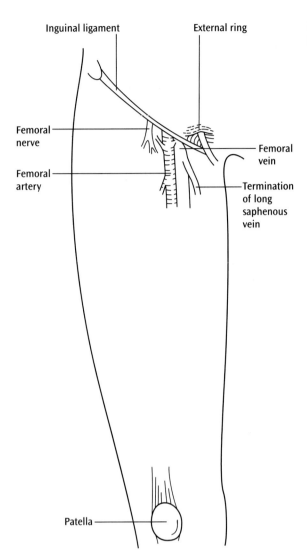

Figure 18.1 *The anatomy of the inguinal area.*

WRIST NERVE BLOCK

The hand distal to the palmar crease may be simply anaesthetized by blocking the terminal branches of the ulnar, median and radial nerves (Figure 18.2).

Anatomy
The ulnar nerve lies lateral to the tendon of flexor carpi ulnaris, adjacent to the ulnar artery. The median nerve lies between the tendons of palmaris longus and flexor carpi radialis. The radial nerve is posterolateral to the brachioradialis.

Technique
Three injections of local anaesthetic are required:

1. Directly lateral to flexor carpi ulnaris (ulnar nerve block).
2. Between palmaris longus and flexor carpi radialis (median nerve block).
3. Subcutaneous infiltration around the dorsolateral aspect of the wrist, lateral to the radial artery (block of superficial branch of radial nerve).

Characteristics of wrist nerve-blocking agents include:

- Dose: 5 ml of 1% lignocaine or prilocaine can be injected at each site
- Onset: 5–10 min
- Duration: 45–60 min.

Blocks of the individual nerves may be considered, depending on the anatomical site of injury.

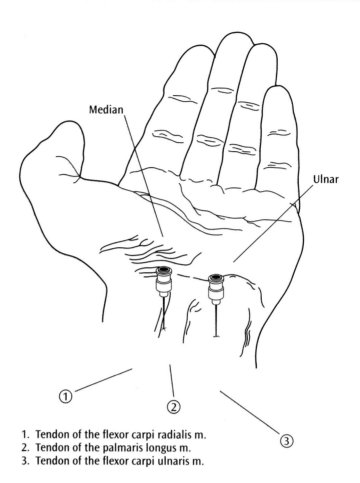

1. Tendon of the flexor carpi radialis m.
2. Tendon of the palmaris longus m.
3. Tendon of the flexor carpi ulnaris m.

Figure 18.2 *Nerve blocks at the wrist.*

DIGITAL NERVE BLOCK

The digital nerves, two dorsal and two palmar, accompany the digital vessels. An aliquot (1–2 ml) of local anaesthetic can be injected at the base of the digit at either side to block these nerves and to anaesthetize the digit. Digital nerve block is usually effective in 5–10 min. A finger tournequet formed from the little finger of a surgical glove can be used, and will significantly increase the effectiveness of the block. Vasoconstrictors must be avoided as digit ischaemia will occur. It is also important to avoid injecting a large volume of anaesthetic agent, as swelling around the nerves may cause distal ischaemia.

> **Lignocaine with adrenaline is absolutely contraindicated in digital nerve blocks**

INTERCOSTAL NERVE BLOCKS

Intercostal nerve blocks are a useful means of providing analgesia for patients with fractured ribs.

Anatomy
The intercostal nerves run in the intercostal groove on the inferior aspect of the rib. For optimum analgesia the nerve should be blocked proximal to the origin of the lateral branch (proximal to the mid-axillary line).

Technique
The patient is positioned either prone, in the lateral decubitus position, or sitting and leaning forwards. The shoulders should be abducted and the arms held forward so that the

scapulae move laterally and aid access to the posterior angle of the ribs. The needle is introduced and advanced until it makes contact with the rib. The needle is then allowed to slip down off the inferior border of the rib. The needle can then be angled at 45° and advanced 0.5 cm inwards towards the intercostal nerve. The patient should be instructed to hold their breath while the injection is taking place in order to avoid penetrating the pleura. Before injection the needle should be aspirated to ensure it is not in a blood vessel.

Characteristics of intercostal nerve-blocking agents include:

- Dose: 3–4 ml of 0.5% bupivicaine, with or without adrenaline, is injected
- Onset of action: 10–20 min
- Duration of action: 4–8 h.

Several intercostal nerves above and below the broken rib will need to be blocked in order to provide effective analgesia.

INTRAVENOUS REGIONAL ANAESTHESIA (IVRA; BIER'S BLOCK)

This technique involves the injection of local anaesthetic into an exsanguinated limb. IVRA is most commonly used in the upper limb in the form of a Bier's block. It is a safe and effective means of providing anaesthesia for short procedures on the hand and forearm. The time limitation of the procedure is related to the discomfort caused by the tourniquet, and is usually limited to no more than 1 h. Tourniquets should be avoided in patients with sickle-cell disease or trait, Raynaud's disease or symptomatic peripheral vascular disease.

IVRA should always be performed by two suitably qualified and experienced operators. The fatalities which have occurred with this technique have been related to single operators and errors with the inflation and release of tourniquets.

A double-cuff tourniquet can be used, so that the area over which the second (lower) cuff lies can be anaesthetized. This requires the upper cuff to be inflated first while the block takes effect. The lower cuff is then inflated and the upper one deflated. Errors in this sequence, however, have led to patients receiving fatal systemic boluses of local anaesthetic. A single-cuff tourniquet is much safer and usually tolerated well by patients.

Technique

Venous access is established in the opposite arm to the injury. A small cannula is also inserted into the back of the hand on the side of the injury. If no suitable venous access is available in the hand, a cannula inserted into the antecubital fossa is an effective alternative.

The next stage is to exsanguinate the arm. Ideally, an Esmarch bandage should be used, but in patients with painful fractures of the forearm, the arm can be elevated gently and pressure applied to the brachial artery.

Once the arm is exsanguinated, the tourniquet is inflated to 100 mmHg above systolic arterial pressure. Prilocaine 0.5% without preservative is the anaesthetic of choice, and it should be injected slowly to prevent it being forced up the arm under the tourniquet and into the systemic circulation. Bupivicaine must never be used for Bier's blocks, as almost all the deaths associated with this technique have used this agent. The normal adult dose is 40 ml, though this may be reduced in frail, elderly patients. The patient may complain of paraesthesia almost immediately, and the skin may appear mottled. The sensory block is usually established in 10 min, and good muscle relaxation is obtained after 20 min.

The tourniquet should be left inflated for at least 20 min; otherwise, once the procedure is complete the tourniquet can be released and the patient closely observed for signs of local anaesthetic toxicity, the signs of which are described above. Careful observation should continue for at least 2 h. Systemic toxicity may occur if the tourniquet is released too soon, and a number of deaths associated with this procedure have been recorded.[18]

> **Intravenous regional anaesthesia is a two-operator technique**

HAEMATOMA BLOCK

Haematoma block is most commonly used for fractures of the wrist. Local anaesthetic is introduced directly into the area of the fracture and its surrounding haematoma.

Technique

The first step is familiarization with the anatomy of the fracture by careful study of the radiographs and comparison with the surface anatomy. The skin over the fracture site is thoroughly cleaned. Using a syringe and green needle, up to 20 ml of 1% lignocaine is then introduced into the area of the fracture and haematoma. Before injection, location of the tip of the needle within the haematoma is confirmed by aspiration of blood. The needle enters the haematoma through the fracture at a site located by comparison of the radiographs and the surface anatomy.

Haematoma block is not suitable for fractures over 24 h old, and levels of analgesia are often not as good as those achieved by Bier's block. Many failures of haematoma blocks could, however, be avoided by waiting until the block can be demonstrated to be effective by gentle movement of the wrist before attempting manipulation.

SEDATION TECHNIQUES FOR TRAUMA PATIENTS

Sedation is a state somewhere along a line which has an awake, conscious patient in full control of their airway at one end, and a fully anaesthetized patient with no airway control at the other end. The drugs used to produce sedation are for the most part the same ones used to produce anaesthesia, but used in smaller doses. The dose of a particular drug that has a defined effect on a patient varies considerably depending on the patient's age, weight and pathophysiological status. Standard doses should only be used as a guide when the patient is undergoing sedation. An ideally sedated patient will be calm and lightly asleep, but will be capable of responding to the operator's voice and obeying commands. Most sedative agents also provide some degree of amnesia, with the result that the patient will usually be unaware of what has occurred while under sedation.

Indications for sedation in trauma patients

Patients with relatively minor trauma who are to undergo a minor procedure in the Emergency Department may benefit from sedation.

Contraindications to sedation in trauma patients include:

- Altered level of consciousness due to:
  - head injury
  - drugs
  - alcohol.
- Haemodynamic instabilty.
- Patients with a full stomach.

Sedation may make it difficult to assess the conscious level of obtunded patients, and precipitate apnoea or loss of airway control. Restlessness due to pain, hypoxia or a full bladder is not an indication for sedation. The cause of the restlessness should be sought, identified and treated.

When undertaking a procedure under sedation the following is recommended:

- The patient should be starved for at least 4 h.
- The patient should receive a full explanation of the procedure, and consent must be obtained.
- There must be two medically qualified people present, one to administer sedation and monitor the patient and one to carry out the procedure. Ideally, both of these doctors should have suitably qualified assistants.
- The patient should be appropriately monitored, including ECG, pulse oximeter and non-invasive blood pressure.
- Intravenous access must be secured before starting sedation.
- The patient should be on a tilting trolley, with full resuscitation equipment available.
- If the patient is to go home after the procedure they should be escorted home and have someone to remain with them, preferably overnight.

- Patients should be advised not to drive, or to perform complicated tasks until the sedation effects have completely worn off.

Drugs used for sedation

BENZODIAZEPINES

These drugs are widely used as sedatives, as they produce anxiolysis and retrograde amnesia. Their main side effect is respiratory depression. These agents are not analgesics, and therefore for painful procedures an appropriate nerve block or small dose of analgesic will be required.

Midazolam

Midazolam is a water-soluble benzodiazepine that may be administered as an intravenous injection. It has a half-life of 2.5 h, and recovery is rapid. The safest way to administer midazolam sedation is to dilute the drug to a 1 mg/ml solution and titrate it as 0.5–1.0 mg aliquots. Elderly patients may require as little as 1–2 mg for sedation, but it may take several minutes to be effective. It is important to wait a few minutes after each small bolus in order to avoid overdose and respiratory depression. The duration of action of midazolam is also prolonged in elderly patients. A young fit patient on the other hand, may require up to 10 mg of midazolam.

Diazepam

Diazepam is often used for sedation. This drug is not particularly water-soluble, and the intravenous preparation is an emulsion (Diazemuls). This should be titrated to reach the appropriate level of sedation. Diazepam has a long half-life, and it may take several hours for its effects to wear off, particularly in the elderly. Diazepam may also be administered orally or rectally as a 5–10 mg dose.

Flumazenil

This is a short-acting benzodiazepine antagonist and may be used to reverse the effects of benzodiazepines. It is given in a dose of 200 µg i.v. over 15 s, then 100 µg every 60 s until effective. The maximum total dose is 1 mg.

The duration of action of flumazenil is about 20 min, and therefore if a patient has had a large dose of benzodiazepine the reversal effects of flumazanil may wear off, allowing the patient to become re-sedated. Flumazenil may cause seizures in epileptic patients. Nausea, vomiting, flushing, agitation and transient increases in heart rate and blood pressure may occur.

OPIOIDS

Opioids may be administered together with benzodiazepines to provide analgesia during sedation. Morphine or pethidine may be used, and they should be titrated as small intravenous boluses. Opioids and benzodiazepines both cause respiratory depression, and when given together their effects are additive. Patients – especially the elderly – need to be closely monitored for several hours after the procedure.

ANAESTHETIC AGENTS

The intravenous anaesthetic agents, propofol and ketamine, may be used to provide sedation. These drugs should only be administered by a doctor who is experienced in their use, as overdose may cause anaesthesia and respiratory arrest.

ANAESTHESIA IN THE EMERGENCY DEPARTMENT

The induction and maintenance of general anaesthesia should ideally be carried out in a properly equipped and staffed operating theatre suite. However, there are circumstances when anaesthesia is required for trauma patients in the Emergency Department. Anaesthesia for trauma patients is complex and requires experienced personnel.

Management of the airway may be made difficult by maxillofacial trauma or suspected cervical spine injuries. Most anaesthetic agents are cardiovascular depressants, thus compounding hypotension in hypovolaemic patients. Guidelines have been laid down by the Association of Anaesthetists of Great Britain and Ireland for the safe provision of anaesthesia, recommended standards of patient monitoring and the requirements for a suitably trained assistant for the anaesthetist.[19–21]

Anaesthesia should only be administered in the Emergency Department by a doctor with suitable training and experience, either a senior anaesthetist or an emergency physician who has undergone anaesthetic training.[22] An in-depth description of trauma anaesthesia may be found elsewhere.[23]

> **Trauma anaesthesia is a specialized field requiring appropriate training and experience**

Monitoring that should be available whenever anaesthesia is induced is outlined in Table 18.4.

Table 18.4 *Monitoring required for administration of general anaesthesia*

Standard monitoring	Additional monitoring
All patients	*(Depending on clinical condition)*
• Oxygen analyser	• Invasive blood pressure
• Pulse oximeter	• Neuromuscular blockade monitoring
• ECG	• Temperature
• Non-invasive blood pressure	• Central venous pressure
• Capnography	
• Ventilator disconnection alarm	

The usual reasons for the administration of a general anaesthetic in the resuscitation room are either to establish a definitive airway or to control a disturbed or aggressive patient in order to facilitate treatment.

Rapid-sequence induction of anaesthesia

All trauma patients are assumed to have a full stomach. Rapid-sequence induction of anaesthesia allows the patient to be anaesthetized and the airway to be secured while reducing the risk of regurgitation and aspiration.[24]

When carrying out rapid-sequence induction of anaesthesia, resuscitation equipment and difficult intubation equipment must be available, and the patient should be on a tilting trolley. Suction must always be available. Appropriate monitoring equipment is required and expert assistance must be to hand.

PROCEDURE FOR RAPID-SEQUENCE INDUCTION

The patient must be pre-oxygenated with high-flow oxygen via a correctly fitting facemask for 3 min, after which anaesthesia is induced with an adequate dose of an induction agent. A variety of anaesthetic agents may be used, including thiopentone and midazolam,[25] but if the patient is cardiovascularly unstable, then etomidate[26] or ketamine are more suitable. The dose of the drug required to produce anaesthesia is estimated on the basis of the patient's weight and given by rapid intravenous injection. Administration of the induction agent is followed immediately by administration of the depolarizing muscle relaxant suxamethonium. Cricoid pressure (Sellick's manoeuvre) is applied as the patient loses consciousness, and is maintained until the airway is definitively protected when it can be removed on the instruction of the intubator.

If cervical spine injury is suspected, an assistant should maintain manual in-line cervical spine immobilization.[27] Rigid cervical collars can impede intubation and should be removed before tracheal intubation is attempted.[28]

Suxamethonium (1–2 mg/kg) is the standard muscle relaxant and provides adequate intubating conditions in approximately 30 s. Before relaxation, muscle fasciculations will occur; when these cease, the patient can be intubated using a cuffed endotracheal tube. Once the position of the tube in the trachea is confirmed, the cuff is inflated and the tube secured, cricoid pressure can be released.[24]

A number of other muscle relaxants, including rocuronium, are available as alternatives to suxamethonium. These drugs should only be used by those who have appropriate experience and expertise.

The side effects of suxamethonium are given in Table 18.5.

Table 18.5 *The side effects of suxamethonium*

- Raised intracranial pressure
- Raised intraocular pressure
- Bradycardia (especially in children or following a second dose)
- Histamine release and anaphylaxis
- Prolonged apnoea in patients who have plasma cholinesterase deficiencies
- Trigger agent for malignant hyperpyrexia

Suxamethonium administration can result in potentially fatal hyperkalaemia in patients with a high spinal cord injury, extensive burns, upper motor neuron lesions or renal failure. This is not a problem in the acute stages immediately following injury.

Once the patient is intubated, the lungs may be ventilated manually or using a ventilator; further sedation and muscle relaxation will be required to maintain anaesthesia.

Intubation may be difficult in trauma patients for several reasons, including:

- facial trauma;
- in-line cervical spine stabilization which may prevent neck extension; and
- incorrectly applied cricoid pressure.

It is therefore essential to assess fully the patient's airway before anaesthetizing and paralysing them. Failure to intubate a patient who was previously maintaining a partial airway and breathing, may be fatal.

If the patient's airway appears to be difficult to intubate, the following paths may be followed.

1. Re-consideration of the need for immediate anaesthesia and intubation.
2. Consideration of awake intubation using local anaesthesia to the airway and either conventional intubation or fibreoptic intubation. Fibreoptic intubation requires a skilled operator, takes time, and may be difficult if there is blood in the airway.
3. Consideration of inhalational induction of anaesthesia to maintain a breathing patient. Laryngoscopy can be performed while the patient is still breathing and before the administration of muscle relaxants. However, this technique still may lead to loss of the airway after administration of muscle relaxant, and the patient will be at risk of regurgitation and aspiration.

If a difficult intubation is anticipated, it is essential that the equipment and expertise required for the formation of a surgical airway is immediately available.

Hypovolaemic patients may develop severe hypotension on administration of induction agents. In these cases a much smaller dose of induction agent is used. Ketamine may also be useful in preventing hypotension.

Tracheal intubation is very stimulating, and large amounts of catecholamines are released which may cause a hypertensive surge. This may be detrimental for patients with head injuries, raised intracranial pressure or cardiovascular system disease. In these patients the rapid sequence induction may be modified to include agents that obtund the pressor response, such as fentanyl,[29] lignocaine,[30] labetolol or esmolol. These drugs should be administered at least 3 min before laryngoscopy if they are to be effective. Such agents may all cause depression of the blood pressure, and therefore the patient must be haemodynamically stable before they are administered.

SUMMARY

Every doctor who deals with the victims of trauma must be capable of providing his/her patients with adequate pain relief. A wide range of methods is described in this chapter, from simple reassurance to rapid-sequence induction of anaesthesia. The best results will be achieved by careful selection of the most appropriate method form modalities which include oral and intravenous analgesia, local, regional and general anaesthesia. Nevertheless, the individual practitioner should recognize that the induction of general anaesthesia, if it is to be safely and effectively accomplished, requires significant skills and experience, and should be administered only by those who possess them.

REFERENCES

1. Subcommittee on Taxonomy. Pain terms: a list with definitions and notes on usage. *International Association for the Study of Pain* 1979; **6**: 249–52.
2. Beecher HK. *Resuscitation and Anesthesia for Wounded Men: The Management of Traumatic Shock*. Springfield, IL: Charles C. Thomas, 1949.
3. Duggan J, Drummond GB. Activity of lower intercostals and abdominal muscle after surgery in humans. *Anesthesia and Analgesia* 1987; **66**: 852–5.
4. Pate JW. Chest wall injuries. *Surgical Clinics of North America* 1989; **69**: 59–70.
5. Austin KL, Stapleton JV, Mather LE. Multiple intramuscular injections: a major source of variability in analgesic response to meperidine. *Pain* 1969; **8**: 47–62.
6. Sawyer RW, Bodai BI, Blaisdell FW, McCourt MM. The current state of intraosseous infusion. *Journal of the American College of Surgeons* 1994; **179**: 353–8.
7. Foster RW (ed.). *Basic Pharmacology (2nd edn)*. Oxford: Butterworths, 1986.
8. Budd K, Langford R. Tramadol revisited. *British Journal of Anaesthesia* 1999; **82**: 493–5.
9. Dahl JB, Kehlet H. Non-steroidal anti-inflammatory drugs: rationale for use in severe postoperative pain. *British Journal of Anaesthesia* 1991; **66**: 703–12.
10. Chapman WP, Arrowwood JG, Beecher HK. The analgesic effect of nitrous oxide compared in man with morphine sulphate. *Journal of Clinical Investigation* 1943; **22**: 871–5.
11. Baskett PJF, Withnell A. Use of entonox in the Ambulance Service. *British Medical Journal* 1970; **284**: 41–3.
12. Moss E., McDowall DG. ICP increases with 50% nitrous oxide in severe head injuries during controlled ventilation. *British Joural of Anaesthesia* 1979; **51**: 757–60.
13. White PF, Way WL, Trevor AJ. Ketamine – its pharmacology and therapeutic uses. *Anesthesiology* 1982; **56**: 119.
14. Shapiro HM, Wyte SR, Harris AB. Ketamine anaesthesia in patients with intracranial pathology. *British Journal of Anaesthesia* 1972; **144**: 1200–4.
15. Desai SM, Bernhard WN, McAlary B. Regional anaesthesia: management considerations in the trauma patient. *Critical Care Clinics* 1990; **6**: 85–101.
16. Wildesmith JAW, Armitage EN (eds). *Principles and Practice of Regional Anaesthesia*. Edinburgh: Churchill Livingstone, 1990.
17. *Advanced Life Support Manual*. Resuscitation Council UK.
18. Heath M. Deaths after intravenous regional anaesthesia. *British Medical Journal* 1982; **285**: 913–14.
19. The Association of Anaesthetists of Great Britain and Ireland 1998. The Anaesthesia Team, London.
20. The Association of Anaesthetists of Great Britain and Ireland 1997. Checklist for Anaesthetic Apparatus.
21. The Association of Anaesthetists of Great Britain and Ireland 1989. Recommendations for Standards of Monitoring during Anaesthesia and Recovery.

22. Walker A, Brenchley J. Survey of the use of rapid sequence induction in the accident and emergency department. *Journal of Accident and Emergency Medicine* 2000; **2**: 95–7.

23. Grande CM. *Textbook of Trauma Anaesthesia and Critical Care*. London: Mosby, 1993.

24. Atkinson RS, Rushman GB, Lee JA (eds). *Accidents, Complications and Sequelae of Anaesthesia. A Synopsis of Anaesthesia*. (10th ed.). Wright, 1987, pp. 318–63.

25. Sivilotti ML, Ducharme J. Randomised, double blind study on sedatives and hemodynamics during rapid-sequence intubation in the emergency department: the SHRED study. *Annals of Emergency Medicine* 1998; **31**: 313–24.

26. Bergen JM, Smith DC. A review of etomidate for rapid sequence intubation in the emergency department. *Journal of Emergency Medicine* 1997; **15**: 221–30.

27. Criswell JC, Parr MJ, Nolan JP. Emergency airway management in patients with cervical spine injuries. *Anaesthesia* 1994; **49**: 900–3.

28. Heath KJ. The effect on laryngoscopy of different cervical spine immobilization techniques. *Anaesthesia* 1994; **49**: 843–45.

29. Cork RC, Weiss JC, Hameroff SR, Bentley J. Fentanyl preloading for rapid sequence induction of anesthesia. *Anesthesia and Analgesia* 1984; **63**: 60–4.

30. Donegan MF, Bedford RF. Intravenous administration of lidocaine prevents intracranial hypertension during endotracheal suctioning. *Anesthesiology* 1980; **52**: 516–18.

19

Trauma intensive care

OBJECTIVES

- To understand the role of the Intensive Care Unit (ICU) in the management of major trauma
- To describe a systematic clinical approach to the trauma patient on the ICU
- To outline the treatment modalities which are used to support organ failure of the types most commonly seen after trauma

INTRODUCTION

Trauma patients constitute a relatively small percentage of patients admitted to most small Intensive Care Units (ICUs) in non-specialist centres, since the incidence of severe trauma in the UK is relatively low [approximately 0.5% of all Accident and Emergency (A&E) attenders in England and Wales].[1] When specialist hospitals are considered, such as those having neurosurgical, thoracic or burns units on site, then the percentage of trauma patients within the ICU population rises to around 20% of total occupancy. Patients with these particular injury patterns may have relatively low injury severity or APACHE scores,[2] but the specific nature of their injury often requires a period of ICU treatment as part of their specialist therapy and carries a high risk of mortality.

The 'third peak'[3] of trauma deaths is often said to occur in ICU as a consequence of multiple organ failure and sepsis. This peak of deaths is unlikely to be diminished by better initial management in the 'golden hour' alone, and the care that the trauma patient receives in ICU will have a direct bearing on their outcome.

The special needs of the trauma patient on the ICU are a consequence of several factors. Admission of trauma patients to the ICU may be direct from the A&E resuscitation room, via the operating theatre, or as direct transfers from other hospitals for specialist care unavailable at the referring hospital. As a consequence the patient may be stable or unstable, and may or may not have had a completed primary survey, secondary survey or a definitive range of investigations specific to their injury.

> **ICU patients may not have completed primary and secondary surveys**

They may have been subjected to therapeutic interventions, which may have been inappropriate or have sown the seeds of iatrogenic complications. Life-saving procedures may have been carried out in circumstances where strict asepsis was impossible, thereby exposing the patient to potential sources of sepsis. Errors of process that may have occurred, either within or without one's own institution, must be identified and corrected. Any stage of the initial assessment and management process that was not completed, due to the need for emergency surgery as part of resuscitation during the primary survey, for example, should be taken to its conclusion to ensure that additional injuries are not missed.

Patients who have suffered multiple trauma will have problems which require input from specialists in several fields, and the ICU team should identify such needs and initiate the appropriate consultations. In order that all these goals are reached, a systematic approach to the initial assessment on admission to ICU is required. Since trauma is a dynamic process with multi-system effects, there is a requirement for a similar detailed review of the patient on a daily basis during their stay on ICU.

ICU ADMISSION ASSESSMENT

The ABCDE approach of the primary survey is well known, but once the trauma patient has arrived on ICU the admission assessment runs virtually from A to Z. Repeating the primary and secondary surveys *de novo* on the moment of admission is a small but vital part of this process. In addition, the presence of established or impending organ failure outside that detected during these surveys is identified, and the appropriate supportive treatment regimes started together with those aimed at pre-empting other organ systems failing. All the data obtained so far must be reviewed, particularly:

- the mechanism of injury;
- resuscitation and other interventions; and
- investigations and imaging.

Everything that may benefit the patient is acted upon. An 'AMPLE' history should be obtained, from the patient's relatives if need be, to determine any co-morbidity that may require specific therapy or modify planned treatment regimes.

A: Airway and cervical spine control

The majority of patients admitted to ICU will have been intubated and ventilated for some reason, or have an airway that is deemed to be 'at risk'. They may also have the potential to develop respiratory failure.

Where the patient arrives already intubated, it is necessary to check that the tube is correctly positioned, and is the right type, size and length for the patient. If the tube was placed in circumstances where sterility may have been compromised, it should be replaced. This must be done safely and appropriate precautions to protect the cervical spine taken – consideration should be given to exchanging the tube over a gum elastic bougie, or airway-exchange catheter rather than by performing direct laryngoscopy. This may be a useful technique for the less experienced or where upper airway anatomy is compromised.

All trauma patients should be assumed to have a full stomach or delayed gastric emptying, and cricoid pressure must be used to prevent aspiration. If the patient has a rigid cervical collar in place, manual in-line stabilization should be applied, the collar removed to optimize the view on laryngoscopy and then replaced after successful intubation. Trauma patients may be very sensitive to the myocardial depressant effects of anaesthetic induction agents, and the dose and choice of agent is determined by the cardiovascular status of the patient. In general, an agent with a high therapeutic ratio, such as etomidate, should be used. The full range of resuscitation drugs and equipment should be immediately available.

If the patient has considerable deformity to the face, the requirement for ventilation is likely to be prolonged or weaning from artificial ventilation likely to be protracted, then consideration should be given to early tracheostomy. The majority of tracheostomies will be performed in ICU using percutaneous dilatational techniques.[4] The one-step forceps technique has theoretical advantages over the Ciaglia technique in the presence of biomechanical instability of the cervical spine, since there is less likelihood that posterior pressure causing flexion of the spine during insertion would occur. Alternatively, if operative fixation of unstable high cervical fractures is undertaken, it may be appropriate that open tracheostomy is performed at that time, although the risk of the tracheostomy becoming infected and sepsis spreading to the metallic fixation must be considered. There is currently no prospective evidence that any one of these methods is safer than the others.

Because of the difficulty in clearing the cervical spine in the unconscious patient,[5] ICU trauma patients frequently have to be managed for long periods with rigid collars *in situ*. This may lead to pressure sores, superficial sepsis, problems with hygiene and, in the case of head-injured patients, may worsen raised intracranial pressure as a consequence of obstructed venous drainage. While the patient is sedated, paralysed and ventilated such collars should be removed, the neck sand bagged and head tape used. The collar should be replaced when the patient is to be woken up or needs to be moved by log-rolling. Efforts to clear the spine radiologically are difficult: computed tomography (CT) scanning and three-dimensional (3D) reconstruction are effective in excluding bony injury, but do not exclude ligamentous instability. The latter problem may be ellucidated by the use of dynamic fluoroscopy of the flexed and extender cervical spine using the C-arm image intensifier in the ICU. The use of magnetic resonance imaging allows identification of cord injury, compression or obvious contusion or damage to ligaments, but is not widely available.

Nosocomially acquired pulmonary sepsis is a major problem in trauma patients, and efficient tracheal toilet to prevent accumulation of secretions is vital, as is the prevention of aspiration. Closed-catheter suction systems and condenser heat and moisture exchanger humidification should be routinely used. Endotracheal tube cuff pressures should be monitored to ensure a balance between optimal protection against overspill of gastric contents or pharyngeal secretions into the trachea and the risk of tracheal mucosal ischaemia.

B: Breathing and ventilation

All patients should receive continuous oxygen saturation monitoring and undergo intermittent arterial blood gas analysis, particularly when ventilatory parameters are adjusted or are changing rapidly.

The precise mode of ventilation should be individualized to the patient, depending upon their diagnosis and their stage within the natural history of the condition producing the need for ventilatory support.

There is no clear strong evidence that one mode of ventilation is better than another in unselected ICU patients. Ventilator-induced lung injury is, however, a recognized entity and efforts should be made to decrease the incidence of pulmonary barotrauma and volutrauma. In general terms this is avoided by the combination of pressure and volume limitation,[6] together with the use of lung recruitment techniques such as positive end-expiratory pressure (PEEP)[7] or the use of intermittent single large tidal breaths with an end-expiratory pause. Such a lung protective ventilatory strategy is particularly important in trauma where the lung may either be damaged directly by thoracic trauma causing lung contusions, or damaged indirectly as a result of pro-inflammatory cytokine activity resulting from the systemic inflammatory response secondary to trauma elsewhere in the body. If there is a known risk factor, i.e. trauma and any evidence of acute lung injury (ALI) or adult respiratory distress syndrome (ARDS), then such strategies should be used from admission. ALI is defined by:

- the presence of bilateral diffuse infiltrates on chest X-ray;
- non-cardiogenic pulmonary oedema (pulmonary artery occlusion pressure <18 mmHg if measured); and
- PaO_2/FiO_2 ratio = <40 kPa

The criteria for ARDS are as defined for ALI, but the PaO_2/FiO_2 ratio = <26 kPa.

The recent US National Heart, Lung and Blood Institute trial into lung protective ventilatory strategies was stopped after 800 of the planned 1000 patients had been enrolled because of a 25% reduction in mortality in the protocol group. This system of ventilation often results in a raised CO_2 – so-called permissive hypercapnia – which will provoke raised intracranial pressure in unstable head-injured patients. Additional ventilatory modes such as tracheal gas insufflation[8] may be required simultaneously to wash out the dead space in order to minimize CO_2 retention. The complete range of ventilatory support systems available is beyond the scope of this chapter, and reference may be made to the further reading (see p. 271).

If pulmonary barotrauma occurs, then all pneumothoraces must be drained until low-pressure assisted spontaneous breathing or low-pressure continuous positive airways pressure is established. When a pneumothorax occurs in a patient undergoing positive pressure ventilation it may progress very rapidly to a tension pneumothorax. Standard needle decompression via the second intercostal space is much less effective than in spontaneously breathing patients, and buys very little time. Sometimes rapid incision, blunt dissection and pleural puncture at the standard chest drain insertion site is needed to relieve cardiovascular collapse while the chest drain and underwater seal is being obtained. Because intrathoracic pressure is always equal to or greater than atmospheric pressure in such circumstances, this temporary open pneumothorax causes no physiological disturbance.

C: Circulation

Trauma patients have frequently had intravenous lines inserted under less than ideal conditions, and asepsis may well not have been possible. Since sepsis is the major late cause of trauma deaths on the ICU, these 'resuscitation' lines should be removed as soon as possible and replaced using a strict aseptic technique. On admission, the ICU doctor should perform a full clinical cardiovascular examination and arrange for a baseline 12-lead ECG to be performed.

Continued haemorrhage, either as a result of uncorrected, uncorrectable or missed 'surgical' bleeding or ongoing coagulopathy, is the commonest cause of cardiovascular instability in the first few hours after admission of the trauma patient to ICU. This may be aggravated by failure to keep pace with ongoing losses and a subsequent fall in pre-load. Because positive-pressure ventilation results in a raised intrathoracic pressure, the adverse cardiovascular consequences of decreased pre-load/hypovolaemia are much greater in the ventilated patient. This is further compounded by the use of myocardial depressant sedative drugs to enable the patient to tolerate ventilation or the presence of any cardiovascular co-morbidity.

For these reasons the trauma patient requires intensive monitoring including:

- continuous ECG;
- pulse oximetry;
- intra-arterial blood pressure monitoring and arterial blood gas (AGB) analysis; and
- central venous pressure monitoring.

Surrogate markers of cardiac output such as urine output, ABG base deficit,[9] blood lactate[10] and peripheral temperature should also be monitored.

If the patient develops an acute dysrythmia, it is important to look specifically for hypoxia, hypercarbia, hypovolaemia, hypokalaemia and acidosis. These are much more common causes than myocardial ischaemia in young trauma patients.

In particularly unstable patients or those where fluid therapy is difficult to control, a more accurate means of measuring pre-load, myocardial contractility and after-load necessitates the use of flow-directed pulmonary artery (Swann–Ganz) catheters[11] or transoesophageal Doppler echocardiography.[12] In some patients, conflicting therapeutic needs (such as fluid restriction in ARDS to minimize transpulmonary capillary leak versus the desire to maintain a high urine output in the face of myoglobinuria secondary to muscle destruction) may also be indications for such invasive monitoring. Haemodynamic data such as cardiac index, systemic vascular resistance index (SVRI), pulmonary vascular resistance index (PVRI), and pulmonary artery occlusion pressure (PAOP or 'wedge pressure') can be derived, depending on which technique is used.

These variables must be measured if the patient requires inotropic support, as in some cases of blunt myocardial injury, or vasopressor support, where vasodilation has occurred in sepsis or systemic inflammatory response. Such methods are used in addition to simple clinical examination, hourly urine output, plasma osmolarity, urine osmolarity and accurate daily fluid balancing.

D: Disability

When the patient is first admitted to the ICU they are generally already anaesthetized or sedated. It is vital to determine and record the pre-sedation Glasgow Coma Score (GCS), pupil status and any lateralizing neurology, as these indicators may have prognostic implications.

> **It is vital to determine and record the pre-sedation GCS, pupil status and any lateralizing neurology before sedative drugs are used**

If sedative drugs are used, the agents and dosage should be documented. The drugs used to achieve sedation or analgesia and to produce tube and ventilator tolerance are not standardized between ICUs, and local protocols should be developed.

The most common regimes use either a combination or midazolam and morphine or propofol and alfentanil. The dose of each drug should be titrated against the patient's response to ensure that excessive sedation does not occur. This requires the use of an objective scoring system such as the Ramsay Sedation Scale[13] (Table 19.1). If the patient is not sedated, then the GCS is used.

Table 19.1 *The Ramsey Sedation Scale*

Ramsay 1	Patient awake, agitated, restless
Ramsay 2	Patient awake, not agitated
Ramsay 3	Eyes closed, but responds to name and opens eyes on request
Ramsay 4	Slow response to voice, responds if tapped on forehead
Ramsay 5	May not open eyes, but shows some response (for example, nods head)
Ramsay 6	No visible response

Standard neurological observations should be performed hourly by the nursing staff and recorded on the main flow chart. Invasive monitoring may be used in patients with severe head injury in specialized ICUs. This may include direct measurement of intracranial pressure (ICP), mean arterial pressure (MAP) and the calculation of cerebral perfusion pressure (CPP) from the equation:

$$CPP = MAP - ICP.$$

This is often measured in conjunction with transcranial near-infrared spectrometry[14] estimations of cerebral blood flow and jugular venous oxygen saturation.[15] Together they can be used to modify treatment aimed at minimizing raised ICP and preserving cerebral blood flow at levels compatible with optimal levels of cerebral oxygen delivery.

Brain electrical activity is measured using a cerebral function analysing monitor (CFAM),[16] particularly if anaesthetic agents are to be used to control persisting epileptic activity. Protocols for the use of such techniques are beyond the scope of this chapter.

E: Equipment

The ICU uses large numbers of monitors, transducers, ventilators, syringe drivers, infusion pumps and other electronic diagnostic equipment. The ICU doctor must be familiar with the range of equipment used on their unit so that they may safely change settings, alarms, rates of infusion and other parameters and be able to ensure the accuracy of all derived data upon which they base any change in the patient's therapy.

F: Fluids

When planning the patient's fluid therapy regime, the ICU doctor must answer the following questions:

- What is the fluid balance for the previous 24 hours, and what is the cumulative balance since injury?
- What is the urine output since injury?
- Is there fluid output from unusual sites such as fistulae, burns, vomit, drains and wounds?
- What fluids have already been given?
- How much and what fluid should be given?

The answer to the last question is determined by the patient's underlying condition and the answers to the other questions. In general terms, normovolaemia should be the fluid resuscitation end-point. Hypovolaemia will predispose to decreased organ perfusion, and hypervolaemia will increase tissue fluid formation in all organ systems where there is increased vascular permeability as a result of the trauma-induced systemic inflammatory response.

> **ICU trauma patients all need invasive cardiovascular monitoring to achieve accurate fluid therapy in the early stages of their admission**

G: Gut

The abdomen must be examined clinically on admission to the ICU and the nature, site, viability and condition of all injuries, operation wounds, drains, fistulae or stomata documented. Since the ICU personnel change shifts and the wounds and stomata may be covered by opaque dressings, the use of a Polaroid or digital photographic record allows sequential monitoring and detection of any adverse changes.

The early detection of splanchnic under-perfusion is vital, as gut ischaemia will allow translocation of bacteria and endotoxins that will rapidly lead to systemic sepsis. In some units, gastric intramucosal pH[17] is monitored as a marker of splanchnic ischaemia. Selective gut decontamination regimes,[18] where oral, enteral and parenteral antibiotics are administered to denude the upper gut of potentially pathogenic organisms in an attempt to prevent ventilator associated pneumonia, are no longer widely used since there is no clear-cut evidence of decreased mortality.[19] Conversely, there is a trend towards preservation of normal gut flora and prevention of translocation by the use of early enteral nutrition[20] and nutritional supplements[21] such as glutamine to promote intestinal mucosal integrity.

H: Haematology

On admission, the trauma patient should have a full range of blood tests including:

- full blood count including platelets;
- coagulation screen;
- electrolytes, urea and creatinine; and
- liver function tests.

Directed investigations determined either by medical co-morbidity or by the nature of the injury may also be required. If blunt myocardial injury is suspected, a troponin screen is of diagnostic value, while for suspected rhabdomyolysis, myoglobin and creatine kinase levels are required.

It is necessary to ensure that adequate supplies of blood and blood products are available, since ongoing haemorrhage is a potential problem. Blood transfusion trigger levels have not been specifically studied in trauma patients, but the general ICU evidence-based trigger of a haemoglobin of 7 g/dl should be used, except in head injury where current consensus guidelines remain at providing a level of haemoglobin of 12 g/dl.

> **All patients should undergo chest X-ray on admission to check for correct endotracheal tube and central venous catheter placement**

I: Imaging

All X-ray requests should be critically assessed in order to see if they are immediately necessary to direct early therapy. Often, the angles and views required are not possible to perform within the confines of the ICU, and the patient should not be exposed to the risk of transfer to the X-ray department unless it is absolutely necessary.

It is best to think in terms of clinical imaging rather than 'X-rays' alone. Other modalities such as ultrasound, transoesophageal Doppler echocardiography, CT scanning, MRI or nuclear medicine studies may offer a more effective means of identifying problems. Whatever the investigation, the image must be reported by senior experienced staff to avoid missed injuries and pathologies.

J: Joints and limbs

Limb injury is very common in multiple trauma. Although not often life-threatening, inadequate treatment may condemn the post-discharge ICU survivor to severe disability and pain. The anecdote concerning the multiple trauma survivor who subsequently seeks compensation for the missed scaphoid fracture which now prevents his/her return to work as a concert pianist is not entirely without foundation! The unconscious sedated ICU patient is unable to complain of pain.

> **Limbs require frequent inspection to exclude compartment syndrome, ischaemia and deep-vein thrombosis**

Fractures and dislocations require definitive treatment as soon as possible, and the appropriate specialist consultation must be arranged. The timing of surgery must be balanced against other conditions present such as severe head injury, severe pulmonary dysfunction or clotting disorder. Deep-vein thrombosis prophylaxis with low-molecular weight heparin must be weighed against the risk of secondary haemorrhage, but must be instigated as soon as possible in all trauma patients.

K: Kelvin

The patient's temperature and temperature chart are vital adjuncts to sepsis surveillance. Blood cultures should be taken at peaks of pyrexia (>38.5°C) to identify any organisms causing bacteraemia.

The majority of trauma patients arrive on ICU with varying degrees of hypothermia. Despite research interest in the role of induced hypothermia in trauma resuscitation, there is currently no convincing evidence base to recommend its use. The goal should be to restore the patient to normothermia.

Surface cooling on the ICU is used in hyperpyrexia to cool to normothermia; this may reduce CO_2 production if this is a problem. Hyperpyrexia is known to worsen the outcome after severe closed head injury, and there is some evidence that induced hypothermia to 34°C may improve outcome.[22] When this is undertaken, the head-injured patient must be fully sedated (Ramsay 6) and paralysed with a neuromuscular blocking agent to prevent shivering.

L: Lines

All lines, intravenous, intra-arterial and others must be monitored:

- When were they placed?
- Where were they placed?
- Are they necessary?
- Do they need replacement or removal?

When lines are removed, the tips must be sent for culture. There are no hard and fast rules for how long lines should be left in before elective replacement; rather, each line should be examined daily and removed as soon as possible, or if there is the slightest suspicion of line sepsis.

Large-bore lines such as quadruple-lumen central lines, pulmonary artery catheters, Swan sheath introducers and double-lumen haemofiltration lines, may cause thrombosis of the veins in which they are placed, particularly if they are a snug fit. Both placement and removal of such lines may result in severe haemorrhage, particularly if there is any co-existing coagulopathy. Clotting should be normal before elective placement and removal, and their insertion is not for the enthusiastic amateur. Whatever site is chosen for insertion, it is necessary to be aware of the potential complications and how to recognize and rapidly treat them if they were to occur. Centrally placed lines must have their position confirmed radiologically before they are used.

M: Microbiology

Sepsis is implicated in approximately 80% of late trauma deaths on ICU. Aggressive microbiological surveillance will help to reduce the incidence of infection, and should be carried out by sending wound swabs, blood cultures, sputum specimens, bronchoalveolar lavage, drain fluid, urine, removed line tips and other samples as appropriate.

Strict asepsis and cross-infection avoidance should be practised. All staff, both visiting and resident, should wear aprons when examining the patient, and follow a strict policy of 'touch a patient – wash your hands'.

Microbiology results must be checked daily, and all samples and results charted. Directed antimicrobial therapy only should be used, as this will help to minimize the risk of developing resistance and the selection of opportunistic infection. A joint daily ward round with a clinical microbiologist will allow:

- rapid communication of results;
- guided changes in antibiotic therapy; and
- advice on treatment duration and dosage and drug levels.

Certain infections are very difficult to treat if they become established in ICU trauma patients, notably methicillin-resistant *Staphylococcus aureus*, *Clostridium perfringens* and *Clostridium tetani*. It is important *never* to assume that a patient is immune to tetanus, and a history of vaccination does not guarantee immunity.

N: Nutrition

All patients need feeding, and unless there is a contraindication, such as gastric or duodenal surgery, enteral nutrition should be commenced in trauma patients from day 1 of ICU admission. A regime of low-volume feeds, increasing dwell time and decreasing frequency of nasogastric tube aspiration allows a build-up to normal-volume feeds (100 ml/h).

Enteral feeding should be discontinued overnight to allow intragastric pH to return to its normal low levels, as this decreases the incidence of nosocomially acquired pneumonia. H_2-receptor antagonists such as ranitidine should not be used for stress ulcer prophylaxis for similar reasons; cytoprotective agents such as sucralfate should be used instead.[23]

Trauma patients may develop gastroparesis, particularly those with high spinal cord lesions or extensive burns. Prokinetic agents such as erythromycin or metoclopramide may facilitate gastric emptying. Where the problem persists, the use of nasojejunal feeding tubes or an operative feeding jejunostomy may be used, with total parenteral nutrition (TPN) being used if all else fails. Percutaneous endoscopic gastrostomy should be considered for patients requiring long-term enteral nutrition if the patient repeatedly removes fine-bore nasogastric tubes or has bulbar dysfunction or a persisting depressed level of consciousness.

If TPN is used, it must be administered through a dedicated line. Consideration should be given to the use of a specific tunnelled feeding line if TPN is a long-term requirement.

If the patient has a prolonged requirement for opiate analgesia, constipation may become a real problem and appropriate stool softeners, aperients or enemata used.

O: Other consultations

Nobody knows everything. . . . It is essential to arrange appropriate specialist opinions and to ensure that the referring team is kept up to date with their patient's progress. The patient's general practitioner and hospital consultant should be informed that one of their patients is on ICU.

P: Pharmacology

Drugs should be prescribed by the appropriate routes, at the correct intervals, and in the right doses; critical illness may alter drug metabolism and excretion. It is important to be constantly alert for the effects of drug accumulation or the development of drug levels in the toxic range. A review of the drug chart should be carried out daily, and doses adjusted accordingly.

Adequate analgesia is essential, as the patient is the only judge of the severity of their pain. Continuous epidural analgesia is useful if the pattern of injury is suitable, notably thoracic epidural analgesia for multiple rib fractures, allowing effective coughing and chest physiotherapy. Epidural abscess formation is a risk, and the catheter should not be left *in situ* for more than 5 days.

Regional anaesthesia should not be used where there is a risk of distal compartment syndrome.

Anaesthesia must not be used as a substitute for effective analgesia. Agitation and confusional behaviour may occur because of inadequate analgesia. One should never forget to talk to the patient! Even if they have a depressed level of consciousness, it is best to assume that they can hear in order to explain procedures simply and carefully, and to use local anaesthesia for practical procedures, even if the patient appears heavily sedated.

Q: Question

If the next management step is unclear, more senior or specialist help should always be sought. It is important never to be afraid to ask questions.

R: Relatives

Relatives must be kept fully informed. In addition, they are a useful source of information regarding the patient's past medical history and normal daily activity.

Discussions should always be held away from the bedside unless the patient is fully aware, autonomous and can participate. The patient's nurse should be present, and conclusions must be documented. Visiting doctors must adhere to the same rules and should be aware of the content of previous discussions.

It is vital not to offer prognoses beyond the extent of one's expertise, and not to guess at possible outcomes. The families of trauma patients frequently ask about functional recovery or permanent disability, and except in exceptional circumstances the ICU is too early in the continuum of care to reach definitive conclusions.

Where a change from aggressive supportive therapy to compassionate, palliative care is planned the relatives must be fully informed and their views must form part of the input to reaching such decisions. Trauma patients often make suitable organ donors, and this should be discussed in a compassionate way, and at the right time, with the relatives.

S: Skin

The skin should be examined for perfusion, wounds, and signs of systemic disease or infection. Pressure area care may be difficult in patients requiring log-rolling, or with limbs immobilized in casts or with external fixators. Specialized rotational therapy,[24] or low-air loss or fluidized beds may be required.

Trauma victims often arrive on the ICU with the dirt picked up at the time of injury still in place, together with blood, secretions and vomit. All are sources of infection and must be removed. Mouth care, hair-washing and skin toilet must not be neglected.

T: Transport

Multi-system trauma patients require multi-disciplinary management, and will often be moved from the ICU to other areas for investigation or operation. Transport of ICU patients within or between hospitals requires the same level of care and monitoring that they receive on the ICU itself, as discussed in Chapter 20.

U: Universal precautions

The plethora of infectious diseases transmitted by blood and other bodily fluids means that all staff should be aware of the necessity for wearing gloves, aprons and occasionally face guards when performing invasive procedures. Where victims are unconscious, consent for HIV testing is not an option, although hepatitis screening is. ICU staff should be immunized against hepatitis as they work in a high-risk environment. All needle-stick injuries must be reported and staff given appropriate treatment.

V: Visitors

These may be the patient's relatives or other medical personnel involved in the patient's care. Visiting colleagues should be treated with respect and courtesy, but ultimately all changes to therapy must be channelled through the ICU medical staff and discussed with the ICU consultant.

W: Wounds

All wounds should hopefully have been cleaned, débrided and dressed before admission, but this is not always the case and appropriate surgical review and intervention is essential. Wound care must be reviewed daily and signs of sepsis treated aggressively. The patient may frequently require to be taken to theatre for further débridement, and re-dressing of delayed primary closure.

Trauma victims will often become involved in forensic proceedings, and all wounds should be documented.

Y: Why?

Every time the patient is reviewed, it is important to ask why the patient was admitted and what their active problems currently are.

Z: Zzzz...

ICU is a stressful 24-hour environment for the patients who are often deprived of rapid eye movement sleep, woken frequently by alarms, new admissions, turning and by painful procedures. It is little wonder that, in addition to acute organic confusional states, frank psychosis or severe depression may occur to the extent where psychotropic drugs are needed. As the trauma patient recovers and becomes more aware of the environment, every effort should be made to establish a normal diurnal pattern of sleep/wake cycles.

SUMMARY

The ICU trauma patient often requires assessment and resuscitation to proceed simultaneously, as in the classical primary survey. It is essential to formulate a plan to deal with the patient's remaining or potential problems. This plan is made after following the steps outlined above; it must be documented clearly in the notes, and discussed with the bedside nurse. Time is an important part of the plan, and regular re-assessment is essential. The plan made in the morning may be obsolete – or even dangerous – by lunchtime.

Parameters must be agreed within which the nurse is able to vary the components of the therapeutic regime according to the patient's response, and outside which medical re-assessment is required.

The patient's condition will vary from day to day, and the process must be repeated daily in the stable patient and at any stage if their condition deteriorates.

Trauma patients requiring admission to ICU usually have a multisystem pattern of injury, and unitary diagnoses are relatively infrequent. It is only by adopting a systematic A to Z approach that the risk of missing injuries and complications occurring or developing can be avoided. If this is achieved, mortality and morbidity will be minimized and the patient's chances of making a good functional recovery enhanced.

REFERENCES

1. Yates DW, Woodford M, Hollis S. Preliminary analysis of the care of injured patients in 33 British hospitals: first report of the United Kingdom major trauma outcome study. *British Medical Journal* 1992; **305**: 737–40.

2. McAnena OJ, Moore FA, Moore EE, Mattox KL, Marx JA, Pepe P. Invalidation of the APACHE II scoring system for patients with acute trauma. *Journal of Trauma* 1992; **33**: 504–7.

3. Trunkey DD, Lim RC. Analysis of 425 consecutive trauma fatalities: An autopsy study. *Journal of the American College of Emergency Physiology* 1974; **3**: 368.

4. Powell DM, Price PD, Forrest LA. Review of percutaneous tracheostomy *Laryngoscope.* 1998; **108**: 170–7.

5. Enderson BL, Maull KI. Missed injuries: the trauma surgeon's nemesis. *Surgical Clinics of North America* 1991; **71**: 399–418.

6. Hickling HG, Henderson HJ, Jackson R. Low mortality associated with low volume pressure limited ventilation with permissive hypercapnia in severe adult respiratory distress syndrome. *Intensive Care Medicine* 1990; **16**: 372–7.

7. Gattinioni L, Pelosi P, Crotti S, Valenza F. Effects of positive end-expiratory pressure on regional distribution of tidal volume and recruitment in adult respiratory distress syndrome. *American Journal of Respiration Critical Care Medicine* 1995; **151**: 1807–14.

8. Barnett CC, Moore FA, Moore EE, *et al.* Tracheal gas insufflation is a useful adjunct in permissive hypercapnic management of acute respiratory distress syndrome. *American Journal of Surgery* 1996; **172**: 518–21.

9. Davis JW, Shackford SR, Mackersie RC, Hoyt DB. Base deficit as a guide to volume resuscitation. *Journal of Trauma* 1988; **28**: 464–7.

10. Baker J, Coffernils M, Kahn RJ, Vincent JL. Serial blood lactate levels can predict the development of multiple organ failure following septic shock. *American Journal of Surgery* 1996; **171**: 221–6.

11. Pulmonary Artery Catheter Consensus Conference. Consensus Statement. *Critical Care Medicine* 1997; **25**: 910–25.

12. Madam AK, UyBarreta VV, *et al.* Esophageal doppler ultrasound monitor versus pulmonary artery catheter in the hemodynamic management of critically ill surgical patients. *Journal of Trauma* 1999; **46**: 607–11.

13. Ramsay MAE, Savage TH, Simpson BRG, Goodwin R. Controlled sedation with alphaxalone and alphadalone. *British Medical Journal* 1974; **2**: 656–9.

14. Kampfl A, Pfausler B, Denchey D, Jaring HP, Schmutzhard E. Near infrared spectrometry (NIRS) in patients with severe brain injury and elevated intracranial pressure. A pilot study. *Acta Neurochirurgica Supplement (Wien)* 1997; **70**: 112–14.

15. Feldman Z, Robertson CS. Monitoring of cerebral hemodynamics with jugular bulb catheters. *Critical Care Clinics* 1997; **13**: 51–77.

16. Sebel PS, Maynard DE, Major E, Frank M. The cerebral function analysing monitor. *British Journal of Anaesthesia* 1983; **55**: 1265–70.

17. Roumen RM, Vreugde JP, Goris RJ. Gastric tonometry in multiple trauma patients. *Journal of Trauma* 1994; **36**: 313–16.

18. Selective decontamination of the digestive tract trialists collaborative group. Meta-analysis of randomised controlled trials of selective decontamination of the digestive tract. *British Medical Journal* 1993; **307**: 525–32.

19. Selective digestive decontamination: a critical appraisal. In: Vincent J-L (ed.). *Yearbook of Intensive Care and Emergency Medicine.* Berlin: Springer-Verlag, 1993, pp. 281–6.

20. Kudsk KA, Croce MA, Fabian TC, *et al.* Enteral verses parenteral feeding. Effects on septic morbidity after blunt and penetrating abdominal trauma. *Annals of Surgery* 1992; **215**: 503–11.

21. Mendez C, Jurkovich GJ, Garcia I, Davis D, Parker A, Maier RV. Effects of an immune enhancing diet in critically injured patients. *Journal of Trauma* 1997; **42**: 933–40.

22. Kirkpatrick AW, Chun R, Brown R, Simons RK. Hypothermia in the trauma patient. *Canadian Journal of Surgery* 1999; **42**: 333–43.

23. Maier RV, Mitchell D, Gentilello L. Optimal therapy for stress gastritis. *Annals of Surgery* 1994; **220**: 353–60.

24. Genitello L, Thompson DA, Tonnessen AS, *et al.* Effect of a rotating bed on the incidence of pulmonary complications in critically ill patients. *Critical Care Medicine* 1988; **16**: 783–6.

FURTHER READING

Hillman K, Bishop G. *Clinical Intensive Care.* Cambridge: Cambridge University Press, 1996.

Craft T, Nolan J, Parr M. *Key Topics in Critical Care.* Oxford: BIOS Scientific Publishers, 1999.

Singer M (ed.) *ABC of Intensive Care.* London: British Medical Journal Books, 1999.

Greaves I, Ryan JM, Porter KM (eds). *Trauma.* Arnold, London 1998. See Riley B. Outcomes of intensive care after trauma. Chapter 20, pp. 227–36.

Riley B. Strategies for ventilatory support. *British Medical Bulletin – Trauma* 1999; **55**: 806–20.

Ravussin P, Bracco D, Moesschler O. Prevention and treatment of secondary brain injury. *Current Opinion in Critical Care* 1999; **5**: 511–16.

20

Patient transfer

'The good work done in the resuscitation room is then undone during the journey…'.[1]

OBJECTIVES

- To understand the indications for intra- and inter-hospital transfer of the trauma patient
- To identify the dangers involved in such transfer
- To appreciate how to plan and perform safe transfer, with particular regard to:
  - communication and planning
  - optimal mode and timing of transport
  - stabilization before transfer
  - equipment and monitoring
  - escorting personnel

INTRODUCTION

Inter-hospital transfer is a potentially dangerous time for the critically ill trauma patient,[2-4] the main risks arising from:

- physical disturbance of the patient;
- lack (or failure) of drugs, equipment and monitoring;
- limited access to the patient;
- difficulty in assessing the patient's condition in transit;
- inexperience of the escorting personnel;
- potential for deterioration due to underlying injuries or medical problems;
- lack of access to specialized help or facilities;
- physical hazards of the out-of-hospital environment;
- unexpected delays in transit; and
- errors in planning or communication.

Many of these risks also apply to patient transport *within* a hospital,[5,6] but here complacency is an added danger. A patient can become extubated just as easily in a hospital corridor as in an ambulance!

Equal care is needed for *intra*-hospital as for *inter*-hospital transfers

Patients should ideally be transported between hospitals by specially trained and equipped retrieval teams, and such teams are used in the USA, Australia and most other European countries. In the UK, only a few such systems exist, mainly for paediatric and neonatal transfers, for which they probably reduce complications.[7,8] However, despite recognition of the risks, critically ill patients are still often transferred by inexperienced doctors with little formal training in patient transfer, and with varying standards of equipment and monitoring.[3]

Guidelines for patient transfer have been published in the UK by the Association of Anaesthetists,[9] the Intensive Care Society,[10] the British Trauma Society[11] and the

Department of Health,[12] and overseas by the American College and Society of Critical Care Medicine[13] and the Australian and New Zealand College of Anaesthetists. This chapter aims to summarize the UK guidelines, and offers a practical guide to safe transfer between and within hospitals.

CLASSIFICATION OF TRANSFERS

The commonest classification of transfers outside hospital is as follows:

- *Primary transfer:* the transfer of the injured patient from the scene of the incident to the receiving hospital. (The protocols for primary transfer in the UK are formulated by the NHS Ambulance Trusts, and are not discussed here.)
- *Secondary transfer:* the movement of the patient from the admitting hospital to another hospital for specialist care.
- *Tertiary transfer:* a transfer for essentially social reasons, such as after completion of a period of specialist care at one hospital to a hospital nearer the patient's home.
- *Category four transfer:* a transfer between hospitals when the local resources have been exhausted, for example due to lack of intensive care beds.

INDICATIONS FOR TRANSFER

Intra-hospital transfer

Transport may be needed at different times for investigation or treatment, between the Accident and Emergency Department, operating theatres, X-radiography department and computed tomography (CT) scanner, intensive care unit (ICU), and high-dependency unit (HDU).

Inter-hospital transfer

This type of transfer may be needed for several reasons:

1. *The injury.* When specialist care is not available at the referring hospital, for example for head, spinal, chest and complex limb or vascular injuries or burns.
2. *The patient.* When specialist care is not available at the referring hospital, for example for paediatric patients or patients with acute renal failure (for haemofiltration or dialysis).
3. *Other considerations.* These include transfer because of intensive care bed shortages, or repatriation for social or economic reasons from another part of the country, or from abroad.

In the UK, head injury is the commonest reason for inter-hospital transfer after major trauma.[14]

DANGERS AND RISKS OF PATIENT TRANSFER

Remember that the dangers of transport apply not only to the patient, but also to the escorting staff (which may include you!), members of the public, and the (often valuable) equipment.

The risks to the patient can be remembered along similar headings to the primary survey. Practically all these dangers apply equally to intra- as well as inter-hospital transfer.

Airway and cervical spine

Dangers here include:

- airway compromise due to:
  - deteriorating level of consciousness
  - increasing airway oedema or haematoma.
- if the patient is intubated, tube obstruction or tube displacement:
  - out of the larynx
  - down into one main bronchus.
- movement, leading to exacerbation of any cervical spine injury.

Breathing

Dangers here include:
- hypoventilation, due to:
  - head injury
  - high spinal cord injury
  - drugs (including those given by the transfer team)
  - inadequate minute volume in the ventilated patient.
- Deterioration in chest injuries, for example:
  - expanding haemothorax
  - tension pneumothorax (especially during air transport).
- 'Accidents' with chest drains:
  - blockage
  - disconnection
  - displacement.
- Complications related to mechanical ventilation (see 'Care of the ventilated patient', Chapter 3), especially:
  - ventilator disconnection
  - ventilator failure.

It should be noted that hypoventilation, hypoxia and hypercarbia are very difficult to detect clinically during transfer. It is particularly important to avoid these complications in head-injured patients.

Circulation

Dangers here include continued bleeding from internal or external injuries (especially if exacerbated by patient movement).

An additional problem is that of displacement of intravascular lines (peripheral venous, central venous or arterial), leading to:

- bleeding;
- loss of drug or fluid effect;
- loss of invasive monitoring;
- air embolism; and/or
- complications of hurried recannulation!

Disability

Disability may manifest as exacerbation of raised intracranial pressure and/or cerebral ischaemia, by:

- hypoxia;
- hypercarbia;
- hypotension;
- coughing or gagging (in the intubated patient, if sedation and paralysis are allowed to wear off); and/or
- acceleration or deceleration forces due to vehicle movement.

Exacerbation of any spinal injury may also occur as a result of patient movement and/or poor patient immobilization.

Exposure

Exposure is seen as a loss of body heat, leading to:

- shivering, with increased oxygen demand; and
- vasoconstriction, with reduced tissue perfusion.

Exacerbation of limb and other injuries may also occur due to movement and inadequate splintage.

Other risks

Additional risks that may be encountered include: (i) injury to patient and staff from unsecured equipment and vehicle movement; (ii) accidents involving the transfer vehicle; and (iii) deterioration of underlying (and perhaps unrecognized) medical problems.

SAFE PATIENT TRANSFER

The key points in arranging safe transfer are summarized in a 'transfer template' (Table 20.1).

Indications and destination

Inter-hospital transfer should only be undertaken if it is essential. Although transfer is often clearly needed for specialist care, every such movement is a potential hazard to the patient. It is vital therefore to consider the risks and benefits carefully, and to think of the resource implications for the hospital and the ambulance service of an unnecessary transfer. Could the specialist care be brought to the patient rather than vice versa?

A secondary transfer should by definition be in the patient's best interest, in that they are being transferred for specialist care. The risk/benefit equation is not so clear for category four transfers, such as when there is no ICU bed available for a trauma patient following resuscitation and surgery. Who should be transferred – the new patient, or an existing ICU patient whose condition is more stable, and who might be less at risk from the stresses of transfer? The answer would ideally be the more stable patient, although this raises difficult ethical issues, as the transfer cannot be justified as being in *his/her* best interests!

In transfers to the most appropriate hospital, cases have occurred where patients have deteriorated after a second and avoidable transfer. For secondary transfers, the appropriate specialist centre is usually obvious. However, it should be noted that some specialist units may be less able to provide general supportive care (surgical, medical and intensive care) than the referring hospital, putting patients with multi-system trauma at increased risk. For transfers due to lack of ICU beds, distance is usually the main consideration, and a national ICU bed information service is available to help locate the nearest available beds (Emergency Bed Service, London: telephone 0207-407 7181).

> **Decisions regarding patient transfer must be taken at consultant level**

Timing

The optimal time for transfer should be chosen for logistical and clinical reasons.

LOGISTICAL FACTORS

For example, in non-urgent cases, a move during 'working hours' allows escorts to be spared more easily from the referring hospital, and may be more convenient for the ambulance service. Weather and daylight conditions are important when considering air transfers.

Table 20.1 *Key points in the safe transfer of trauma patients*

Planning
Indications and destination
(consultant decision)

Referral:
- all relevant information to hand
- consultation/specialist advice on pre-transfer management
- *exact* bed location
- ICU referral also needed?

Transport:
- mode
- timing
- special requirements
- return of staff/equipment

Escorting staff:
- training/experience
- early notification

Preparation
Patient:
- airway secure (*intubate?*)
- breathing/oxygenation adequate
  - *continue O$_2$*
  - *attach transport ventilator early and check blood gases*
  - *chest drain needed?*
- cardiovascularly stable
  - *bleeding controlled*
  - *good i.v. access*
  - *consider arterial line*
- splinting/immobilization
  - *spine*
  - *limbs*
- sedation/analgesia
- nasogastric tube/catheter
- all tubes, lines, drains secure

Equipment:
- oxygen
  - *portable cylinder*
  - *ambulance reserves*
- ventilator   ⎤ *early application*
- infusion pumps (and spare) ⎬ *batteries checked*
- monitors   ⎦
- airway, intravenous and other kit
- drugs, fluids, blood

Escorting staff:
- fully briefed
- equipped, clothed and insured
- hospital duties covered
- return arrangements
- documentation (notes, X-rays, results, etc.)

Transfer
Before departure:
- crew briefed
- vehicle oxygen and equipment checked
- bed availability and ETA confirmed
- notes, X-rays, etc. packaged
- patient still stable
In transit:
- access and monitoring
- equipment and staff safety
- immobilization/splinting
- temperature control
- physiological stability

Handover:
- reassess A,B,Cs and priorities
- face-to-face handover
- notes, X-rays, etc.
- retrieve all equipment

CLINICAL FACTORS

Transfer should be delayed when possible, if this would reduce the risk of patient deterioration. For example, in cervical spinal cord lesions, there is a risk of delayed diaphragmatic paralysis due to ascending cord oedema.[15] If intensive care facilities are not available in the specialist unit, the transfer may be best delayed until this risk has passed.

Mode of transport

Inter-hospital transfer may be by either:

- land ambulance (either 'front-line', or a dedicated and specially adapted transfer vehicle);
- helicopter; or
- fixed-wing aircraft.

The choice of transport depends on the indications, urgency and distance of transfer, the time taken to arrange transport, the weather and traffic conditions, the training of the escorting personnel, and the cost. For all modes of transport, a list of contacts should be available in advance. For air transport, because of the very different environment and the legal requirements of the Civil Aviation Authority, the accompanying personnel should ideally have been trained specifically for this role. Aeromedical transport is considered in more detail below.

LAND AMBULANCE

This is the commonest method in the UK, and is usually fastest over distances of up to 50 miles. Land ambulances are generally low-cost, quickly mobilized, and operate over 24 hours and in most weather conditions. Compared with aircraft they generally allow better access to the patient, and are more familiar to most hospital staff. Crucially, they are able to *stop* if necessary for procedures to be performed.

HELICOPTER

Helicopters are generally faster over distances greater than 50 miles, and are also useful when road access would be difficult. However, many hospitals do not have helicopter landing facilities directly outside. Therefore over shorter distances, helicopters may *not* be faster if the patient must be loaded on and off a land ambulance at either end of the journey! Their disadvantages include expense, limited availability, and possible restrictions at night or in poor weather conditions. They are also very noisy, unpressurized, prone to vibration, and may provoke air-sickness (even in experienced personnel used to fixed-wing aircraft). If intervention is needed in transit, they cannot stop.

FIXED-WING AIRCRAFT

These are most suitable for distances greater than 200 miles. In common with helicopters they are expensive and of limited availability. However, they are often more spacious, and less affected by movement, noise and vibration. They may or may not be pressurized, and will almost always need relay land ambulances at either end of the journey.

Route and speed

Most transfers in the UK are by road, and a smooth journey is usually more important than breakneck speed. The ambulance crew will usually plan the route, but rough roads and speed-bumps are best avoided, especially for spinal injuries. The tradition of transporting spinal injury patients at walking pace is rarely justified, as the suspensions of most ambulances function best at moderate speeds.[16] For longer journeys across urban areas, consider requesting police help to provide an escort, and to stop traffic at successive road junctions.

Communication

Good communication is vital, and is needed at several points in the transfer process.

INITIAL REFERRAL

With regard to communication at the initial referral:

- It is important to communicate at senior (ideally consultant) level with the medical staff at the receiving hospital, as soon as the need for transfer is recognized.
- All relevant information must be to hand: 'a neurosurgeon will ask predictable questions'.[1,14]
- If available, CT scans can be transmitted over a digital image link.
- The accepting specialist may give advice about management and stabilization, including surgery, before transfer.

- If the patient needs intensive care, the ICU consultant at the receiving hospital must accept the referral, as well as the appropriate consultant surgeon.
- the *exact* location of, and access to, the bed at the receiving hospital should be clearly established.
- For the accepting specialist, consideration should be given to using the A&E department as a 'single portal of entry' for initial re-assessment, in case of patient deterioration and unrecognized injuries.[17]

AMBULANCE CONTROL

At ambulance control, or at any other transport agency, *they* will need to know:

- the patient's details and diagnosis;
- the patient's exact location and destination;
- the degree of urgency and predicted timings;
- the name of the accepting doctor;
- the mode of transport required;
- which personnel will accompany the patient; and
- any specific requirements (equipment, immobilization, police escort, etc.).

As the transferring doctor, it is necessary to know the estimated arrival time of the transport, and whether the return of the transfer team is guaranteed!

THE TRANSFER TEAM

The transfer team must be fully briefed, and notified in enough time to familiarize themselves with the case, assess and prepare the patient, and check all equipment.

THE PATIENT

If the patient is conscious, an attempt should be made to explain and reassure, despite the transport possibly being uncomfortable and unpleasant.

RELATIVES

It is vital to ensure that relatives are aware of the transfer, and know the receiving unit's location and contact details. It is also vital to check how they will travel and for them to note their own contact details for the receiving unit.

AT DEPARTURE

Just before departure, it is important to establish communications with:

- *the receiving hospital*, to confirm that the bed is still available, and to notify the expected time of arrival; and
- *the transport crew*, to ensure that they are aware of the destination and requirements, and that enough oxygen and equipment are available.

IN TRANSIT

During the transfer, it is essential to remain in contact with the receiving unit, especially if the patient's condition deteriorates.

Escorting personnel

Apart from the transfer vehicle's crew, patients with critical illness or major trauma should be accompanied by two escorts: one a doctor, and the other either a nurse, operating department practitioner (ODP), paramedic, technician or another doctor.[10,11] Both escorts should be:

- appropriately experienced (see below);
- specifically trained in (and have supervised experience of) patient transfer;

- familiar with the relevant equipment, drugs and documentation;
- physically fit for the task;
- not susceptible to motion sickness; and
- insured for personal injury.

The escorting doctor should be competent in resuscitation, airway management and ventilation, and should have at least 2 years' experience in anaesthesia, intensive care medicine or another 'equivalent speciality'.[9,10] An accompanying nurse 'should be qualified to ENB100 or equivalent level, with 2 years' intensive care experience'.[10] Both should have training and experience of major trauma management.

All escorting staff must have minimum standards of training and experience

Ideally, the team should have the opportunity to train together, and should have repeated exposure to transfers to prevent the decay of skills. They should be familiar in advance with the layout of their local ambulance service vehicles, particularly the oxygen supply and connections, suction, and electrical supply and outlets.

The welfare and safety of the transfer team is usually forgotten! Ambulances are sometimes prone to leaving them 'stranded' after the journey, and staff should take suitable outdoor clothing, money and credit cards. Advance arrangements must be made for their safe return, either in the transport vehicle or by some other means.

PATIENT PREPARATION

The patient should be fully resuscitated and stabilized before departure. A patient who is persistently shocked should never be transferred; time may be saved by not identifying and treating the cause, but the patient will suffer in transit and death or multiple organ dysfunction secondary to hypoperfusion will occur. For patients with head injuries in particular, hypoxia, hypercarbia and hypotension *must* be corrected (Table 20.2). Surgery to control internal bleeding may be needed before transfer, and external bleeding (e.g. from the scalp) can be underestimated and may also need surgical control.[18]

The patient must be stabilized fully before transfer

Table 20.2 *Indications for intubation and ventilation after head injury (Modified from Ref. 1, and reproduced with permission.)*

Immediately:
- Coma (not obeying commands, not speaking, not eye opening, i.e. GCS ≤8)
- Loss of protective laryngeal reflexes
- Ventilatory insufficiency as judged by blood gases:
  - hypoxaemia (Pa_{O_2} <13 kPa on oxygen)
  - hypercarbia (Pa_{CO_2} >6 kPa)
- Spontaneous hyperventilation causing Pa_{CO_2} <3.5 kPa
- Respiratory arrhythmia

Before the start of the journey:
- Significantly deteriorating conscious level, even if not in coma
- Bilateral fractured mandible
- Copious bleeding into the mouth
- Seizures

An intubated patient must be ventilated with muscle relaxation, and should receive sedation and analgesia.
Aim for a PaO_2 >13 kPa, $PaCO_2$ 4.0–4.5 kPa.

Despite this, some assessments may be delayed if the transfer is urgent; for example, there may not have been time for a full secondary survey or spinal clearance. It is important to record and communicate what has *not* been done as well as what has, so that these things can be done at the receiving unit.

The transfer team must be given time to familiarize themselves with the mechanism of injury, findings on primary and secondary survey, and the investigations and treatment carried out. They must assess the patient's condition independently before departure, in order to ensure that resuscitation has been optimal. Although no time can be wasted if the transfer is urgent, there is often a tendency for preparations to be rushed, especially when the ambulance crew arrives! If the patient has deteriorated the team should not be afraid to delay departure, even if the transport has to be re-booked when the problem has been treated.

In particular:

- The airway must be secure: it is best to intubate electively *before* transfer if there is any doubt, as this may be very difficult in transit.

> **Intubate before transfer if the airway is at risk**

- Ventilation and oxygenation must be adequate: clinically, and by pulse oximetry, blood gas measurement and capnography if appropriate (Table 20.2).
- There must be large-bore venous access, and objective evidence of cardiovascular stability: systolic blood pressure >120 mmHg, pulse <120 beats/min, urine output >40 ml/h unless contraindicated.
- Spinal immobilization (if indicated) must be adequate for the transfer: a spinal board or vacuum mattress with cervical immobilization may be used. (Hanging-weight traction systems for spinal and other injuries are dangerous and impractical, especially with air transport. Traction splints and spinal traction frames are more suitable.[19,20])
- Known or suspected pneumothoraces should be drained before transfer. Diagnosis and treatment of an expanding or tension pneumothorax is very difficult in transit.
- All tubes entering the patient, be they endotracheal, chest drainage, venous or arterial lines must be *firmly* secured. Whenever the patient is moved they are easily pulled out, and once on the road or in the air they can be very difficult to replace.
- ICU patients usually have multiple infusions, and any not essential during the transfer may be temporarily discontinued. This reduces clutter, and lessens the risk of line displacement.
- The patient must have adequate sedation and analgesia, or be anaesthetized if appropriate.
- A nasogastric tube and urinary catheter should be inserted and left on free drainage. (Head-injured patients who have been given mannitol should be catheterized and the bag emptied before leaving!)
- Wounds or burns must be dressed with non-constrictive dressings, and fractures stabilized.
- Notes, blood results, X-rays, and blood or blood products should be obtained and packaged before transfer.

EQUIPMENT

When possible, the 'pro-active use' of monitoring and equipment is recommended.[14] If the monitor, ventilator and infusion pumps used in the resuscitation room are chosen in advance to be suitable for transfer, they can be kept attached for the entire journey. Equipment function can then be checked before departure, ventilator settings optimized by checking blood gases, and drug infusions continued without interruption. This reduces the risk of instability at the time of departure, when equipment is often changed (and sometimes found not to work) at the last minute! 'Proactive use' demands that batteries are kept fully charged in advance, and equipment is used on mains back-up until ready to leave.

The patient should be stabilized on transfer equipment as early as possible

If separate transfer equipment is used, it must be 'ring-fenced' so that it is instantly available, and kept in one place so that the entire package is ready to go. It should be well maintained, with batteries and back-ups always being fully charged. (It is useful to note that battery life may be severely shortened in older syringe pumps, which may fail early during transfer.[21]) If the equipment and monitors differ from those normally used in the hospital, then the transfer team should be fully trained in their use. Even if separate equipment is used, it should still be applied as early as possible.

Monitors

The standard of monitoring should be identical to that required during general anaesthesia and routine intensive care.[22] The monitors themselves must accompany the patient at all stages of the journey. It is pointless providing high standards of monitoring in the resuscitation room if the patient is then wheeled down a long corridor to the CT scanner, without monitoring, before they are connected to another set of monitors.

The ideal transport monitor should be:

- portable, robust, compact and lightweight;
- multimodal (ideally with all desired variables monitored by one unit);
- resistant to vibration artefact,;
- battery-powered, with a long battery life, a battery charge indicator, and mains back-up facility;
- easy to operate;
- visible from various angles, and in varying light conditions (some screens are only clear if viewed from a single direction);
- fitted with visible as well as audible alarms, in case of likely background noise in transit;
- fitted with a facility for data storage, and downloading or printing;
- free from sharp edges, and with a protective case or cover; and
- trolley-mountable (ideally, to fit a purpose-built transfer trolley, some of which are available commercially).

The following modes of monitoring should be available, ideally in a single unit:

- ECG
- Non-invasive blood pressure (NIBP)
- Invasive pressure channels: ideally two (one to monitor direct arterial blood pressure, and the second for central venous or other pressures)
- Pulse oximetry
- Capnography
- Inspired oxygen percentage
- Temperature (e.g. by aural probe)

ECG, NIBP and pulse oximetry should be monitored in all patients, although these are prone to vibration artefact in moving vehicles. It is essential to have a low threshold for using an arterial line, which allows continuous and more reliable blood pressure monitoring in transit.[23] An arterial line should be used in any ventilated patient, and in any trauma patient with potential cardiovascular instability.

Use arterial line monitoring in 'critical' patients during transit

Central venous pressure can also be monitored with a second invasive pressure channel. If a patient is transferred with a pulmonary artery ('Swan–Ganz') catheter *in situ*, there is a risk of unrecognized 'wedging' and pulmonary infarction. To avoid this, either the pulmonary arterial pressure trace should be monitored, *or* the catheter temporarily withdrawn into the superior vena cava.

Capnography should be used to monitor the adequacy of artificial ventilation, particularly to avoid hypercarbia in head-injured patients. (Pulse oximetry alone does *not* detect hypoventilation.) It is important to note that end-tidal CO_2 will underestimate arterial $PaCO_2$,[24] especially with ventilation–perfusion mismatch, and capnography should be checked against blood gases before departure.

Urine output and neurological status (including Glasgow Coma Score) should also be monitored.

Oxygen

Oxygen therapy should be continued during transfer. It is vital to check how much oxygen is carried on the vehicle: this must be enough for the whole journey at the *maximum* flow rate, with a 1- to 2-h reserve (oxygen cylinder contents are given in Table 20.3). This is easy to calculate for self-ventilating patients: for transport ventilators, the ventilator's *maximal* oxygen consumption should be checked (see below). The correct spanner to turn on replacement cylinders should always be available! A small D-size cylinder will be needed for loading and unloading.

Table 20.3 *Oxygen cylinder sizes and contents*

	Cylinder size					
	C	D	E	F	G	J
Height (inches)	14	18	31	34	49	57
Capacity (litres)	170	340	680	1360	3400	6800

> **Check oxygen cylinder supplies against patient requirements**

Ventilators

Portable transport ventilators are needed for intubated patients, who should normally be ventilated for the transfer.[10] Although ambulances may carry such ventilators, it is best not to rely on these. Referring units should have their own transport ventilators with which medical staff should be familiar. The patient should be stabilized *early* on ventilation before departure, guided by blood gases. The safest ventilation mode for transfer is *volume control*, since pressure control may lead to undetected hypoventilation. The ventilator's maximal oxygen consumption (on 100% O_2) must be known, and this is often little more than the preset minute volume.[25] A self-inflating (Ambu-type) bag should always be carried in case of oxygen or ventilator failure.

> **Always take a self-inflating bag on *every* transfer**

Transport ventilators may be gas-driven, or powered electrically from rechargeable batteries and mains back-up. They should provide:

- airway pressure monitoring;
- alarms for high pressure and low pressure/disconnection;
- high-pressure cut-out facility;
- variable oxygen percentage;
- positive end-expiratory pressure (PEEP); and
- variable respiratory rates, ratios and tidal volumes.

Other equipment

A suggested list of equipment and drugs is given in Table 20.4. Again, it is best to take (and be familiar with) one's own equipment rather than relying on what might be on the ambulance. Infusion pumps should be refilled before departure, any drugs which might be required should be drawn up in clearly labelled, capped syringes, and needles and ampoules discarded safely.

There must be enough space for all this during the transfer, and while it is tempting to 'pack the kitchen sink', too much equipment can impede access to the patient. Simplicity is important and a checklist of minimal/maximal equipment is useful. Patients have other needs, and simple things such as blankets, pillows and cleaning swabs are often forgotten.

Table 20.4 *Suggested adult transfer drug and equipment list (This is a general list which may need modification according to patient needs, transport vehicle equipment, and transport distance.)*

Intravenous
syringes: 2, 5, 10 and 20 ml
needles: 21, 23 and 25 G
syringe caps
i.v. cannulae: 14, 16, 18 and 20 G
alcohol swabs
tourniquet
dressings, tape and bandages
arm splints
i.v. giving sets
pressure infusion device
fluids:
• Hartmann's solution: 1000 ml × 2
• Haemaccel/Gelofusine: 500 ml × 2
• 5% dextrose: 1000 ml × 1
• Mannitol 10%: 500 ml × 1

Drugs
Resuscitation (Minijets):

• adrenaline 1: 10 000, 10 ml, × 5
• atropine 1 mg in 5 ml, × 3
• lignocaine 1%, 10 ml, × 2
• sodium bicarbonate 8.4%, 50 ml, × 1
• calcium chloride 10%, 10 ml, × 1
• glucose 50%, 50 ml, × 1

Anaesthetic/sedative/analgesic:
• etomidate
• propofol (enough for infusion if needed)
• midazolam
• suxamethonium (stored in fridge)
• vecuronium
• morphine
• fentanyl

Other:
• naloxone
• flumazenil
• saline/sterile water for dilution
• GTN spray
• lignocaine 1% (for infiltration)
• salbutamol nebulizer solution
• adenosine
• aminophylline
• hydrocortisone
• chlorpheniramine
• metoclopramide
• labetalol
• frusemide

Airway
oxygen mask (non-rebreather reservoir-type)
facemasks (anaesthetic-type)
airways:
• oropharyngeal: sizes 2, 3, 4
• nasopharyngeal: sizes 6, 7, 8
self-inflating bag (Ambu-type) with reservoir
O_2 tubing
laryngoscopes: two (one with large blade)
spare bulbs and batteries
tracheal tubes: sizes 7.0, 8.0, 9.0
lubricating jelly
10-ml syringe
intubating bougie or stylet
Magill's forceps
tape or tie
laryngeal mask airway: size 3 and/or 4
portable O_2 cylinder
breathing system filter/heat and moisture
    exchanger
tracheal suction catheters
cricothyrotomy kit with pre-prepared connectors
    (see Chapter 3)

Electrical/gas-powered
transport ventilator
monitors
infusion pumps (and spare)
defibrillator (if not on vehicle)

Miscellaneous
portable suction
disposable gloves
blood glucose strips
adhesive tape
blades/sutures
dressings/bandages
scissors
stethoscope
disposable razors
chest drain equipment
manual sphygmomanometer (mercury-free)

PRE-DEPARTURE CHECKLIST

Safe transfer requires the coordination of many aspects of patient care, and no-one has an infallible memory. Therefore, just before departure the entire 'process' should be physically ticked off on a checklist.

* Transfer team members appropriate and completed final patient check?
* Equipment, batteries, oxygen, fluids and drugs checked?
* Transfer vehicle ready and waiting?
* Reception at receiving hospital confirmed with named doctor, giving estimated time of arrival?
* Confirmed bed still available, and its exact location?
* All case notes, X-rays, results, referral letter collected?
* Contact numbers and phone?
* Return arrangements checked?
* Relatives informed of departure?
* Is the patient still stable after transfer to the trolley?
* Equipment, infusions and monitors still attached and functioning?

All lines and tubes should be secured firmly, and *re-checked* whenever the patient is moved

---

MANAGEMENT DURING TRANSFER

The following points should be monitored during transfer:

* *Access and visibility:* it should be possible to see the patient, the monitors, the ventilator, the syringe pumps and infusions, and the doctor must be in a position to actively treat the patient if required.
* *Immobilization:* adequate stabilization of spinal and other injuries must be continued in transit.
* *Equipment:* all equipment must be secured so that it is not hazardous to staff or patient.
* *Reassessment:* as in the resuscitation room, the patient's 'A,B,Cs' should be re-assessed regularly, and monitored to the same standard.
* *Team roles:* team members should carry out their predefined tasks as normal.
* *Temperature:* drops in transit are difficult to avoid, but the patient should be kept covered as far as access and monitoring allow, and the inside of the vehicle must be kept warm.
* *Attendant safety:* a moving vehicle is potentially hazardous; attendants should stay seated as much as possible, kneeling in a stable position if it is necessary for patient treatment.
* *Intervention:* if major treatment interventions are needed, then in road transfers it is usually best to stop at the first *safe* opportunity (as best judged by the vehicle crew).
* *Record keeping:* with good preparation most transfers go smoothly, but recording the patient's condition during transfer is vital, for the benefit of the receiving hospital as well as for medicolegal reasons. A pre-prepared transfer sheet should be used to include a checklist for all things previously mentioned, and a record of patient data in transit.

AEROMEDICAL TRANSPORT

The transfer of patients by air has its own specific problems,[26] and requires specialized training and experience beyond the scope of this chapter. Without this, the transfer team may become a danger to the patient, themselves and the aircraft. Even more than for land transport, it is vital to ensure that the patient is stable and that any intervention that may possibly be needed is performed before departure. The equipment, patient and escort weight should be calculated in advance.

Specific problems of aeromedical transport

PRESSURE

The major problem of this type of transport is pressure and pressure changes. Atmospheric pressure falls with increasing altitude, and the effects depend on the aircraft used. Helicopters are usually unpressurized, but fly at low altitude and thus such problems are normally avoided; fixed-wing aircraft are often pressurized, but to a lower cabin pressure [equivalent to up to 8000 feet (2400 m)] than at sea level. Decreased pressure causes:

- a fall in partial pressure of atmospheric oxygen, with increasing risk of hypoxia and the need for oxygen supplementation.
- expansion of closed gas-containing structures according to Boyle's law. This affects:
  - pneumothoraces: a small pneumothorax will expand by 20% when climbing from sea level to 6000 feet (1850 m). All pneumothoraces should be drained before transfer.
  - gas-containing organs (consider a nasogastric tube).
  - pneumoperitoneum or pneumocephalus.
  - air-filled tracheal tube cuffs (inflate with saline instead of air before departure).
  - nasogastric, catheter and other drainage bags.
  - air splints, leading to compartment syndrome.
  - vacuum mattresses, leading to ineffective immobilization.
  - air trapped under encircling limb plasters (bivalve before transfer).

OTHER PROBLEMS

- *Temperature:* temperature also falls with increasing altitude, and this is a problem in unpressurized aircraft.
- *Humidity:* air at altitude is less humid, and airway complications may occur if humidification is not provided[27] (for example, via a heat and moisture exchanger for intubated patients).
- *Vibration and noise:* especially in helicopters, these cause difficulty with communication, monitoring and the performance of tasks. Helmets and earphones will be needed by the escorts, and ear-protectors for the patient.
- *Access and visibility:* some helicopters in particular are very cramped, and access to the patient can be very limited.
- *Equipment:* may interfere with aircraft electrical systems. The installation of monitors, defibrillators and similar equipment must be approved by the Civil Aviation Authority, and other equipment should only be carried exceptionally.[24,28,29]

INTRA-HOSPITAL TRANSFER

The same standards of equipment, monitoring and escorting staff training should apply for *intra*-hospital transfers as for those between hospitals. It is essential to avoid the temptation to 'cut and run', even for short distances! However the journey time is shorter and more predictable, and help is more readily available. Drugs, equipment and oxygen supplies may therefore be 'scaled down' accordingly – always allowing for unexpected delays, the most serious of which is being stuck in a lift.

Key points for intra-hospital transfer

THE BED/TRANSFER TROLLEY

This should have:

- smooth wheels;
- cot sides;
- a firm base for cardiopulmonary resuscitation (CPR);

- the ability to tip head-down; and
- the facility to attach pumps, monitors, oxygen, suction, etc.

ESCORTING STAFF

These should be *properly trained*, and should *not* have to push the bed/trolley themselves.

ROUTE PLANNING

As with inter-hospital transfers, the *best route* should be chosen (the shortest may not be the quickest or smoothest). It should be arranged for people to *hold doors and lifts open ahead*.

COMMUNICATION

Ensure that the receiving department is ready *before you leave*.

ARRIVAL AND HANDOVER

Unloading the patient from the vehicle is just as dangerous as loading, perhaps more so, since the relief of arrival may cloud the judgement of the less experienced. Standards of monitoring and vigilance must be maintained until arrival at the previously agreed handover point, where the receiving team should take over the patient's care. In the ventilated patient sedation must be continued, and 'top-up' doses of muscle relaxant may be needed before unloading in order to prevent coughing.

The transfer team

A number of points should be adhered to by the transfer team:

- Standards of care should be maintained until handover.
- Handover should be directly to the receiving team: a 'handover template' is useful[14] (Table 20.5).
- The patient's condition on arrival should be documented and the following documents handed over:
  - notes
  - transfer records
  - investigation results
  - X-rays
  - relatives' details
  - any other documents

Table 20.5 *Handover template (Modified from Ref. 14.)*

A. Immediate information
1. Personnel: introduce yourselves
2. Patient: introduce your patient
3. Priority: indicate any major problem that needs immediate attention

B. Case presentation
1. Presentation: mechanism and time of injury
2. Problems: list of injuries, and other problems (medical conditions, drugs, allergies)
3. Procedures: list of major interventions and investigations (including those awaited or still to be done)
4. Progress: system review
   - respiratory (e.g. oxygenation and ventilator settings)
   - circulatory (e.g. haemodynamic status and blood transfused)
   - neurological (e.g. conscious level and sedation/paralysis)
   - metabolic (e.g. urine output and glucose level)
   - host defence (e.g. temperature, antibiotics, steroids)

- cross-matched blood (if available)
- contact details of referring team, in case of later queries.
- It is important never to be coerced into providing treatment, tests, anaesthesia or further transfer to other parts of the hospital because of unfamiliarity with the layout, equipment, and local emergency procedures at the receiving hospital.
- All your equipment should be retrieved before leaving.

The receiving team

Likewise, the receiving team should adhere to the following guidelines:

- The 'A,B,C,D,Es' should be immediately re-assessed and tubes and lines checked, while care and monitoring continue.
- A verbal handover should be taken from the transfer team.
- It is essential to ensure that all notes, X-rays, other details, and cross-matched blood have been received.
- As the monitors and equipment are exchanged, assisting the transfer team to retrieve theirs will be appreciated.
- The transfer team should be offered facilities for rest and refreshment.
- If the transfer has been conducted poorly, this should be pointed out politely. However, high-handed criticism of junior staff should be avoided: the real fault may lie elsewhere. It is best to raise serious concerns later at senior level.
- Don't forget to say thank you!

ORGANIZATION, PLANNING AND AUDIT

At present, the paucity of funding means that responsibility for patient transfer services is likely to remain with referring hospitals for the forseeable future. It remains a reasonable goal that regional retrieval teams could eventually be developed and funded, and this would allow concentration of expertise, equipment and training.

Until such time, each hospital should develop clear guidelines and channels for communication regarding transfer. They should analyse their most commonly used transfer 'networks', and ensure that receiving hospitals all agree to standard procedures, documentation, training standards, supervision and audit. Lead clinicians should be designated at each site to be responsible for the supervision of the service. Hospitals should maintain a database of appropriate transfer personnel, using the most rather than the least experienced staff, and there should be advance planning to cover their absence on escort duties. Adequate insurance cover, in addition to professional indemnity cover, is vital for those involved. Currently the only means of achieving this is through membership of the Association of Anaesthetists of Great Britain and Ireland or the Intensive Care Society, or through individual policies specifically including this risk.

The provision of transfer services is costly in terms of equipment, training and staffing. These costs must be included when the hospital negotiates funding from purchasing authorities, and this should include provision for consultant involvement in transfer-related duties.

Details of all transfers undertaken, together with copies of the transfer records, should be kept for subsequent audit. This allows monitoring of standards, assistance with training, and aids the modification and improvement of transfer protocols. As an aspect of clinical governance and risk management, the consultant with overall responsibility for transfers should look specifically for any shortfall from the agreed standards and ensure that this is rectified. Where there have been problems with agencies outside his or her own institution, then the appropriate authority must be informed. Where local transfer networks have been established, arrangements should be made for sessions allowing discussion of cases and feedback to both referring and receiving hospitals together with the transfer team and outside agencies. Ideally, this should form part of each hospital's regular trauma audit.

SUMMARY

Transfer of patients within and between hospitals will continue for the forseeable future. Whatever the reason for moving trauma patients, they are placed at increased risk during this process. The use of consistent guidelines and protocols by adequately trained and funded transfer teams represents the best way of minimizing this risk. If regional transfer teams are developed in the future it is to be hoped that they will work to nationally agreed standards. In the absence of such teams each hospital has the responsibility of providing funding, facilities and training to facilitate safe and effective transfer of trauma patients.

REFERENCES

1. Gentleman D, Dearden M, Midgley S, Maclean D. Guidelines for resuscitation and transfer of patients with serious head injury. *British Medical Journal* 1993; **307**: 547–52.
2. Gentleman D, Jennett B. Audit of transfer of unconscious head-injured patients to a neurosurgical unit. *Lancet* 1990; **335**: 330–4.
3. Lambert SM, Willett K. Transfer of multiply-injured patients for neurosurgical opinion: a study of the adequacy of assessment and resuscitation. *Injury* 1993; **24**: 333–6.
4. Hicks IR, Hedley RM, Razis P. Audit of transfer of head injured patients to a stand-alone neurosurgical unit. *Injury* 1994; **25**: 545–9.
5. Andrews PJD, Piper IR, Dearden NM, Miller JD. Secondary insults during intrahospital transport of head-injured patients. *Lancet* 1990; **335**: 327–30.
6. Venkataraman ST. Intrahospital transport of critically ill children – should we pay attention? *Critical Care Medicine* 1999; **27**: 694–5.
7. Britto J, Nadel S, Maconochie I, Levin M, Habibi P. Morbidity and severity of illness during interhospital transfer: impact of a specialised paediatric retrieval team. *British Medical Journal* 1995; **311**: 836–9.
8. Mok Q, Tasker R, Macrae D, James I. Impact of specialised paediatric retrieval teams. *British Medical Journal* 1996; **312**: 119.
9. *Recommendations for the transfer of patients with acute head injuries to neurosurgical units.* London: Association of Anaesthetists of Great Britain and Ireland, 1996.
10. *Guidelines for the transport of the critically ill adult.* London: Intensive Care Society, 1997.
11. Oakley PA. Setting and living up to national standards for the care of the injured. *Injury* 1994; **25**: 595–604.
12. *Guidelines on admission to and discharge from intensive care and high dependency units.* Department of Health, 1996.
13. American College of Critical Care Medicine. Guidelines for the transfer of critically ill patients. *Critical Care Medicine* 1993; **21**: 931–7.
14. Oakley PA. Interhospital transfer of the trauma patient. *Trauma* 1999; **1**: 61–70.
15. Highland T, Salciccioli G, Wilson RF. Spinal cord injuries. In: Wilson RF, Walt AJ (eds). *Management of Trauma* (2nd ed.). Baltimore: Williams & Wilkins, 1996, pp. 203–24.
16. Fairhurst R. Transport in pre-hospital care. In: Greaves I, Porter K (eds.). *Pre-hospital Medicine.* London: Arnold, 1999, pp. 647–50.
17. O'Connor PM, Steele JA, Dearden CH, Rocke LG, Fisher RB. The accident and emergency department as a single portal of entry for the reassessment of all trauma patients transferred to specialist units. *Journal of Accident and Emergency Medicine* 1996; **13**: 9–10.
18. Fitzpatrick MO, Seex K. Scalp lacerations demand careful attention before interhospital transfer of head injured patients. *Journal of Accident and Emergency Medicine* 1996; **13**: 207–8.
19. Fairhurst RJ, Ryan J. Stabilisation and transport. In: Driscoll P, Skinner D (eds). *Trauma Care: Beyond the Resuscitation Room.* London: BMJ Books, 1998, pp. 283–93.
20. Davies G. Aeromedical evacuation. In: Greaves I, Porter K (eds). *Pre-hospital Medicine.* London: Arnold, 1999, pp. 651–9.

21. Tatman A, Brunner H, Stokes M. Premature failure of battery-powered syringe pumps. *Anaesthesia* 1996; **51**: 1041–2.

22. *Recommendations for standards of monitoring during anaesthesia and recovery.* London: Association of Anaesthetists of Great Britain and Ireland, 1994.

23. Runcie CJ, Reeve WG, Reidy J, Dougall JR. Blood pressure measurement during transport. *Anaesthesia* 1990; **45**: 659–65.

24. Morley AP. Prehospital monitoring of trauma patients: experience of a helicopter emergency medical service. *British Journal of Anaesthesia* 1996; **76**: 726–30.

25. Elliot JM. Airway management. In: Greaves I, Porter K (eds). *Pre-hospital Medicine.* London: Arnold, 1999, pp. 27–48.

26. Martin T. Aviation medicine. In: Greaves I, Porter K (eds). *Pre-hospital Medicine.* London: Arnold, 1999, pp. 661–74.

27. Armitage JM, Pyne A, Williams SJ, Frankel H. Respiratory problems of air travel in patients with spinal cord injuries. *British Medical Journal* 1990; **300**: 1498–9.

28. Bristow A. Medical helicopter systems – recommended minimum standards for patient management. *Journal of the Royal Society of Medicine* 1991; **84**: 242–4.

29. Colvin AP. The use of defibrillators in helicopters. *Journal of the British Association for Immediate Care* 1992; **15**: 35–7.

21

Triage

OBJECTIVES

- To understand that triage is the process in which patients are sorted to ensure optimal care and use of resources. It operates at many levels, especially in circumstances with large numbers of casualties and limited resources
- To appreciate that triage systems cannot be applied to single patients
- To realize that triage is a dynamic process and must be repeated regularly
- To recognize that triage systems must be simple and swift but also reliable and reproducible
- To understand that senior staff should be used as triage officers and triage decisions must be recorded
- To acknowledge that triage should never be allowed to delay treatment

INTRODUCTION

The campaigns of the Napoleonic wars saw battles that created huge numbers of killed and wounded soldiers over a single day. At Borodino on 7th September 1812, the worst of these battles resulted in 80 000 French and Russian soldiers being killed. In addition the Russians inflicted 35 000 wounded on the French side.[1] During these campaigns Baron Dominique Larrey (1766–1842), Chief Surgeon to Napoleon Bonaparte, introduced a system of sorting the casualties arriving at his field dressing stations. His primary objective was the swift return of fit men to action, and so minor wounds were treated early, but thereafter his priorities were similar to those in use today. Larrey used senior military surgeons as triage officers, finding that experienced doctors produced more accurate triage.

Triage is the process of sorting patients into priorities in order to establish an order for treatment and evacuation. The term originated from the selection of coffee beans, and is derived from the French *'trier' – to sort or to sieve*. Triage now takes many different forms, and operates at a number of different levels, but its overall aim at all times is to give the right patient the right care at the right time in the right place. In certain circumstances this may also mean 'doing the most for the most'.

$$\boxed{\text{Trier – to sort or to sieve}}$$

Triage must be a simple procedure that is swift, but reliable and reproducible. There are many systems in use world-wide depending on the scenario and the end-point required. A surgeon deciding which of three patients to operate on first will employ a different system to a doctor faced with 80 casualties at a major incident.

The condition of any patient is dynamic and liable to change. This is especially true of the seriously injured. Time or medical intervention may change a patient's priority. An unconscious patient with a minor isolated head injury may die if their airway is not supported but once conscious can be simply observed. This patient's priority is at first high, but after intervention becomes low. To reflect this, triage is a dynamic process and must be repeated on a regular basis.

When does triage take place?

In pre-hospital medicine triage is used not only to assign treatment and evacuation priorities to casualties but also to determine which hospital the patient goes to, how they get there, and what sort of team meets them on arrival. Triage of the emergency call at Ambulance Control can also determine the type and speed of the ambulance crew that responds to that call. Prioritized despatch is a common practice in the United States and Europe, but is a relatively recent innovation in the United Kingdom.

Triage to assign treatment and evacuation priorities must take place whenever casualties outnumber the skilled help and other resources available. A two-man ambulance crew attending a two-car road traffic accident (RTA) could have six casualties to deal with. Initially, the crew must assess all those involved, identify those with life-threatening and serious injuries, and develop a plan of action for treatment and transport both before and as other help becomes available.

Within an Emergency Department the same six trauma patients may arrive in a short period of time. Unless the hospital encounters this scenario on a regular basis, it is unlikely that the resuscitation room will have a bay and a full trauma team available for each patient. Using triage principles will help the team leader to determine how to allocate his/her staff and decide which patients are seen in the resuscitation room. Ideally, ambulance control will have triaged some of the patients to other local hospitals, but this may not be possible for geographical reasons. Once the resuscitation has been completed, patients may need further triage for transfer to specialist centres such as neurosurgical or burns units.

Where does triage take place?

Before there is any patient contact, triage at the Ambulance Control Centre may have determined the type of response despatched. Once at the scene, the ambulance crew will triage the patient or patients to determine the mode of transport to hospital and the destination hospital. In most areas of the UK there is little choice other than movement by road to the nearest major Accident and Emergency Department. As the use of helicopter ambulances spreads, this will become a more widely available option. In the United States triage will determine whether the receiving hospital is a trauma centre or a general hospital.

During a major incident involving multiple casualties, triage takes place at the scene in order to determine initial priorities for treatment and transport to the Casualty Clearing Station. The patients may be re-triaged for treatment priorities on arrival at the Casualty Clearing Station and again for transport priorities to hospital after treatment. At the hospital another round of triage will take place at the doors of the Accident and Emergency Department to re-assign treatment priorities. After initial resuscitation, priorities for surgery will be determined.

In accordance with the Patients' Charter, UK Accident and Emergency Departments should carry out triage of all patients on arrival. These circumstances are obviously very different from those pre-hospital or at a major incident, but the same principles of triage apply. Immediately life-threatening conditions and injuries must be treated without delay. Serious problems must be identified and given a higher priority than minor ones. Triage principles have also been used successfully in 'hospital tents' at mass gatherings such as rock festivals and sporting events,[2] to ensure the best use of limited resources.

Who performs triage?

The exact nature of the incident and the timing and site of triage will determine the identity of the triage officer or officers. Whenever possible, triage should be performed by experienced senior staff. Although at first sight this might seem to be a waste of a valuable resource better employed in direct resuscitation, accurate triage will help to ensure optimal use of all staff and resources to achieve the best care for all the casualties. Overtriage – awarding a higher priority to a patient than appropriate – will consume staff and resources and dilute or divert them from other high-priority patients. Undertriage will result in the patient receiving the lower priority getting delayed or inadequate care.

Triage should be performed by experienced senior staff

PRIORITIES

Different systems of triage are used in the UK, depending on the situation. A working knowledge of the common systems and categories will assist trauma teams to appreciate what may have happened to the patient earlier.

UK pre-hospital triage priorities

The two common pre-hospital systems in use in UK civilian practice are summarized in Table 21.1. They are the Priority 'P' system and the Treatment 'T' system.[3] The significant difference is the inclusion of the expectant priority in the 'T' system. The importance and use of this priority is discussed below. Each triage priority is conventionally assigned a particular colour.

Table 21.1 *UK pre-hospital triage priorities*

Description	System P	System T	Colour
Immediate	1	1	Red
Urgent	2	2	Yellow
Delayed	3	3	Green
Expectant		4	Blue
Dead	Dead	Dead	White

Immediate priority:	Red	casualties requiring immediate procedures to save life. e.g. airway obstruction, tension pneumothorax
Urgent priority:	Yellow	casualties requiring medical treatment within 4–6 h. e.g. compound fractures
Delayed priority:	Green	casualties with injuries that can wait for treatment until after 4–6 h. e.g. small cuts and contusions, minor closed fractures
Expectant priority:	Blue	see below
Dead:	White	dead casualties must be identified and clearly labelled as such to avoid re-triage

EXPECTANT PRIORITY

This priority is given to casualties with non-survivable injuries, or whose injuries are so severe and their chances of survival so small that their treatment would divert medical resources, thus compromising the survival of other casualties. This priority should only be invoked in a 'mass casualty' situation, where the number of casualties completely overwhelms the medical resources available, and rescuers must 'do the most for the most'. The decision to use the expectant priority is taken by the Medical and Ambulance Incident Officers acting in concert at the scene. To date, it has not been needed in any major incident in the UK. As a concept, the use of this priority goes against the instincts of all trauma carers, but its appropriate use will save lives and inappropriate avoidance will cost them. Severe (>80%) burns or a comatose patient with a compound skull fracture are examples of patients for whom this priority would be appropriate in a declared mass casualty situation. These patients should still be given analgesia and be made comfortable.

The International Committee of the Red Cross (ICRC) often needs to triage patients arriving at their hospitals in war zones.[4] The categories used are shown in Table 21.2.

Table 21.2 *ICRC triage categories*

Category I:	Patients for whom urgent surgery is required and for whom there is a good chance of reasonable survival.
Category II:	Patients who do not require surgery. This includes those for whom reasonable survival is unlikely.
Category III:	Patients who require surgery, but not urgently.

Accident and Emergency triage

A five-category system is used in most A&E departments in the UK (see Table 21.3). The Manchester Triage system provides a framework to guide the triage personnel in selecting the right category for an individual patient.[5]

Table 21.3 *Accident and Emergency triage categories*

Description	Priority	Colour	Target time
Immediate	1	Red	On arrival
Very urgent	2	Orange	Within 10 min
Urgent	3	Yellow	Within 1 h
Standard	4	Green	Within 2 h
Non-urgent	5	Blue	Within 4 h

SYSTEMS

Triage systems may use anatomical or physiological data, as well as information regarding the mechanism of injury. Accurate triage using an anatomical system requires a full secondary survey of an undressed patient. This is so that all injuries are identified and assessed, individually and collectively, before a priority is given. Anatomical systems require experienced operators, time, and a warm, well-lit environment – all of which will be lacking at the scene of an incident. Once the incident has occurred, a patient's injuries will not change. As a result, anatomical systems are static and are only of use in a hospital and with a small number of patients to assess. Pre-hospital, obvious injuries may be used as criteria for trauma team activation. Anatomical information may be used to modify other triage systems, if senior staff with sufficient experience are the triage officers.

Systems using the mechanism of injury help promote a high index of suspicion for occult injury. By recognizing and reporting a mechanism of injury associated with a high chance of serious injury the pre-hospital carers draw the attention of the trauma team to the likely problems. These systems are not of use when dealing with a large number of casualties. In this situation, the mechanism will have been broadly similar for all, and small variations between individuals – such as position within a railway carriage – will not be clear early on. With small numbers of patients, these systems allow the identity of the receiving hospital and activation of a trauma team to be determined.[6] The mechanism-based criteria for activation of a trauma team are shown in Table 21.4. Occasionally, the trauma team will receive a patient without a serious injury when the activation has been based solely on the history.[7] While the disruption is annoying for all concerned, this is a necessary evil if all serious occult injury is to be detected. Some trauma centres use a two-tier graded response to incoming trauma to minimize the nuisance effects and cost of overtriage.[8,9] The pre-hospital information is triaged for either a full or modified trauma call. A senior doctor still leads the modified team, and the response can be upgraded to a full trauma call at any time. The criteria for full and modified responses are shown in Table 21.5.

Table 21.4 *Trauma team activation criteria*

Anatomical	>1 long-bone fracture – unilateral radius and ulna count as one
	>1 anatomical area injured
	Penetrating injury to head, thorax or abdomen
	Traumatic amputation or crush injury
Mechanism	Fall >6 m
	Pedestrian or cyclist hit by car
	Death of other occupant in same vehicle
	Ejection from vehicle/bicycle
	Major vehicular deformity or significant intrusion into passenger space
	Extrication time >20 min
	Vehicular roll-over
Physiological	Respiratory rate >29/min
	Pulse rate <50 or >130 beats/min
	Systolic blood pressure <90 mm Hg
	GCS <13

GCS, Glasgow Coma Score.

Table 21.5 *Criteria for full and modified trauma calls*

Full	Modified
Anatomical	
• traumatic pneumothorax	
• traumatic amputation or degloving	
• all obvious major vascular injuries	
• open fractures (except hands and feet)	
• burns >15% BSA, or airway involvement	
• electrical burn	
Mechanism	
• penetrating injury to head or torso	
• all shotgun wounds	
• fall >20 ft or two stories	
• pedestrians and motorcyclists	
• RTA with death in same vehicle	
• ejection from vehicle	
Physiological	All patients not specified opposite
• SBP <90 mmHg	
• pulse <50 or >120 beats/min	
• RR <10 or >30/min	
• head injury with GCS <13	
• deterioration of stable patient	

BSA, body surface area; RR, respiration rate; SBP, systolic blood pressure.

Physiological systems give the best indication of a patient's current condition, although they do not allow for the compensatory mechanisms of children and young adults. When undertriage occurs, it is usually due to the physiological parameters being ignored. Ideally, the triage officer should employ a physiological system and use their experience to modify the priority assigned if anatomical or mechanical considerations demand it. This is why the triage officer should be as experienced in dealing with trauma as possible. The most sensitive triage tools combine aspects of all three types of systems, but are harder to use in the field.

The Triage Sieve[3] (Table 21.6)

This is a fast, snap-shot assessment of the patient that can be used at the scene of a major incident. It is based on mobility, followed by a simple assessment of ABC. The capillary refill time (CRT) is preferred for circulatory assessment as it gives an indication of peripheral perfusion and is simple and rapid to ascertain. The environmental conditions, especially dark and cold, may make the use of CRT difficult. If this is the case the pulse should be used. This system will overtriage normally non-mobile patients at the extremes of age, and will undertriage a mobile but severely injured patient. A paediatric triage tape, similar to the Broslow tape, displaying triage sieves adjusted for length has been developed to address the triage of young children. The severely injured but mobile patient (for example, a patient with 40% burns) will eventually cease to be mobile and be re-triaged. In the meantime, this casualty may have been able to evacuate him/herself to an area where more help is available, and a more sophisticated triage system can be used which will recognize the significance of his/her injury.

Table 21.6 *The Triage Sieve*

Mobility	Can the patient walk?		yes			$\rightarrow$	*P3 Delayed*
			no			$\rightarrow$	assess A and B
Airway and breathing	Is the patient breathing?		no	$\rightarrow$	open airway, breathing now?		
				no		$\rightarrow$	*Dead*
				yes		$\rightarrow$	*P1 Immediate*
			yes	$\rightarrow$	assess rate		
				< 10 or > 29		$\rightarrow$	*P1 Immediate*
				10–29		$\rightarrow$	assess C
Circulation		CRT	> 2 s				
			or pulse > 120 beats/min			$\rightarrow$	*P1 Immediate*
		CRT	< 2 s				
			or pulse < 120 beats/min			$\rightarrow$	*P2 Urgent*

CRT = Capillary refill time.

The simple triage and rapid treatment system[10] (START) and the triage trauma rule[11] are alternative systems to the triage sieve which are in use in the United States (see Tables 21.7 and 21.8).

Table 21.7 *The simple triage and rapid treatment system (START)*

Is the patient breathing?	no	$\rightarrow$	open airway, breathing now?	
		no	$\rightarrow$ *Dead*	
		yes	$\rightarrow$ *Immediate care*	
	yes	$\rightarrow$	assess rate	
			> 30	$\rightarrow$ *Immediate care*
			< 30	$\rightarrow$ check radial pulse
Radial pulse present?	no	$\rightarrow$	control haemorrhage	
		$\rightarrow$	*Immediate care*	
	yes	$\rightarrow$	assess mental state	
Following commands	no	$\rightarrow$	*Immediate care*	
	yes	$\rightarrow$	*Urgent care*	

Table 21.8 *The trauma triage rule*

Major trauma victim =	Systolic blood pressure <85 mmHg
	motor component of GCS <5
	penetrating trauma to head, neck or torso

After the rapid and simple first triage, a more sophisticated triage tool can be used. This is often referred to as the 'triage sort'. The Triage Revised Trauma Score (TRTS) is the system currently recommended for this use.

Triage Revised Trauma Score

This modification of the Revised Trauma Score[12] (RTS) allows rapid physiological triage of multiple patients in the field. It uses the unweighted sum of the RTS values to allocate priorities (Table 21.9). This system is used once the patients have been moved from the immediate scene of the incident and a more thorough assessment can be made, for example at the Casualty Clearing Station. The TRTS was first developed in the United States to help paramedics determine which patients should be taken to a trauma centre and which to a general hospital. The triage officer should also carry out a limited anatomical assessment to avoid the problem of undertriaging patients with serious injuries but currently stable parameters.

Table 21.9 *Triage priorities using TRTS*

Respiratory rate (per min)	0	1–5	6–9	30+	10–29
Points	0	1	2	3	4
Systolic blood pressure (mmHg)	0	1–49	50–75	76–89	90+
Points	0	1	2	3	4
GCS (total)	3	4–5	6–8	9–12	13–15
Points	0	1	2	3	4

Total score		Priority	
12		T3/P3	Delayed
10–11		T2/P2	Urgent
1–9		T1/P1	Immediate
0		Dead	

Prioritized despatch

This is a concept that has recently been introduced in the UK. Studies in the United States have shown that prioritized despatch – dividing calls into priorities by using questions about the patient's respiratory and neurological state – improves the efficiency of the ambulance service.[13,14] The two systems in use are the Advanced Medical Priority Despatch system (AMPDS) and Criteria-Based Despatch (CBD). Both use a fixed sequence of questions to determine the priority. AMPDS sorts calls into four categories, and CBD into three.

As well as ranking emergency calls by urgency, prioritized despatch allows the Ambulance Control to determine the type and level of response. The target of one paramedic per crew has almost been achieved throughout the country, so the choice between the paramedic crew and the all-technician crew is less relevant. Helicopter ambulances are now becoming more widespread and therefore available for despatch. In France, there is always a doctor in the Ambulance Control Room to monitor calls, and another doctor available to respond to pre-hospital emergencies when despatched. In areas of the UK with a British Association for Immediate Care (BASICS) scheme, a doctor may be requested to attend a scene by Ambulance Control, or a mobile medical team requested from a nearby Accident and Emergency Department.

Triage for destination

There are very few specialized trauma centres in the UK at the present time. Nearly all seriously injured patients will therefore be taken to the nearest Accident and

Emergency Department. The use of alternative trauma systems for the UK is still under review. One alternative is the regionalization of trauma services recommended in the report on major trauma by the Royal College of Surgeons of England in 1988.[15] This would be a similar system to that in use in the United States. Paramedics need triage tools to help them determine which patients can safely be taken to the local district hospitals, and which must bypass them and be taken to the trauma centres. There are many different triage systems in use based on separate or combined anatomical, mechanical and physiological criteria. Unfortunately, there is little agreement as to the 'gold standard'.

The TRTS (Table 21.9) was developed from the Trauma Score and the Revised Trauma Score (see Chapter 22). Just one point dropped from any of the three parameters signifies increased mortality, and is an indication for the patient to be taken to a trauma centre. Some 97% of all trauma deaths will be identified using this method, the missed deaths being patients with serious injury whose compensatory mechanisms still allow their physiological parameters to remain normal when the first readings are taken by the ambulance crew. This will occur most often when the patient is young and the ambulance arrives quickly. To avoid this problem, the American College of Surgeons' Committee on Trauma devised a Triage Decision Scheme[16] (Table 21.10) which assesses physiological, anatomical, mechanical and pre-morbid factors.

Table 21.10 *Triage decision scheme*

Measure vital signs and level of consciousness

Step 1.	RR <10 or >29 SBP <90 GCS <13	Yes →	Take to trauma centre Alert trauma team
	(i.e. drop one point on TRTS)	No →	Assess anatomy of injury (Step 2)
Step 2.	Flail chest 2+ proximal long-bone fractures Amputation proximal to wrist/ankle All penetrating trauma unless distal to elbow and knee	Yes →	Take to trauma centre Alert trauma team
	Limb paralysis Pelvic fractures Combination trauma with burns	No →	Evaluate mechanism of injury (Step 3)
Step 3.	Ejection from vehicle/bicycle Death in same vehicle Pedestrian thrown or run over or >5 m.p.h. impact speed Motorcycle RTA speed >20 m.p.h. (30 k.p.h.) Car RTA speed >40 m.p.h. (64 k.p.h.)	Yes →	Contact medical control Consider taking to trauma centre Consider alerting trauma team
	Major vehicular deformity or intrusion into passenger space Extrication time >20 min Vehicular roll-over Falls > 6 m	No →	Assess pre-morbid state (Step 4)
Step 4.	Age <5 or >55 years Pregnancy Immunosuppressed patients Cardiac or respiratory disease	Yes →	Contact medical control Consider taking to trauma centre Consider alerting trauma team
	IDDM, cirrhosis Coagulopathy, morbid obesity	No →	Re-evaluate with medical control

When in doubt, take to a trauma centre.

IDDM, insulin-dependent diabetes mellitus; GCS, Glasgow Coma Score; RR, respiration rate (per min); SBP, systolic blood pressure (mmHg)

LABELLING

Once the casualty is in hospital, a patient number and notes will be assigned. Clinical information and decisions can and must be properly recorded. Before arrival in hospital, clinical data and triage decisions also need to be recorded. The patient report form is a valuable source of information for the trauma team leader during and after a resuscitation. The form does not, however, replace listening to the ambulance crew at the handover. In an incident involving a large number of casualties, once a triage priority has been assigned, the triage officer must label the patient appropriately. This prevents duplication of effort and confusion among other rescuers as to which patients need treatment and evacuation first.

Unfortunately, there are many different labelling systems available, and there is no accepted national or international standard. This does not matter as long as everyone who is likely to use the local system is familiar with it. Problems are most likely to arise when staff move areas or are operating out of their local region. A labelling system must be dynamic and allow the patient to get better and worse. It should also be simple to use and easily recognized. Part of the label should allow clinical data to be recorded and updated as the patient moves along the chain of care. Labels should be easily visible and robust enough to be of use in dark and wet environments, and must be easily attached to the patient. Ideally, each label should have an identifying number that allows the triage officer to know how many patients have been triaged, and to give the casualty an identifying number by which they can later be traced through the course of the incident.

There is no agreed convention on labelling the expectant priority. Blue is commonly used, but both red and green cards annotated 'expectant' are alternatives. If the cruciform cards are in use, the triage officer can fold the corners of the green card back, showing the red behind. Whatever local alternative is in use, all those who may need to know must be informed as part of major incident planning and preparation.

Many labelling systems use single, coloured cards. Clinical information is recorded on one side of each card. These systems are not ideal as they are not dynamic. If a patient changes priority, a new card needs filling out with the clinical data. This wastes time and there is an attendant risk of transposition errors. As more patients change priority and receive a second card, the triage officer will lose track of the exact number of casualties. If the out-of-date card is thrown away, vital information may be lost, but if it is left with the patient then confusion may occur as to which of the cards is the current one.

The Mettag label is a commonly used system that falls between the single priority and the multiple priority cards. It is a plain white label for clinical information, which has coloured strips at the base of the card that can be ripped off to denote the priority. This system has two major drawbacks. First, it is difficult to tell what category the patient is without going close up to them, and second the category can only be changed by tearing off further strips in order to indicate a worse category. If the patient improves, a new form is required.

The multiple category card systems are currently the best types available. Data is recorded on the card, which is then folded and replaced in a clear plastic envelope so that only one colour is visible. There is plenty of room for clinical information, and if the category changes then the card is simply refolded. The cards can be tricky to fold and replace in the envelope if the operator is unfamiliar with them. Another disadvantage is that patients might change their own category to ensure earlier evacuation. These cards are relatively expensive, and it is this that has prevented their wider use.

SUMMARY

Triage is the process in which patients are sorted to ensure optimal care and use of resources. It operates at many levels, especially in circumstances with large numbers of casualties and limited resources. Triage systems cannot be applied to single patients. Triage is a dynamic process and must be repeated regularly; therefore triage systems must be simple and swift, as well as reliable and reproducible. Ideally, senior staff should be used as triage officers, and triage decisions must be recorded. It is vital to remember, therefore, that the overall aim at all times is to give the right patient the right care, at the right time, and in the right place.

REFERENCES

1. Rignault D, Wherry D. Lessons from the past worth remembering: Larrey and Triage. *Trauma* 1999; **1**: 86–9.
2. Kerr GW, Parke TRJ. Providing 'T in the Park': pre-hospital care at a major crowd event. *Pre-Hospital Immediate Care* 1999; **3**: 11–13.
3. Advanced Life Support Group. *Major Incident Medical Management and Support – The Practical Approach*. London: BMJ Publishing Group, 1995.
4. Coupland RM, Parker PJ, Gray RC. Triage of war wounded: the experience of the International Committee of the Red Cross. *Injury* 1992; **23**: 507–10.
5. Manchester Triage Group. *Emergency Triage*. London: BMJ Publishing Group, 1997.
6. Hodgetts TJ, Deane S, Gunning K. *Trauma Rules*. London: BMJ Publishing Group, 1997.
7. Simon BJ, Legere P, Emhoff T, *et al*. Vehicular trauma triage by mechanism: avoidance of the unproductive evaluation. *Journal of Trauma* 1994; **37**: 645–9.
8. Ochsner MG, Schmidt JA, Rozycki GS, Champion HR. The evaluation of a two-tier trauma response system at a major trauma center: is it cost effective and safe? *Journal of Trauma* 1995; **39**: 971–7.
9. Tinkoff GH, O'Connor RE, Fulda GJ. Impact of a two-tiered trauma response in the Emergency Department: promoting efficient resource utilisation. *Journal of Trauma* 1996; **41**: 735–40.
10. Super G, Groth S, Hook R. *START: Simple Treatment and Rapid Treatment Plan*. Newport Beach, CA: Hoag Memorial Presbyterian Hospital, 1994.
11. Baxt WG, Jones G, Fortlage D. The trauma triage rule: a new resource-based approach to the pre-hospital identification of major trauma victims. *Annals of Emergency Medicine* 1990; **19**: 1401–6.
12. Champion HR, Sacco WJ, Copes WS, *et al*. A revision of the Trauma Score. *Journal of Trauma* 1989; **29**: 623–9.
13. West JG, Gales RH, Cazaniga AB. Impact of regionalisation. The Orange County Experience. *Archives of Surgery* 1983; **18**: 740.
14. Culley L. Increasing the efficiency of emergency medical services by using criteria based despatch. *Annals of Emergency Medicine* 1994; **24**: 867–72.
15. Royal College of Surgeons of England. *Commission on the provision of surgical services. Report on the working party on the management of patients with major injuries*. London: Royal College of Surgeons of England, 1988.
16. American College of Surgeons' Committee on Trauma. *Advanced Trauma Life Support for Doctors – Course Manual*. Chicago, Illinois: American College of Surgeons, 1997.

22

Trauma scoring

OBJECTIVES

- To understand the principles of trauma scoring
- To understand the importance of trauma scoring in auditing and developing best practice

INTRODUCTION

No one trauma patient is exactly the same as another. Patterns of injury have been defined and should be recognized, so that a high index of suspicion for occult injuries is maintained. There is an almost infinite variety of separate and combined injuries that may result from trauma. Other variables, such as the age of the patient, will also affect the outcome. New interventions and changes to the structure of trauma care must be shown to be clinically beneficial and cost-effective. Trauma scoring systems are tools to allow analysis and comparison of individual patients and groups. The uses that these tools can be put to are shown in Table 22.1.

Table 22.1 *Uses of trauma scoring*

• Epidemiology
• Research
• Triage
• Outcome prediction
• Anatomical and physiological evaluations of injury severity
• Intra- and inter-hospital evaluation of trauma care
• Trauma registers
• Planning of and resource allocation within trauma systems

Trauma scoring first developed in the United States during the 1960s, and has become increasingly sophisticated. The overall usefulness and validity of trauma scoring is dependent on personnel within trauma teams ensuring adequate and accurate data collection. Any scoring system must be accurate, valid, reproducible, and free from observer bias.

Scoring systems are based on anatomical or physiological data, or combine both. Anatomical systems have the advantage in that the amount of tissue damage is open to clinical examination and radiological, operative or post-mortem findings. In addition, the findings are usually constant after the initial injury, as opposed to physiological systems which rely on data that will change constantly during a resuscitation. The initial set of observations in the resuscitation room is currently used for calculations, but may not reflect the true nature of the situation. The physiological data used in the calculation of a trauma score may be collected before the compensatory mechanisms of a pregnant or young casualty are exhausted, causing an overestimation of the probability of survival. Despite this, physiological systems can give a more accurate reading of the overall condition of the patient. This is particularly seen in closed head injuries. Combined systems that use both sets of data are the most accurate, but are the most complicated to use.

ANATOMICAL SYSTEMS

Abbreviated Injury Scale (AIS)[1]

This system was developed by the Association for the Advancement of Automotive Medicine and was first introduced in 1971. It assigns a six-figure code and a severity score to individual penetrating and blunt injuries. The most recent revision in 1990 (AIS 90) lists over 1200 injuries. The code allows easier computer entry and retrieval of data. The severity score ranges from 1 to 6 (Table 22.2) and is non-linear, as the differentials between each point are not the same. The Maximum AIS (MAIS) – the highest single AIS of a multiply injured patient – has been used as an expression of overall severity, and is still used for research into the design of safer vehicles.

Table 22.2 *Severity scores in the Abbreviated Injury Scale*

1 – Mild	Example	450212.1	single rib #
2 – Moderate		450220.2	2–3 rib # 's, stable chest
3 – Serious (non-life-threatening)		450230.3	>3 rib # 's one side, #3 rib # 's on other side, stable chest
4 – Severe (life-threatening)		450260.4	unilateral flail chest
5 – Critical		450266.5	bilateral flail chest
6 – Fatal		413000.6	bilateral obliteration of large portion of chest cavity

The presence of a haemothorax and/or pneumothorax adds a point to the injuries scoring 1–4.

Organ injury scaling

Scaling systems for injuries to individual organs have been developed by the American Association for the Surgery of Trauma. The scales, like the AIS, run from 1 to 6, with 6 being a mortal injury.

Injury Severity Score (ISS)[2,3]

All the patient's injuries are coded with AIS 90 and divided into six body regions (Table 22.3). The highest severity score from each of the three most seriously injured regions is taken and squared. The sum of the three squares is the ISS, which has a range of 1 to 75. Table 22.4 shows an example of an ISS calculation. A score of 75 is incompatible with life, and therefore any patient with an AIS 6 injury in any one region is awarded a total score of 75.

Since the ISS is based on the AIS it is also a non-linear measure. In addition, certain scores are common and others impossible. The non-linearity is a disadvantage as a patient with an isolated AIS 5 injury is more likely to die than a patient with both an AIS 4 injury and an AIS 3 injury. However, both patients will have an ISS of 25.

An ISS >15 signifies major trauma, as a score of 16 is associated with a mortality rate of 10%.

Table 22.3 *The six ISS body regions*

- Head and neck
- Face
- Chest
- Abdomen and pelvic contents
- Extremities and bony pelvis
- External (skin)

New Injury Severity Score (NISS)[4]

This system takes the three highest AIS severity scores, regardless of body area. The scores are squared and added (see Table 22.4). Again, a range of 1 to 75 is produced, and any single AIS of 6 gives a total score of 75. This system is simpler to calculate and is more sensitive than the ISS, as multiple injuries to one body area are given their full weight. For example, a patient with bilateral closed femoral shaft fractures can exsanguinate into his/her thighs and is obviously more seriously injured than a patient with a single fracture, but both would have an ISS of 9. With both injuries counting in NISS the score is 18. Similarly, severe closed head injuries may be underscored by ISS. At present, NISS is unlikely to replace ISS completely because of the key role of the latter in Trauma and Injury Severity Score (TRISS) methodology.

Table 22.4 *An example of ISS and NISS calculation*

Patient S.W., 45-year-old female cyclist hit by car

Head and neck

depressed parietal skull #	150404.	3	*squared*	*9*
small subdural haematoma	140652.	**4**	***squared***	***16***

Face

abrasions	210202.	1

Chest

# 3 ribs R chest, stable chest	450220.	**2**	**squared**	**4**

Abdomen and pelvic contents
nil

Pelvis and extremities

open # radius	752804.	**3**	***squared***	***9***
open # ulna	753204.3			

External (skin)
nil

ISS = 16 + 4 + 9 = 29
NISS = 16 + 9 + 9 = 34

International Classification of Disease Injury Severity Score (ICISS)[5–7]

This system has developed since the early 1990s. Although it is based on the International Classification of Disease 9th edition (ICD-9), it has recently been validated for ICD-10 codes.[8] The calculation of Survival Risk Ratios (SRRs) for all possible injuries is central to this method (see Table 22.5), and operative procedures have also been coded. Other injuries are disregarded in the SRR calculation. The SRRs were determined from large trauma registries in the USA. The ICISS is the product of the SRRs for each of the patient's ten worst injuries (Table 22.5). The ICISS claims improvements in predictive accuracy over ISS and TRISS (see below), especially when combined with factors allowing for physiological state and age, but has yet to be adopted on a widespread basis. Since patients are already coded for the ICD, it is also considered that this reduces the effort required in assigning AIS values.

Table 22.5 *International Classification of Diseases Injury Severity Score (ICISS)*

Survival Risk Ratio (SRR) for injury ICD code $= \dfrac{\text{Number of survivors with injury ICD code}}{\text{Number of patients with injury ICD code}}$

ICISS = SRR (injury1) × SRR (injury2) × .... × SRR (injury 10)

Where injury 1 is the injury with the lowest SRR in that patient

Wesson's criteria[9]

This is a crude calculation for assessing the effectiveness of a trauma system (Table 22.6). It provides a simple expression of performance based on ISS scores. Major trauma cases (ISS >15) are taken, and those with an ISS >60 or a head injury AIS of 5 are excluded. Those left are considered 'salvageable'. It is an easier calculation than those produced in the TRISS methodology.

Table 22.6 *Wesson's criteria*

$$\frac{\text{Salvageable patients* who survived} \times 100}{\text{All salvageable patients}}$$

*Salvageable patient = ISS <15 but >60, No head injury AIS of 5

PHYSIOLOGICAL SYSTEMS

Glasgow Coma Score (GCS)[10]

This was first introduced in 1974 as a research tool for studying head injuries. Its full details and paediatric modifications are dealt with in Chapter 8.

Trauma score (TS)[11]

This assesses five parameters, awarding weighted points, to give a score of 1 to 16 (Table 22.7), but has been superseded by the Revised Trauma Score (RTS).

Table 22.7 *The Trauma score*

Parameter	Score*	Parameter	Score*
Respiratory rate (per min)		**Total GCS points**	
10–24	4	14–15	5
25–35	3	11–13	4
36+	2	8–10	3
1–9	1	5–7	2
0	0	3–4	1
Respiratory expansion		**Systolic blood pressure (mmHg)**	
Normal	1	90+	4
Shallow	0	70–89	3
None	0	50–69	2
		1–49	1
		0	0
Capillary refill			
Normal	2		
Delayed	1		
None	0		

*Unweighted score

The Revised Trauma Score (RTS)[12]

This records only three parameters – respiratory rate, systolic blood pressure, and GCS. Each parameter scores 0–4 points, and this figure is then multiplied by a weighting factor (Table 22.8). The resulting values are added to give a score of 0 to 7.8408. The percentage probability of survival (Ps) for the nearest whole number is shown in Table 22.9. The weighting factor allows the RTS to take account of severe head injuries without systemic injury, and be a more reliable indicator of outcome. In America, an unweighted value of less than 4 in any one parameter is an indication for evacuation to a definitive trauma centre.

Table 22.8 *The Revised Trauma Score (RTS)*

Respiratory rate (RR; per min)	0	1–5	6–9	30+	10–29	
Score	0	1	2	3	4	
	score		$\times 0.2908$			$= \alpha$
Systolic blood pressure (SBP; mmHg)	0	1-49	50–75	76–89	90+	
Score	0	1	2	3	4	
	score		$\times 0.7326$			$= \beta$
GCS (total)	3	4–5	6–8	9–12	13–15	
Score	0	1	2	3	4	
	score		$\times 0.9368$			$= \chi$

$$RTS = \alpha + \beta + \chi$$

Example: Patient S.W., 45-year-old female cyclist hit by car; injuries as Table 22.4
First observations in resuscitation room – RR 28, SBP 140, GCS – E1 M4 V2 = 7
$RTS = (4 \times 0.2908) + (4 \times 0.7326) + (2 \times 0.9368) = 1.1632 + 2.9304 + 1.8736 = 5.9672$

Table 22.9 *Probability of survival against RTS*

Nearest whole number	Ps (%)
8	99
7	97
6	92
5	81
4	61
3	36
2	17
1	7
0	3

Triage Revised Trauma Score (TRTS)

This modification of the RTS allows rapid physiological triage of multiple patients. It uses the unweighted sum of the RTS values to allocate priorities (Table 22.10). This system is currently used by many ambulance services.

Table 22.10 *The Triage Revised Trauma Score (TRTS)*

Respiratory rate (RR; per min)	0	1–5	6–9	30+	10–29	
Score	0	1	2	3	4	
	Unweighted score					$= A$
Systolic blood pressure (SBP; mmHg)	0	1–49	50–75	76–89	90+	
Score	0	1	2	3	4	
	Unweighted score					$= B$
GCS (total)	3	4–5	6–8	9–12	13–15	
Score	0	1	2	3	4	
	Unweighted score					$= C$

$$TRTS = A + B + C$$

Example: Patient S.W., 45-year-old female cyclist hit by car; injuries as Table 22.4
First observations in resuscitation room – RR 28, SBP 140, GCS – E1 M4 V2 = 7

$$TRTS = 4 + 4 + 2 = 10$$

Table 22.11 *Triage priorities using Triage Revised Trauma Score (TRTS)*

TRTS	Priority	
12	3	Delayed
10–11	2	Urgent
1–9	1	Immediate
0	Dead	

The Paediatric Trauma Score (PTS)[13,14]

The RTS has been shown to underestimate injury severity in children. The PTS (Table 22.12) combines observations with simple interventions and a rough estimation of tissue damage. The PTS tends to overestimate injury severity, but is used as a paediatric pre-hospital triage tool in the USA.

Table 22.12 *The Paediatric Trauma Score*

	Paediatric Trauma Score		
	+2	+1	−1
Weight (kg)	>20	10–20	<10
Airway	Normal	Simple adjunct	ET tube/surgical
Systolic blood pressure (mmHg)	>90	50–90	<50
Conscious level	Alert	Decreased/history of loss of consciousness	Coma
Open wounds	None	Minor	Major/penetrating
Fractures	None	Minor	Open/multiple
	Total range −6 to 12		

COMBINED SYSTEMS

TRauma score-Injury Severity Score (TRISS)[15]

This uses the RTS and ISS as well as the age of the patient. Different weighting factors are used for blunt and penetrating trauma. The equation for Ps is shown in Table 22.13. Different study groups may use their own coefficients to take account of the characteristics of the trauma seen in their populations. By convention, patients with a Ps of <50% who survive are 'unexpected survivors' and those with a Ps >50% that die are 'unexpected deaths'. TRISS is not valid for children under the age of 12 years.

Table 22.13 *TRISS equation*

$Ps = 1 / 1 + e^{-b}$
where $b = b_0 + b_1 (RTS) + b_2 (ISS) + b_3 (age\ coefficient)$
$b_0 - b_3$ = coefficients for blunt and penetrating trauma (will vary with the trauma system being studied)

Original coefficients	b_0	b_1	b_2	b_3
Blunt trauma	−1.2470	0.9544	−0.0768	−1.9052
Penetrating trauma	−0.6029	1.1430	−0.1516	−2.6676

e = 2.718282 (base of Naperian logarithm)
RTS and ISS = calculated scores for RTS and ISS
age coefficient = 0 if ≤ 54, 1 if ≥ 55

Example: Patient S.W., 45-year-old female cyclist hit by car; injuries and observations as before.
RTS = 5.9672, ISS 2
$b = b_0 + b_1 (RTS) + b_2(ISS) + b_3 (age\ factor)$
$b = -1.2470 + (0.9544 \times 5.9672) + (-0.0768 \times 29) + (-1.9052 \times 0)$
$b = 2.2209$

$Ps = 1/1+e^{-b} = 1/1.1085 = 0.9021$ or 90.21%

It must be stressed that the Ps is a mathematical expression of the probability of survival, and not an absolute statement of the patient's chances. One in four patients with Ps 75% will still be expected to die. While these cases may be highlighted for audit to see if there are any lessons to be learned, conclusions about performance should not be drawn from single patients. Other calculations can be made from TRISS values that better reflect a unit's results against the regional or national standards (see Table 22.14).

Table 22.14 *TRISS – Definitive outcome-based evaluation*

M statistic

This examines the injury severity match between the study group and the baseline group. The range is 0–1. A good match is shown by a figure near 1. A good match is needed to ensure that the groups being compared are alike and that any conclusions drawn are valid. Values less than 0.88 are unacceptable for further analysis. This prevents a centre that regularly receives more seriously injured patients than the rest of the centres within a study group being unfairly singled out for criticism.

Ps range category	Fraction in range		
	Baseline group % in each category (a)	Study group (b)	Smaller figure of a or b
0.96–1	0.828	n	S1
0.91–0.95	0.045	o	S2
0.76–0.90	0.044	p	S3
0.51–0.75	0.029	q	S4
0.26–0.50	0.017	r	S5
0–0.25	0.036	s	S6

n – s are the percentages of patients in each Ps range from the study group being compared to the baseline group. If n is smaller than 0.828, S1 = n, if n is larger than 0.828, S1 = 0.828

$$M = S1 + S2 + S3 + S4 + S5 + S6$$

Z statistic

This is a measure of the difference between actual and expected survivors (or deaths) for a unit against the current normal level within that trauma system. Values greater than 1.96 or less than −1.96 suggest a significant difference in outcome to that expected.

$$Z = A - E/\sqrt{\text{sum of } Pi\,(1 - Pi)}$$

where Pi = predicted Ps for each patient (from baseline)
         A = actual number of survivors
         E = expected number of survivors

W statistic

This allows a clinical value to be placed on trauma care. The value is the number of survivors more or less than expected per 100 patients.

$$W = \frac{A - E}{n/100}$$

where   A = actual number of survivors
         E = expected number of survivors
         n = number of patients analysed

A Severity Characterization Of Trauma (ASCOT)[16]

This is a more recent system first described in 1990. ASCOT has proved more reliable than TRISS in predicting outcome in both blunt and penetrating trauma. ASCOT provides a more accurate assessment of a patient's anatomical and physiological injury status than TRISS,[17] but is a more complicated calculation (Table 22.15). ASCOT takes account of all injuries classified as serious by AIS (scores 3–5). TRISS is flawed because of its reliance on using ISS, which only counts the worst injury within a single body region and ignores other serious ones. ASCOT also has a better classification which takes more account of the age of the patient.

Table 22.15 *The ASCOT calculation*

$Ps = 1/1 + e^{-k}$
where $k = k0 + k1(GCS) + k2(SBP) + k3(RR) + k4(A) + k5(B) + k6(C) + k7(age)$
k0–7 are fixed coefficients for blunt or penetrating trauma

Original coefficients	k0	k1	k2	k3	k4	k5	k6	k7
Blunt trauma	−1.1570	0.7705	0.6583	0.2810	−0.3002	−0.1961	−0.2086	−0.6355
Penetrating trauma	−1.1350	1.0626	0.3638	0.3320	−0.3702	−0.2053	−0.3188	−0.8365

e = 2.718282 (base of Naperian logarithm)
GCS, SBP and RR are coded values (0–4) as per RTS
A = √(sum of the squares of all AIS codes 3, 4 or 5 in the head and rear of neck)
B = √(sum of the squares of all AIS codes 3, 4 or 5 in the chest and front of neck)
C = √(sum of the squares of all AIS codes 3, 4 or 5 in all other body areas)
   age = coded value for defined age ranges
       0 = 0–54 years, 1 = 55–64, 2 = 65–74, 3 = 75–84, 4 = 85+

Example:
Patient S.W., 45-year-old female cyclist hit by car; injuries and observations as before.
A = (9 + 16) = 5, depressed parietal skull fracture AIS 3, small subdural haematoma AIS 4
B = (0)
C = (9 + 9) = 4.2426, open fracture radius AIS 3, open fracture ulna AIS 3

K = k0 + k1(GCS) + k2(SBP) + k3(RR) + k4(A) + k5(B) + k6(C) + k7(age)
k = −1.1570 + (0.7705 × 2) + (0.6583 × 4) + (0.2810 × 4) + (−0.3002 × 5) + (−0.1961 × 0) + (−0.2086 × 4.2426) + (−0.6355 × 0)
k = 1.7552
Ps = 1/1+e⁻ᵏ = 1/1.1729 = 0.8526 or 85.26%

MULTICENTRE STUDIES

The Major Trauma Outcome Study (MTOS) started in the United States during the early 1980s,[18] and is now established internationally. MTOS expanded into the United Kingdom in 1988 following the report of the Royal College of Surgeons criticising trauma care. Now called the UK Trauma Audit Research network (UK TARN), it is based at the North West Injury Research Centre. Around 50% of UK hospitals that receive trauma contribute data to UK TARN. The initial aim of MTOS was to develop and test coefficients and Ps values to increase the predictive accuracy of scoring systems, and to give feedback to contributing trauma units. The data collected have become more detailed. Pre-existing morbidity, mechanism of injury, operations, complications and the seniority of staff are all included as the patient is followed from the scene of injury through the Emergency Department and hospital to discharge. The feedback allows audit and comparison of performance over time and between units. The approach to the injured patient has changed as a result, with the introduction of trauma teams and increasingly, senior staff leading them.

Entry criteria for the MTOS are shown in Table 22.16.

Other studies are also in progress in the UK, for example, the Scottish Trauma Audit Group (STAG). Each study group may develop different coefficients for TRISS and ASCOT to reflect their own trauma populations.

Table 22.16 *Entry criteria for trauma patients into MTOS*

- Admitted to hospital for 3+ days
- Died in hospital
- Intensive care required
- Inter-hospital transfer required for specialist care

Exclude patients with fractures of distal radius and single pubic ramus

FUTURE DEVELOPMENTS

None of the systems developed so far is perfect, but succeeding systems are continually improving reliability and predictive performance. New systems are under development to take the process further.

Measuring mortality rates and calculating survival probabilities only looks at one outcome for the trauma patient. For every patient killed, another two suffer residual problems. Measuring the degree of these problems is difficult, especially in relation to musculoskeletal injuries. An Injury Impairment Scale is currently undergoing evaluation, and the UK TARN study assesses morbidity at 3 months. The ICISS can generate expected results for the cost and length of hospital stay.

The pre-morbid condition of the patient is not currently taken into account. In the previously hypertensive patient a normal systolic blood pressure may indicate substantial blood loss. A previously fit and independent patient is likely to cope with injury better than one of the same age with chronic disease processes. Studies into this issue have been published, and are continuing.[19]

Pre-hospital care is a developing field with increasing medical input alongside the paramedics. Currently physiological and combined scoring systems, by convention, use the first set of observations after arrival in the resuscitation room as this is a relatively 'fixed point'. Evidence is required as to the value of pre-hospital medical care, and different strategies such as 'stay and play' versus 'scoop and run' could be evaluated by extending scoring to cover the pre-hospital environment.

SUMMARY

Trauma care teams must be able to show that they are providing as good a service as possible. The optimal organization of trauma care in the UK is still a matter of debate, and any new systems need to be based on good evidence, and trialled. The time, effort and skill that teams bring to patient care may be wasted without proper analysis of their results. In this way good practice can be recognized and spread, and lessons learned from poor outcomes. Trauma scoring systems provide the data to allow this analysis to be made. Trauma teams must appreciate the importance of scoring, and ensure adequate and accurate data collection.

REFERENCES

1. Association for the Advancement of Automotive Medicine. *The Abbreviated Injury Scale, 1990 Revision*. Des Plaines, Illinois, 1990.
2. Baker SP, O'Neill B, Haddon W, Long WB. The Injury Severity Score: a method for describing patients with multiple injuries and evaluating emergency care. *Journal of Trauma* 1974; **14**: 187–96.
3. Baker SP, O'Neill B. The Injury Severity Score: an update. *Journal of Trauma* 1976; **16**: 882–5.
4. Osler T, Baker S, Long W. A modification of the Injury Severity Score that both improves accuracy and simplifies scoring. *Journal of Trauma* 1997; **43**: 922–6.
5. Rutledge R, Fakhry S, Baker C, Oller D. Injury severity grading in trauma patients: a simplified technique based upon ICD-9 coding. *Journal of Trauma* 1993; **35**: 497–507.
6. Rutledge R. Injury severity and probability of survival assessment in trauma patients using a predictive hierarchical network model derived from ICD-9 codes. *Journal of Trauma* 1995; **38**: 590–601.
7. Rutledge R, Osler T, Emery S, Kromhout-Schiro S. The end of the Injury Severity Score (ISS) and the Trauma and Injury Severity Score (TRISS): ICISS, an International Classification of Diseases, ninth revision-based prediction tool, outperforms both ISS and TRISS as predictors of trauma patient survival, hospital charges and hospital length of stay. *Journal of Trauma* 1998; **44**: 41–9.

8. Yoon Kim, Koo Young Jung, Chang-Yup Kim, *et al*. Validation of the International Classification of Diseases 10th Edition-based Injury Severity Score (ICISS). *Journal of Trauma* 2000; **48**: 280–5.

9. Wesson D, *et al*. *Journal of Trauma* 1988; **28**: 1226–31.

10. Teasdale G, Jennett B. Assessment of coma and impaired consciousness: a practical scale. *Lancet* 1974; **1**: 81–4.

11. Champion HR, Sacco WJ, Carnazzo AJ, *et al*. The Trauma Score. *Critical Care Medicine* 1981; **9**: 672–6.

12. Champion HR, Sacco WJ, Copes WS, *et al*. A revision of the Trauma Score. *Journal of Trauma* 1989; **20**: 623.

13. Tepas JJ, Mollitt DL, Bryant M. The Paediatric Trauma Score as a predictor of injury severity in the injured child. *Journal of Paediatric Surgery* 1987; **22**: 14–18.

14. Kaufmann CR, Maier RV, Rivara P, Carrico CJ. Evaluation of the Paediatric Trauma Score. *Journal of the American Medical Association* 1990; **263**: 69–72.

15. Boyd CR, Tolson MA, Copes WS. Evaluating trauma care: the TRISS method. *Journal of Trauma* 1987; **27**: 370–8.

16. Champion HR, Copes WS, Sacco WJ, *et al*. A new characterisation of injury severity. *Journal of Trauma* 1990; **30**: 539–46.

17. Champion HR, Copes WS, Sacco WJ, *et al*. Improved predictions of severity characterisation of trauma (ASCOT) over Trauma and Injury Severity Score (TRISS): results of an independent evaluation. *Journal of Trauma* 1996: **40**: 42–8.

18. Champion HR, Copes WS, Sacco WJ, *et al*. The major trauma outcome study: establishing national norms for trauma care. *Journal of Trauma* 1990; **30**: 1356–65.

19. Hannan EL, Mendeloff J, Farrell LS, Cayten CG, Murphy JG. Multivariate models for predicting survival of patients with trauma from low falls: the impact of gender and pre-existing conditions. *Journal of Trauma* 1995; **38**: 697–704.

USEFUL ADDRESS

North Western Injury Research Centre
University of Manchester
Hope Hospital
Salford M6 8HD,
United Kingdom

Imaging in trauma

INTRODUCTION

An increasingly wide range of imaging modalities is now available in the majority of hospitals called upon to deal with trauma patients. Nevertheless, the cornerstone of effective immediate management of the trauma victim remains the appropriate ordering and systematic interpretation of plain radiographs supplemented by the appropriate use of more complex modalities taking into account the patient's clinical condition. This chapter offers a system which will aid the logical use and interpretation of the various forms of imaging.

PRIMARY SURVEY: ABC

Imaging during the primary survey should be strictly limited to investigations which will produce results which change the *immediate* management of the patient. These investigations must complement and not compromise the patient's management. These investigations will include plain radiography of the chest, pelvis, and cervical spine, together with imaging modalities designed to identify the presence of blood in the abdomen, thorax or retroperitoneum.

A supine chest X-ray should be the first investigation, and should be performed as soon as possible after the patient has arrived in hospital. It is important that the patient is fully exposed, not rotated, and in the middle of the trolley (and film!). A systematic approach to the interpretation of all X-rays, in particular the supine trauma chest radiograph, is essential (Figure 23.1, Table 23.1). If the patient is fully alert and there is no suggestion or suspicion of a spinal injury, an erect anteroposterior (AP) chest X-ray should be performed first.

Depending on the mechanism of injury, the patient should also have a supine pelvic film which is best considered to be part of C, as a method of determining the presence of life-threatening or potentially life-threatening haemorrhage (Figure 23.2; Table 23.2).

The patient should not be rotated and the iliac crests should be included in an adequate pelvic X-ray. Failure to perform an adequate examination here will lead to missed fractures, which could be potentially fatal. The presence of fractures should be correlated with clinical findings. Pubic fractures are associated with urethral and bladder injuries, while major pelvic ring fractures are associated with vascular injuries.

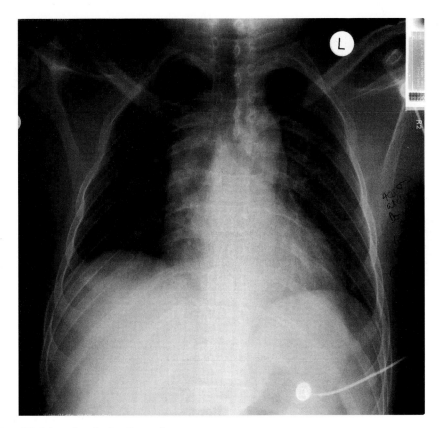

Figure 23.1 *A supine chest radiograph.*

Table 23.1 *Interpretation of a supine chest X-radiograph*

A. Airway
- check trachea is central and not deviated
- is the airway patent?
- is the endotracheal tube correctly sited (above the aortic arch or 3.5–5.5 cm above the carina)?
- are there any loose teeth or foreign bodies?
- check all other lines and tubes (for example, particular central lines and nasogastric tube)

B. Breathing
- exclude a pneumothorax or haemothorax
- check there is no 'flail' segment
- check there are no fractured ribs
- check that both lungs are well aerated

C. Circulation
- check heart size
- check mediastinal size
- is the mediastinal contour normal?
- is the aortic arch clearly visible?

D. Diaphragm
- can both diaphragms be seen?
- are the diaphragms in the correct position?
- is there any evidence of a diaphragmatic injury clinically or radiologically?
- look under the diaphragm, in particular for free air

E. Edges
- are the pleural spaces clear?
- is there any possibility of a subtle pneumothorax or haemothorax?

F. Soft tissues
- is there any evidence of surgical emphysema?
- is there any evidence of gross soft-tissue swelling?
- are the paravertebral/paraspinal lines normal (right measures 3 mm max, left measures 10 mm max)?

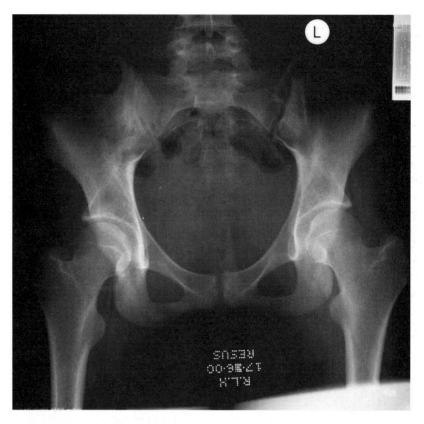

Figure 23.2 *A radiograph of the pelvis.*

Table 23.2 *Interpretation of the pelvic radiograph*

A. Alignment
- are the sacroiliac (SI) joints and the pubis symmetrical?

B. Bones
- the pelvis has three rings, one major and two minor (see Figure 23.2). In general, if a fracture is seen in one ring there is usually a second fracture in the same ring
- look at the iliac crests
- look at the lower lumbar spine
- look at the hip joints and greater trochanter (you may need a bright light)

C. Cartilage
- look at the sacroiliac (SI) joints and pubis. Make sure that the joint spaces are intact and the joint margins are parallel

S. Soft tissues
- look at the soft-tissue planes, in particular the perivesical, and psoas fat planes

During the primary survey, as part of C, ultrasound may be carried out by a 'trauma radiologist' or an 'ultrasound-trained' emergency physician,[1-7] and the chest should be included as part of the study[8] by looking for a haemothorax and pericardial fluid.[9] Ultrasound is faster and cheaper than diagnostic peritoneal lavage, is non-invasive, and is comparable in its accuracy in detecting free fluid in the abdomen. In many hospitals, urgent out-of-hours trauma ultrasonography is not yet available. Diagnostic peritoneal lavage (DPL) is a suitable alternative in haemodynamically unstable patients or in patients who cannot undergo computed tomography (CT) for other reasons (for example, neurologically unstable patients).

If the patient is neurologically and haemodynamically stable and the mechanism of injury suggests the possibility of cervical spine injury, a single cross-table lateral cervical spine (C/S) radiograph should be performed. However, it has been conclusively demonstrated that an alert asymptomatic individual with a normal examination, who does not have a distracting injury, does not require imaging.[10–16]

Employing only a lateral C/S radiograph will result in a significant number of undetected injuries with a false-negative rate of 13–42%.[17–22] A significant portion of missed injuries will result if a meticulous systematic approach is not used (Figure 23.3; Table 23.3), and if the C7/T1 junction is not clearly seen on the lateral. A swimmer's view may adequately show the C7/T1 junction if conventional lateral views are inadequate. Repeated unsuccessful attempts at lateral films should be avoided.

If the patient is not intubated and is cooperative, supplementary open-mouth peg and AP views will significantly improve the detection rate to 93–99%.[18,22] The use of the trauma oblique C/S views in this group of patients is debatable. CT of suspicious or inadequately visualized levels,[20,23–25] such as the craniocervical junction[26–30] or the cervicothoracic junction,[30] will increase the sensitivity and accuracy to over 95%.

Once any life-threatening injury has been identified and treated, if the initial cervical spine radiographs are normal and the patient is conscious, cervical immobilization can be removed and the patient re-examined.

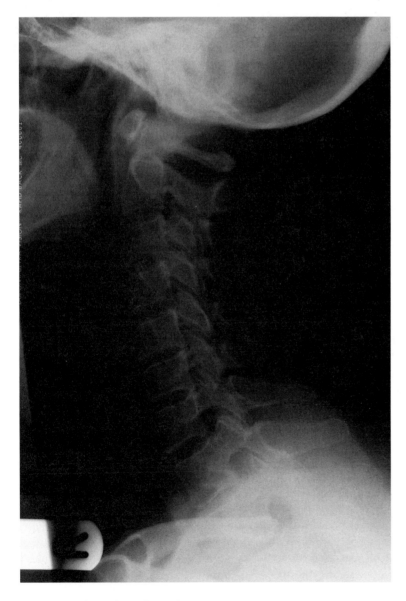

Figure 23.3 *Lateral cervical spine radiograph.*

Table 23.3 *Interpretation of the lateral cervical spine radiograph*

A. Alignment
- alignment of the anterior vertebral body line
- alignment of the posterior vertebral body line
- alignment of the spinolaminar line
- alignment of the odontoid peg and C2 body

B. Bones
- check the vertebral bodies
- check all the posterior elements, in particular the spinous processes

C. Cartilage
- check that the disc spaces are similar at all levels

S. Soft tissues (pre-vertebral space 3 × 7 rule)
- pre-odontoid space 3 mm (5 mm in children)
- C3 less than 7 mm (approximately half width of the adjacent vertebra)
- C6/7 equal to 21 mm (approximately the width of the adjacent vertebra)
- sphenoid sinus – look for a fluid level

N.B. These measurements are only useful in non-intubated patients

If there are no clinical suspicions of a cervical spine injury, then the cervical spine can be 'cleared'. A small proportion of these patients will however complain of persisting localized pain. These patients should be referred for specialist opinion with a view to obtaining flexion and extension views which may reveal additional injuries.[31,32] It is essential that these views are performed only in fully alert patients and under the auspice of a specialist to minimize the risk of further neurological damage. A proportion of flexion and extension views are inadequate due to pain and spasm leading to insufficient movement.[33,34] These patients should be kept in a collar and reviewed by the specialist. If there are any symptoms or signs of neurological damage at this stage, then magnetic resonance imaging (MRI) should be performed, but only after plain radiography, CT of suspicious areas and specialist referral. MRI will provide valuable information on all the soft tissues, especially traumatic disc herniation, ligamentous injuries, paravertebral collections, cord oedema or haemorrhage and cord compression.[35]

In the unconscious intubated patient, an open-mouth PEG view and often the AP are difficult to perform and interpret due to the presence of all the overlying equipment (for example, the endotracheal tube, oxygen mask or tubing and collar). However, as these patients often require a head CT, the craniocervical junction can be included as part of the scan. The evidence regarding the clearance of the C/S in this unconscious group of patients is very limited. In those patients who are expected to recover consciousness within 24–48 h, cervical immobilization can be maintained, although head blocks and tape should be used without a cervical collar due to the risk of raised intracranial pressure associated with prolonged wearing of a cervical collar. In these circumstances, there are several options on how to image and clear the spine:

- Lateral C/S and AP and routine CT of the craniocervical junction (CCJ).
- Lateral and two trauma obliques and routine CT of CCJ.
- Lateral C/S and spiral CT of the whole C/S.
- Any of the above combinations and MRI.

The practice of performing flexion and extension views in the unconscious patient is considered dangerous, and is definitely not recommended.

A significant number of injuries will be detected by CT of the CCJ.[26,29] Supine trauma obliques will help to assess alignment of the posterior bony elements and characterize injuries. However, they are relatively difficult to perform, are time-consuming, and have not been shown to improve sensitivity.[36] The advent of spiral CT means that the whole of the C/S can be imaged in thin sections with multiplanar reconstruction in under 1 minute. This is time-saving, and the analysis and results of several studies are awaited with interest. MRI of the whole C/S in all obtunded patients would theoretically be the best option, but is unrealistic in practice. The MRI environment is neither safe nor friendly to trauma patients. In addition, MRI is not readily accessible, may not necessarily exclude all unstable injuries, and may 'overcall' significant numbers of injuries, leading to patients being over-investigated. Overall, it is important to take into account the mechanism of injury and likelihood of injuries in determining how much imaging is necessary. It is essential to emphasize that 'clearance of the C/S' is not based on imaging but on clinical examination on an alert patient. However, every Accident and Emergency (A&E) Department should have a recommended imaging protocol for clearance of the C/S (Figure 23.4).

Once the primary survey is finished, it is imperative that a significant head injury is ruled out if the patient is haemodynamically stable and has an altered Glasgow Coma Score (GCS) or any clinical evidence of a head injury. Skull X-rays (SXR) have a very limited role in head injury and the only indications are:

- suspected depressed skull fracture;
- penetrating injury, for example gunshot wounds or stabbings;
- detection of foreign bodies; and/or
- suspicion of non-accidental injury in young children.

Over 50% of trauma deaths are associated with head injury. It is estimated that over 30% of trauma deaths are unnecessary,[37] and a significant number of these are due to poor management of head injuries. There is little that one can do for the primary injury, but secondary insults due to poor management are unacceptable. It has been demonstrated that delay in treatment of subdural haematomas (SDH) and extradural haematomas (EDH) has a deleterious effect on outcome.[38,39] More specifically, a delay of greater than 3 h from time of injury to time of surgery in EDH[40] and 4 h in SDH[41] results in greater morbidity and mortality. Therefore, all haemodynamically stable patients with a reduced GCS should have a CT scan of the head as soon as possible to rule out a potentially fatal injury.

Therefore, it is critical that after resuscitation, a haemodynamically stable patient with a known or suspected head injury should have a CT scan performed without undue delay. Apart from EDH and SDH, CT will detect subarachnoid blood with a sensitivity of greater than 90%.[42] Although sub-arachnoid haemorrhage (SAH) itself does not require surgical intervention, it is a risk factor of poor outcome.[43–45]

The intra-axial lesions include cortical contusions, diffuse axonal injury (DAI) and deep cerebral grey matter and brainstem injuries. Cortical contusions and DAI are a result of sheer-stress injuries, and are important causes of morbidity in head-injury patients. The initial scan may be negative and the true extent of the injury may only be evident at 24–48 h, with 20% of contusions appearing after a delay.[46,47] CT is far less sensitive at demonstrating the diffuse axonal injury seen at the grey–white matter interface, corpus

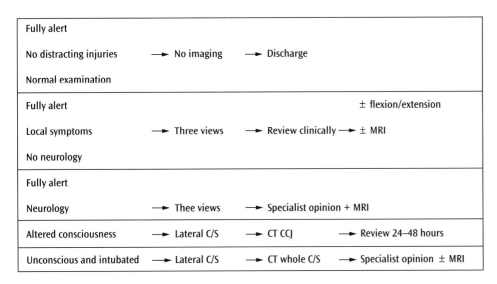

Figure 23.4 *Protocol for clearance of the cervical spine (C/S) in trauma.*

callosum and the upper brainstem, with only 20–50% of patients having an abnormality on the admission CT.[48,49] All these abnormalities should be looked for in a systematic manner (Table 23.4).

Table 23.4 *Interpretation of a head CT scan*

1. Always review the scanogram at the start as it may provide clues to other problems difficult to visualize on CT, for example craniotomy, burr holes, gunshot and foreign bodies.
2. Check position and symmetry of ventricles.
3. Check that the 3rd and 4th ventricles are in the midline.
4. Compare the two cerebral and cerebellar hemispheres – look for asymmetry.
5. Check that the sulci can be clearly seen, and are symmetrical.
6. Look for blood in the ventricular system and subarachnoid spaces.
7. Look for blood in the peripheral edges of the cerebral and cerebellar hemispheres.
8. Look at the brainstem.
9. Look at the grey–white matter differentiation.
10. Look at the sinuses for air fluid levels.
11. Ask for bone windows and assess soft tissues and bones.

ROLE OF MRI

The MRI environment is not trauma-friendly, as scanning patients takes a lot longer than CT scanning, and acute haemorrhage can be missed. There is also an inherent lack of bone detail and images may be severely degraded by uncooperative patients. In addition, MRI scanners are on the whole sited away from the A&E Departments and an emergency service is not always available. Therefore, at present, this investigation has no role in acute trauma. In the future, with the advent of open scanners, and MRI becoming more readily accessible, there is no doubt that it will have a role. In particular, it may be a better indicator of long-term prognosis and functional outcome.

IMAGING OF THE THORACIC AND LUMBAR SPINE

Conscious patients with symptoms or signs of a thoracic or lumbar spine injury should have routine AP and lateral views. If the upper thoracic spine is poorly visualized, then further views may be necessary.[50,51]

The mechanism of injury should also raise suspicion of an injury to the thoracic spine and lumbar spine. In particular, direct or penetrating trauma, lap belt injuries, injuries sustained from jumps or falls and the presence of distracting injuries should alert the physician to the possibility of spinal injuries.[52] Other associated injuries with a high risk of spinal trauma, such as calcaneal,[51] scapular or sternal[53,54] fractures also warrant imaging of the thoracic and lumbar spine. Any patient who has a spinal injury detected should have the rest of the spine very meticulously looked at in view of the high incidence of multiple-level injuries. In practice, there should be a low threshold for imaging the thoracic and lumbar spine in patients who are unconscious and who have been involved in significant trauma. Thoracic and lumbar spine injuries may be very subtle on plain X-rays, and careful review of the imaging is essential with special attention to the paraspinal lines (Figure 23.5; Table 23.5).

If an abnormality is detected or even if there is a hint (no matter how small) of a possible injury, CT should be performed from the superior end plate of the vertebral body above, to the inferior end plate of the vertebral body below. However, the imaging of the thoracic and lumbar spine should only be performed when the patient is haemodynamically stable. CT will help to show the injury clearly and to characterize the lesion, in particular the integrity of the posterior elements and protrusion of disc or bone fragments into the canal. This is especially important in the thoracic spine, where the cord occupies a proportionally greater

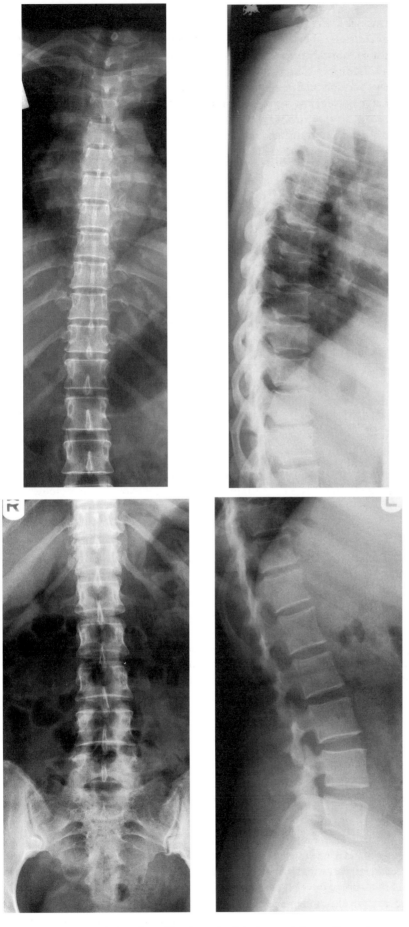

Figure 23.5 *Interpretation of thoracic and lumbar spine injuries on plain X-radiograph.*

area of the canal than in the C/S or lumbar spine (L/S). Multiplanar reconstruction in sagittal and coronal planes should always be made available.

Detection of thoracic spine (T/S) and in particular L/S injuries or multiple level injuries warrants an abdominal CT to exclude associated abdominal injuries. MRI of the thoracic and lumbar spines should be requested by a specialist. Indications include patients with neurological symptoms and signs, when an injury to the cord, disc or ligament is suspected, and cases where an abnormality which the specialist feels is unstable has been detected on a plain radiograph and confirmed on CT.

Table 23.5 *Interpretation of thoracic and lumbar spine radiographs*

A. Alignment
- check for the normal spinal curvature (thoracic kyphosis and lumbar lordosis)
- look for the alignment of the anterior margin of the vertebral bodies
- look at the alignment of the posterior margin of the vertebral bodies
- look on the AP view to check that the spine is straight and the vertebral bodies are aligned

B. Bones
- check each vertebral body carefully
- make sure that the height of the anterior and posterior elements of the vertebral bodies are the same
- check that the pedicles are clearly visible on the AP and lateral views
- look out for abnormal separation of the pedicles and spinous processes
- look carefully at the transverse processes and the posterior ribs

C. Cartilage
- check that the height of the intervertebral disc spaces are the same (they gradually get slightly bigger)
- look out for subtle loss of joint space

S. Soft tissues
- make sure that the paraspinal lines are normal in the thoracic spine (the right should measure less than 3 mm, and the left less than 1 cm)
- check that the psoas shadows are visible on the lumbar spine X-radiographs, and that they are symmetrical

LIMB INJURIES

In general, the management and imaging of extremity injuries in polytrauma patients is similar to those with single-limb injury, except that the management of life-threatening injuries will take priority. As a consequence, limb injuries are often ignored, missed, poorly imaged and badly treated. Delayed or poor management of relatively minor limb injuries will often lead to delay in recovery, significant morbidity and litigation. It is not within the scope of this chapter to cover the full range of limb injuries, but some general rules are included (Table 23.6).

ROLE OF CT IN TRAUMA

CT provides a unique way of identifying injuries in the head, chest, abdomen and pelvis. Technological advances and the advent of multislice spiral CT have led to scans of the entire chest, abdomen and pelvis being performed in under 1 minute once the patient is on the CT couch.

CT is unique in that it can be used to:

- diagnose injuries accurately;
- detect occult injuries which may be life-threatening (in particular, occult pneumothoraces);
- detect solid-organ injuries, which may then be treated conservatively;
- diagnose vascular injuries which may be amenable to treatment by surgery or interventional radiology, for example traumatic aortic injury and aortic stenting or liver, renal and splenic lacerations treated with embolization; and/or

- follow-up patients treated conservatively or those submitted to surgery or an interventional procedure.

Table 23.6 *Helpful tips for limb radiography*

1. Check that the radiograph belongs to the correct patient.
2. Check the hospital number.
3. Check the labels, date, and sidemarker.
4. Check the quality of the radiograph (for example, for exposure and centering).
5. One view is one view too few.
6. Two views is one view too few if it does not fit the clinical history (hence four views for the scaphoid).
7. Always get two views at right-angles to each other.
8. Always get a dedicated view of the joint above and below if there is midshaft injury to a long bone.
9. Ask the radiographers which additional views are necessary.
10. Ask the radiographers to interpret the radiographs (including red dot).
11. Use a systematic approach to interpretation.
12. Ask a senior colleague or the radiologist for further advice on imaging and management, e.g. role of isotopes, CT or MRI.

In effect, any haemodynamically stable patient suspected of a significant head, chest, abdominal or pelvic injury should have spiral CT. Radiologists should be consulted early so that appropriate facilities and expertise can be made available.

CT is also extremely helpful in identifying occult fractures of the pelvis and excluding vascular and visceral injuries such as bladder, rectal and vaginal injuries. Fractures which involve major joints and complicated fractures of the ankle and feet should also have thin-section CT scans, using a bone algorithm with multiplanar and 3D reconstruction. While 3D images may not reveal any additional injuries, they are extremely helpful in selected cases in deciding on the extent of injury and the orthopaedic approach.

ROLE OF CONTRAST STUDIES, ANGIOGRAPHY AND INTERVENTIONAL RADIOLOGY IN TRAUMA

Advice should be obtained as soon as possible from the radiologist whenever a contrast examination or interventional procedure is necessary. The various procedures and their indications are summarized in Table 23.7. However, it is not within the scope of this chapter to give details of the specific indications.

Table 23.7 *Indications for contrast studies and interventional procedures*

Condition	Contrast study/intervention
Chest	
Ruptured oesophagus	Contrast swallow
	Oesophageal stenting
Traumatic aortic injury	Aortogram
	Aortic stenting
Ruptured diaphragm	Contrast via chest drain
Abdomen/pelvis	
Urethral rupture	Urethrogram
Bladder rupture	Cystogram
Rectal injuries	CT, MRI or contrast enema
Pelvic bleeding	Angiography and embolization
Solid-organ injury	Selective angiography and embolization
Limbs	
Active bleeding	Angiography

SUMMARY

In the initial stages of the acute management of major trauma, the mainstay of imaging remains the appropriate use of a limited range of plain radiographs chosen, taking into account the patient's clinical condition and mechanism of injury. Appropriate use of techniques such as ultrasound scanning and CT scanning will aid in the diagnosis of internal haemorrhage. A wide range of other modalities is also available for the elucidation, and in some cases treatment of specific images. The key to the correct use of all these more complex procedures is to ensure that they do not put the patient at further risk. No image is worth dying for.

REFERENCES

1. Nordenholz KE, Rubin MA, Gularte GG, *et al*. Ultrasound in the evaluation and management of blunt abdominal trauma. *Annals of Emergency Medicine* 1997; **29**: 357–66.
1a. Ma OJ, Mateer JR, Ogata M, *et al*. Prospective analysis of a rapid trauma ultrasound examination performed by emergency physicians. *Journal of Trauma* 1995; **36**: 879–85.
2. Ingeman JE, Plewa MC, Okasinski RE, *et al*. Emergency physician use of ultrasonography in blunt abdominal trauma. *Academic Emergency Medicine* 1996; **3**: 931–6.
2a. Schlager D, Lazzareschi G, Whitten D, *et al*. A prospective study of ultrasonography in the emergency department by emergency physicians. *American Journal of Emergency Medicine* 1994; **12**: 185–9.
3. Thomas B, Falcone RE, Vasquez D, *et al*. Ultrasound evaluation of blunt abdominal trauma: program implentation, initial experience and learning curve. *Journal of Trauma* 1997; **42**: 384.
3a. McKenney M, McKenney K, Compton R, *et al*. Can surgeons evaluate emergency ultrasound scans for blunt abdominal trauma? *Journal of Trauma* 1998; **44**: 649–53.
4. Board of Faculty of Clinical Radiology. *Guidance for training of medical non-radiologists*. London: Royal College of Radiologists, March 1997.
4a. Ma OJ, Mateer JR, Scalea TM, *et al*. Trauma ultrasound examination versus chest radiography in the detection of hemothorax. *Annals of Emergency Medicine* 1997; **29**: 312–16.
5. Plummer D, Brunette D, Asinger R, *et al*. Emergency department echocardiography improves outcome in penetrating cardiac injury. *Annals of Emergency Medicine* 1992; **21**: 709–12.
6. Fischer RP. Cervical radiographic evaluation of alert patients following blunt trauma. *Annals of Emergency Medicine* 1984; **13**: 905–7.
7. Mirvis SE, Diaconis JN, *et al*. Protocol driven radiological evaluation of suspected cervical spine injury: efficacy study. *Radiology* 1989; **170**(3 Pt 1): 831–4.
8. Gbaanador GB, Fruin AH, *et al*. Role of routine emergency cervical radiography in head trauma. *American Journal of Surgery* 1986; **152**: 643–8.
9. Hoffman SR, Shriger DL, *et al*. Low risk criteria for cervical spine radiography in blunt trauma: a prospective study. *Annals of Emergency Medicine* 1992; **21**: 1454–60.
10. McNamara RM, Heine E, *et al*. Cervical spine injury and radiography in alert, high risk patients. *Journal of Emergency Medicine* 1990; **8**: 177–82.
11. Roberge RJ, Wears RC, *et al*. Selective application of cervical spine radiography in alert victims of blunt trauma: a prospective study. *Journal of Trauma* 1988; **28**: 784–8.
12. Saddison D, Vanek VW, *et al*. Clinical indications for cervical spine radiographs in alert trauma patients. *American Surgeon* 1991; **57**: 366–9.
13. Bachulis BL, Long WB, *et al*. Clinical indications for cervical spine radiography in traumatised patients. *American Journal of Surgery* 1987; **153**: 473–8.
14. MacDonald RL, Schwartz ML. Diagnosis of cervical spine injury in motor vehicle crash victims: how many x-rays are enough? *Journal of Trauma* 1990; **30**: 392–7.
15. Cohn SM, Lyle WG, *et al*. Exclusion of cervical spine injury: a prospective study. *Journal of Trauma* 1991; **31**: 570–4.

16. Ross SE, Schwab CW, *et al*. Clearing the cervical spine: initial radiographic evaluation. *Journal of Trauma* 1987; **27**: 1055–60.

17. Shaffer MA, Davis PE. Limitation of the cross table lateral view in detecting cervical spine injuries: a retrospective analysis. *Annals of Emergency Medicine* 1981; **10**: 508–13.

18. Streightwieser DR, Knopp R, *et al*. Accuracy of standard radiographic views in detecting cervical spine fractures. *Annals of Emergency Medicine* 1983; **12**: 538–42.

19. Borock EC, Gabram SG, *et al*. A prospective analysis of a two year experience using CT as an adjunct for cervical spine clearance. *Journal of Trauma* 1991; **31**: 1001–5.

20. Mace SE. Emergency evaluation of cervical spine injuries: CT versus plain radiographs. *Annals of Emergency Medicine* 1985; **14**: 973–5.

21. Schleehan K, Ross SE, *et al*. CT in the initial evaluation of the cervical spine. *Annals of Emergency Medicine* 1989; **18**: 815–17.

22. Kirshenbaum KJ, Nadimpalli SR. Unsuspected upper cervical spine fractures associated with significant head trauma: role of CT. *Journal of Emergency Medicine* 1990; **81**: 183–98.

23. Blacksin MF, Lee HJ. Frequency and significance of fractures of the upper cervical spine detected by CT in patients with severe neck trauma. *American Journal of Roentgenology* 1995; **165**: 1201.

24. Link TM, Schuierer G, *et al*. Substantial head trauma: value of routine CT examination of the cervicocranium. *Radiology* 1995; **196**: 741.

25. Hadley-Rowe R, Easty M, Coates TJ, Chan O. Significance of craniocervical junction injuries in polytraumatised patients. *RSNA* 1998; **209**: 314.

26. Tehranzadeh J, Bonk R, *et al*. Efficacy of limited CT for non-visualised lower cervical spine in patients with blunt trauma. *Skeletal Radiology* 1994; **23**: 349–52.

27. Davis JW, Park SN. Clearing the cervical spine in obtunded patients: the use of dynamic fluoroscopy. *Journal of Trauma* 1995; **39**: 435–8.

28. Lewis LM, Docherty M. Flexion-extension views of the evaluation of cervical spine injuries. *Annals of Emergency Medicine* 1991; **20**: 117–21.

29. Wang JC, Hatch JD. Cervical flexion and extension radiographs in acutely injured patients. *Clinical Orthopedics* 1999; **365**: 111–16.

30. Wilberger JE, Maroon JC: Occult post traumatic cervical ligamentous instability. *Journal of Spinal Disorders* 1990; **3**: 156.

31. Beers GJ, Raque GH. Magnetic resonance imaging in acute cervical spine trauma. *Journal of Computer Assisted Tomography* 1988; **12**: 755–61.

32. Goldberg AL, Rothfus WE, *et al*. The impact of magnetic resonance on the diagnostic evaluation of acute cervicothoracic spinal trauma. *Skeletal Radiology* 1988; **17**: 89–95.

33. Katzberg RW, Benedetti P. Acute cervical spine injuries: prospective MR imaging assessment at a Level 1 trauma centre. *Radiology* 1999; **213**: 203–12.

34. Freemyer B, Knopp R, *et al*. Comparison of five view and three view cervical spine series in the evaluation of patients with cervical trauma. *Annals of Emergency Medicine* 1989; **18**: 818–21.

35. Rose J, Valtonen S, Jennett B. Avoidable factors contributing to death after head injury. *British Medical Journal* 1977; **2**: 615–18.

36. Mendelow AD, Karmi MZ. Extradural haematoma: effect of delayed treatment. *British Medical Journal* 1979; **1**: 1240–2.

37. Seelig JM, Becker DP, Miller JD, *et al*. Traumatic acute subdural haematoma: major mortality reduction in comatose patients treated within four hours. *New England Journal of Medicine* 1981; **304**: 1511–18.

38. Davis JM, Ploetz J, Davis KR, *et al*. Cranial CT in subarachnoid haemorrhage. Relationship between blood detected by CT and lumbar puncture. *Journal of Computer Assisted Tomography* 1989; **4**: 794–8.

39. Patel HC, Hutchinson PJ, Pickard JD. Traumatic subarchnoid haemorrhage. *Hospital Medicine* 1999; **60**: 697–9.

40. Levy LM, Rezai A, *et al*. The significance of subarachnoid haemorrhage after penetrating craniocerebral injury: correlations with angiography and outcome in a civilian population. *Neurosurgery* 1993; **32**: 532–40.

41. Kakarieka A; Braakman R; Schakel. Clinical significance of the finding of subarachnoid blood on CT scan after head injury. *Acta Neurochirurgica* 1994; **129**: 1–5.

42. Hesselink JR, Dowd CF, *et al*. MR imaging of brain contusions: a comparative study with CT. *American Journal of Neuroradiology* 1988; **9**: 269–87.

43. Gentry LR, Gordersky JC, Thompson B. MR imaging of head trauma: review of distribution and radiopathologic features of traumatic lesions. *American Journal of Neuroradiology* 1988; **9**: 101–10.

44. Gentry LR, Gordersky JC, *et al.* Prospective comparative study of intermediate-field MR and CT in the evaluation of closed head trauma. *American Journal of Neuroradiology* 1988; **9**: 91–100.

45. Kelly AB, Zimmerman RD, *et al.* Head trauma: comparison of MR and CT – experience in 100 patients. *American Journal of Neuroradiology* 1988; **9**: 699–708.

46. El-Khoury GY (ed.) *Imaging of Orthopaedic Trauma*. The Radiologic Clinics of North America, 1997.

47. Harris JH Jr, Harris WH, Novelline RA (eds). *The Radiology of Emergency Medicine*. (3rd edn). Baltimore: Williams & Wilkins, 1993.

48. American College of Surgeons Committee on Trauma. *Advanced Trauma Life Support: Instructor Course Manual.* Chicago, 1997.

49. Hills MW, Delprado AM, *et al.* Sternal fractures: associated injuries management. *Journal of Trauma* 1993; **35**: 55–60.

50. Jones HK, McBride GG. Sternal fractures associated with spinal injury. *Journal of Trauma* 1989; **29**: 360–4.

51. Meyer S. Thoracic spine trauma. *Seminars in Roentgenology* 1992; **27**: 254–61.

52. Bohlman H. Treatment of fractures and dislocations of the thoracic and lumbar spine. *Journal of Bone and Joint Surgery* 1985; **67-A**: 165–9.

53. Rabinovici R, Ovadia P. Abdominal injuries associated with lumbar spine fractures in blunt trauma. *Injury* 1999; **30**: 471–4.

54. Young PC, Petersilge CA, *et al.* MR imaging of the traumatised lumbar spine. *Magnetic Resonance Imaging Clinics of North America* 1999; **7**: 589–602.

Index